Biotechnology of Blood Proteins
Purification, Clinical and Biological Applications

Biotechnologie des protéines du sang
Purification, applications cliniques et biologiques

Colloques INSERM
ISSN 0768-3154

Other *Colloques* published as co-editions by John Libbey Eurotext and INSERM

133 Cardiovascular and Respiratory Physiology in the Fetus and Neonate. *Physiologie Cardiovasculaire et Respiratoire du Fœtus et du Nouveau-né.*
Scientific Committee : P. Karlberg,
A. Minkowski, W. Oh and L. Stern;
Managing Editor : M. Monset-Couchard.
ISBN : John Libbey Eurotext 0 86196 086 6
INSERM 2 85598 282 0

134 Porphyrins and Porphyrias. *Porphyrines et Porphyries.*
Edited by Y. Nordmann.
ISBN : John Libbey Eurotext 0 86196 087 4
INSERM 2 85598 281 2

137 Neo-Adjuvant Chemotherapy. *Chimiothérapie Néo-Adjuvante.*
Edited by C. Jacquillat, M. Weil and D. Khayat.
ISBN : John Libbey Eurotext 0 86196 077 7
INSERM 2 85598 283 7

139 Hormones and Cell Regulation (10th European Symposium). *Hormones et Régulation Cellulaire (10ᵉ Symposium Européen).*
Edited by J. Nunez, J.E. Dumont and R.J.B. King.
ISBN : John Libbey Eurotext 0 86196 084 X
INSERM 2 85598 284 7

147 Modern Trends in Aging Research. *Nouvelles Perspectives de la Recherche sur le Vieillissement.*
Edited by Y. Courtois, B. Faucheux, B. Forette, D.L. Knook and J.A. Tréton.
ISBN : John Libbey Eurotext 0 86196 103 X
INSERM 2 85598 309 6

149 Binding Proteins of Steroid Hormones. *Protéines de liaison des Hormones Stéroïdes.*
Edited by M.G. Forest and M. Pugeat.
ISBN : John Libbey Eurotext 0 86196 125 0
INSERM 2 85598 310 X

151 Control and Management of Parturition. *La Maîtrise de la Parturition.*
Edited by C. Sureau, P. Blot, D. Cabrol, F. Cavaillé and G. Germain.
ISBN : John Libbey Eurotext 0 86196 096 3
INSERM 2 85598 311 8

Suite page 317
(Continued p. 317)

Biotechnology of Blood Proteins
Purification, Clinical and Biological Applications

Biotechnologie des protéines du sang
Purification, applications cliniques et biologiques

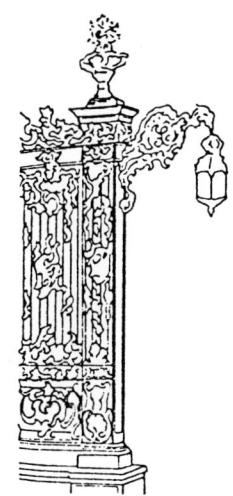

Proceedings of the 2nd International Symposium held in Nancy, November 16-18, 1992

Sponsored by INSERM (Institut National de la Santé et de la Recherche Médicale)

Edited by

Claude Rivat
Jean-François Stoltz

John Libbey EUROTEXT

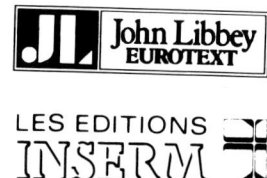

British Library Cataloguing in Publication Data

A catalogue record for this book
is available from the British Library

ISBN 2 7420-0007-0
ISSN 0768-3154

First published in 1993 by

Editions John Libbey Eurotext
6 rue Blanche, 92120 Montrouge, France. (33) (1) 47 35 85 52
ISBN 2-7420-0007-0

John Libbey and Company Ltd
13 Smiths Yard, Summerley Street, London SW18 4HR,
England.
(44) (81) 947 27 77

Institut National de la Santé et de la Recherche Médicale
101 rue de Tolbiac, 75654 Paris Cedex 13, France.
(33) (1) 44 23 60 00
ISBN 2-85598-515-3

ISSN 0768-3154

© 1993 Colloques INSERM/John Libbey Eurotext Ltd,
All rights reserved
Unauthorized publication contravenes applicable laws

Acknowledgments/*Remerciements*

CONSEIL REGIONAL DE LORRAINE   The organizers thank very greatly the Région de Lorraine for the realization of the project.

Les organisateurs remercient chaleureusement la Région de Lorraine pour l'aide qu'elle a bien voulu apporter à la réalisation de ce projet.

They do want to express their gratitude to the District Urbain de Nancy and to the various firms wich gave their aid:

Ils tiennent également à exprimer leur gratitude au District Urbain de Nancy et aux diverses sociétés qui ont apporté leur soutien :

Centre Régional de Transfusion Sanguine de Lille, Cuno Europe, Flobio, Merck Clevenot, Millipore, Pharmacia Bioprocess, Quality Biotech, Sepracor.

With the sponsorship of
Avec le soutien de

Ministère de la Recherche et de l'Espace
INSERM (Institut National de la Santé et de la Recherche Médicale)
EPFA (European Plasma Fractionation Association)
Région de Lorraine
District de l'Agglomération Nancéienne
Université de Nancy I
Institut National Polytechnique de Lorraine
Faculté de Médecine de Nancy

President/*Président*

J.-F. Stoltz

Scientific Secretary/*Secrétaire scientifique*

C. Rivat

Scientific Committee/*Comité scientifique*

E. Boschetti

T. Burnouf

M. Grandgeorge

B. Horowitz

J.-J. Huart

C. Rivat

J.-F. Stoltz

W.G. van Aken

List of participants
Liste des participants

Adenot Nicole, CRTS Lyon-Beynost, 01704 Beynost, France

Afeyan Noubar, Perceptive Biosystems Inc., 38 Sidney Street, Cambridge, MA 02139, États-Unis

Alexandre P., CRTS, avenue de Bourgogne, 54500 Vandœuvre, France

Allgaier Hermann, Birkendorfer Strasse 65, 7950 Biberach/Rib, Allemagne

Allioux Catherine, Sepracor/IBF, 35, avenue Jean-Jaurès, 92390 Villeneuve-la-Garenne, France

Andrieu Jean-Claude, Baxter Biotech., Boulevard Branquart 80, Hyland Division, 7860 Lessines, Belgique

Armstrong D., NBTS, P.O. Box 2356, 4000 Durban, Afrique du Sud

Askildsen Arne, National Institute of Public Health, 0462 Oslo, Norvège

Balstrup Flemming, Statens Serum Institute, 5 Artillerivej, 2300 Copenhagen, Danemark

Beer Hans-Jorg, Armour Pharma, Grüberstrasse 46 A, 8011 München, Allemagne

Begue Stéphane, CRTS Lyon-Beynost, 01704 Beynost, France

Bengio Sylvio, Sepracor/IBF, 35, avenue Jean-Jaurès, 92390 Villeneuve-la-Garenne, France

Berezenko Stephen, Delta Biotechnology, 59 Castle Boulevard, NG7 1FD Nottingham, Royaume-Uni

Berglöf Jan, Pharmacia BioProcess Technology, S-75187 Uppsala, Suède

Birkenmeier Gerd, University of Leipzig, Institute of Biochemistry, Liebigstrasse 16, D-7010 Leipzig, Allemagne

Bos Octaaf, Blood Transfusion Service, Plesmanlaan 125, Central Laboratory, 1066 CX Amsterdam, Pays-Bas

Boschetti Egisto, Sepracor/IBF, 35, avenue Jean-Jaurès, 92390 Villeneuve-la-Garenne, France

Boyeldieu Denis, Hôpital Cochin, Centre des Hémophiles, 27, rue du Faubourg Saint-Jacques, 75014 Paris, France

Briquel M.E., CRTS, avenue de Bourgogne, 54500 Vandœuvre, France

Brodniekicz Teresa, Haemacure, 245, boulevard Hymus, H9 Rigg Point Claire, Canada

Brunko Patricia, Commission des Communautés Européennes, DGIII/C/3, B-1049 Bruxelles, Belgique

Burnouf Thierry, CRTS, 21, rue Camille-Guérin, 59012 Lille, France

Burnouf-Radosevich Mirjana, CRTS, 21, rue Camille-Guérin, 59012 Lille, France

Burton Steven J., Affinity Chromatography Ltd, 307 Huntingdon Road, Cambridge CB3 CJX, Royaume-Uni

Cambou Bernard, Rhône-Poulenc Rorer, Recherche et Développement, B.P. 14, 94403 Vitry-sur-Seine, France

Capolino Ugo, Baxter, via le Tiziano 25, 00195 Roma, Italie

Chtourou Sami, CNTS, 3, avenue des Tropiques, B.P. 100, 91943 Les Ulis Cedex, France

Cidda Claudio, Schiapparelli Diag. SpA, Via Castagneta n° 7, 00040 Pomezia, Italie

Clar Manfred, DRK-Blutspendedienst, Burgweg 5-7, Rheinland-Pfalz, 6550 Bad Kreuznach, Allemagne

Closs Brigitte, 6, rue Charles-Brun, B.P. 213, 19100 Brive, France

Coadou Yvette, INSERM, Bureau des Colloques, 101, rue de Tolbiac, 75654 Paris Cedex 13, France

Conradie J.D., NBTS, P.O. Box 2356, 4000 Durban, Afrique du Sud

Conradson M., Pharmacia BioProcess Technology, S-75187 Uppsala, Suède

Cook Anne, British Biotechnology Ltd, Watlington Road, Cowley, Oxford OX45 SLY, Royaume-Uni

Cox David, 8, rue Maurice-Nogues, 78960 Voisins-le-Bretonneux, France

Curling John, Swedenborgsgatan 3-5, S-75334 Uppsala, Suède

Darling Allan, Quality Biotech Ltd, 6 04 Kelvin Campus, Glasgow G20 OSP, Royaume-Uni

Dazey Bernard, CRTS, place A. Raba-Léon, B.P. 24, 33035 Bordeaux, France

De Wael Luc, Rue J.-Stallaert 5, 1060 Bruxelles, Belgique

Delaplace Brigitte, Sepracor, 35, avenue Jean-Jaurès, 92395 Villeneuve-la-Garenne Cedex, France

Dellacherie Edith, CNRS, URA 494, ENSIC, B.P. 451, 54001 Nancy Cedex, France

Derlemans Conny, Blood Transfusion Service, Plesmanlaan 125, 1066 AX Amsterdam, Pays-Bas

Bernis Dominique, CRTS, 21, rue Camille-Guérin, B.P. 2018, 59012 Lille, France

Devantie Olesen Charlotte, Novo Nordisk, Biopharma Division, Niels Steensensvej 1, 2820 Gentofte, Danemark

Donner M., INSERM, Plateau de Brabois, C.O. 10, 54500 Vandœuvre Cedex, France

Dusch M., INSERM, Plateau de Brabois, C.O. 10, 54500 Vandœuvre Cedex, France

Engman Lena, Kabi Pharmacia, Plasma Products, S-11287 Stockholm, Suède

Eran Henry, 10046 Ruffner Avenue, Granada Hills, California, États-Unis

Evans David, 94 Isis Avenue, Bicester OX6 8GS, Royaume-Uni

Evers Théo, Red Cross Transfusion Service, Plesmanlaan 125, Central Laboratory, 1066 CX Amsterdam, Pays-Bas

Falksveden Lars, National Bacteriology Laboratory, 105 21 Stockholm, Suède

Fauchille Sylvain, CNTS, 3, avenue des Tropiques, B.P. 100, 91943 Les Ulis, France

Feldman Peter A., Bio Products Laboratory, Dagger Lane, Elstree WD6 3BX, Royaume-Uni

Fernandez Jesus, Instituto Grifols S.A., C/Co Guasch s/n, Poligono Levante, 08150 Barcelona, Espagne

Fouron Yves, Sepracor/IBF, 35, avenue Jean-Jaurès, 92390 Villeneuve-la-Garenne, France

Friedli Hans, 2LB Xankdorfstrasse 10, 3000 Bern, Suisse

Galatioto Leonardo, Serum and Vaccine Institute, P.O. Box 3001, Berne, Suisse

Garg Vipin, Forestal Centre, 303 B College Road East, SIer DNX, Princeton, NJ 08540, États-Unis

Geschier C., CRTS, avenue de Bourgogne, 54511 Vandœuvre, France

Graafland Hubert, Institut d'Hématologie, Centre Régional de Transfusion Sanguine, 240, avenue Emile-Jeanbrau, 34000 Montpellier, France

Grace Ulrich, Blutspendedienst, Feithstrasse 180, D-5800 Hagen, Allemagne

Grandgeorge Michel, Pasteur Mérieux, 1541, avenue Marcel-Mérieux, 69280 Marcy-L'Etoile, France

Grosse-Wilde Hans, Universitätsklinikum, Institut Immunologie, 4300 Essen, Allemagne

Gucek V., INSERM, Plateau de Brabois, C.O. 10, 54500 Vandœuvre Cedex, France

Guéant Jean-Louis, Hôpital de Brabois, Biochimie des Protéines, 54511 Vandœuvre Cedex, France

Guillerm Jean, Société Biologique, 59, rue P.-Curie, Allée G.-Voisin, 78370 Plaisir, France

Guyot Alain, Sepracor/IBF, 35, avenue Jean-Jaurès, 92390 Villeneuve-la-Garenne, France

Hagberg Roland, Kabi Pharmacia, Plasma Products, S-112 87 Stockholm, Suède

Harbers Anne, Pharmacia Biotech., 4 Byfield Street, North Ryde NSW, 2113 Sydney, Australie

Herrington Robert W., CSL Limited, 45 Poplar Road, Parkville, Victoria 3052, Australie

Hessing Martin, Blood Transfusion Service, Central Laboratory, Plesmanlaan 125, 1066 CX Amsterdam, Pays-Bas

Hiemstra Harry, CLB, Plesmanlaan 125, 1066 CX Amsterdam, Pays-Bas

Horaud Florian, Laboratoire de Virologie Médicale, Institut Pasteur, 75724 Paris Cedex 15, France

Horowitz Bernard, Blood Center, 310 E 67th Street, New York, NY 10021, États-Unis

Hory Dieter, Biotest Pharma, D-6072 Dreieich, Allemagne

Huart Jean-Jacques, CRTS, 21, rue Camille-Guérin, 59012 Lille, France

Jagschies Günter, European Consultancy, Pharmacia Biosystems Gmbh, W-7800 Freiburg, Allemagne

Jensen Anni, Novo Nordisk, Biopharma Division, Niels Steensens Vej 1, 2820 Gentofte, Danemark

Jensen Lisbeth, Statens Seruminstitut, 5, Artillerivej, 2300 Copenhague, Danemark

Johannig Detlef, Pharmacia Biosystems, BioProcess Technoloy, Munzinger Strasse 9, D-7800 Freiburg, Allemagne

Johansson M., Pharmacia, 751 82 Uppsala, Suède

Kjeldal Allan, Novo Nordisk, Niels Steensensvej 1, 2820 Gentofte, Danemark

Kluge Matthias, Boehringer Mannheim Gmbh, Abteilung GB-PZI, 8122 Penzberg, Allemagne

Knevelman Anne, Bloodbank Friesland, Jelsumerstraat 41-A, 8901 BV Leeuwarden, Pays-Bas

Koops Koos, Bio-Intermediair B.V., P.O. Box 454, 97000 AL Groningen, Pays-Bas

Kosow David, Baxter Biotech., 4501 Colorado boulevard, Los Angeles, CA 90039, États-Unis

Lang Jean, Pasteur Mérieux, 1541, avenue Marcel-Mérieux, 69280 Marcy-L'Etoile, France

Latour Guy, CRTS Lyon-Beynost, 01704 Beynost, France

Laub Ruth, Rue J.-Stallaert 5, 1060 Bruxelles, Belgique

Laurian Yves, CNTS, 3, avenue des Tropiques, B.P. 100, 91943 Les Ulis Cedex, France

Leaute Jean-Baptiste, CNTS, 3, avenue des Tropiques, B.P. 100, 91943 Les Ulis Cedex, France

Linnau Yendra, Industrie 67, A-1220 Wien, Autriche

Linssen Paul J.M., Blood Transfusion Service, Central Laboratory, Plesmanlaan 125, 1066 CX Amsterdam, Pays-Bas

Ljunqovist Ake, Kabi Pharmacia, Plasma Products, S-11287 Stockholm, Suède

Löf Anna-Lena, Kabi Pharmacia AB, S-11287 Stockholm, Suède

Lutsch Charles, Pasteur Mérieux, 1541, avenue Marcel Mérieux, 69280 Marcy-L'Etoile, France

MacBain Wendy, Quality Biotech Ltd, 6 04 Kelvin Campus, Glasgow G20 OSP, Royaume-Uni

MacLeod Alex, Protein Fraction Centre, 21 Ellen's Glen Road, Edinburgh EH17 7QT, Royaume-Uni

MacNaughton Malcolm, Inveresk Research International Ltd., Tranent EH33 2NE, Royaume-Uni

Manach Michel, Sepracor/IBF, 35, avenue Jean-Jaurès, 92390 Villeneuve-la-Garenne, France

Mangin Christian, 117, avenue des Nations, B.P. 60079, 95973 Roissy Cedex, France

Marrs Stephen, Blood Transfusion Service, P.O. Box 9326, Johannesburg, Afrique du Sud

Marshall P.J., Bio Products Laboratory, Dagger Lane, Elstree WD6 3BX, Royaume-Uni

Maugras M., INSERM, Plateau de Brabois, C.O. 10, 54500 Vandœuvre, France

Michalski Catherine, CRTS, 21, rue Camille-Guérin, 59012 Lille, France

Micucci Vito, CSL Limited, 45 Poplar Road, Parkville, Victoria 3052, Australie

Mohr Harald, Blutspendedienst, Niedersachsen, Eldagsener Strasse 38, D-3257 Springe 1, Allemagne

Montreuil Jean, Université des Sciences et Techniques de Lille, Laboratoire de Chimie Biologique, UMR n° 11 du CNRS, 59655 Villeneuve-d'Ascq, France

More John, Bio Products Laboratory, Dagger Lane, Elstree WD6 3BX, Royaume-Uni

Morgenthaler Jean-Jacques, Laboratoire Central, Service de Transfusion, Wankdorfstrasse 10, 3000 22 Berne, Suisse

Moriot A., INSERM, Plateau de Brabois, C.O. 10, 54500 Vandœuvre Cedex, France

Movshovitz Rina, Engineers and Consultant Ltd, 8, Uziel Street, Givat Shmuel, 51905 Israël

Mskine Malika, Faculté de Médecine, Hématologie, Plateau de Brabois, 54500 Vandœuvre, France

Muller Daniel, L.R.M., avenue J.B. Clément, 93430 Villetaneuse, France

Ng Paul K., Miles Inc., Cutter Labs, P.O. Box 1986, Berkeley, CA 94701, États-Unis

Nicoud R.-M., Separex, 5, rue J.-Monod, 54250 Champigneulles, France

Noël Jean-Marie, Baxter Biotech., Boulevard Branquart 80, Hyland Division, 7860 Lessines, Belgique

Norichafi Nadia, Faculté de Médecine, Hématologie, Plateau de Brabois, 54500 Vandœuvre, France

Nouaille-Degorge Julien, DRET-DGA, 4, rue de la Porte-d'Issy, 00460 Paris Armées, France

Over Jan, Blood Transfusion Service, Central Laboratory, Plesmanlaan 125, 1066 CX Amsterdam, Pays-Bas

Pere Maurice, Institut Pasteur-Texcell, 25, rue du Docteur-Roux, 75724 Paris Cedex 15, France

Petersen Ignatius Peter, 10 Connaught road, Beaconvale, 7500 Parow, Afrique du Sud

Pfister M., INSERM, Plateau de Brabois, C.O. 10, 54500 Vandœuvre Cedex, France

Piquet Yves, CRTS, place A. Raba-Léon, B.P. 24, 33035 Bordeaux, France

Polsler Gerhard, Immuno AG, Uferstrasse 15, 2304 Wien, Autriche

Poplavsky Jean-Louis, Rue J.-Stallaert 5, 1060 Bruxelles, Belgique

Prowse Christopher, Royal Infirmary, Blood Transfusion Service, Edinburgh EH3 9HB, Royaume-Uni

Rasolo Jean-Louis, Faculté de Médecine, CRITT-GBM, 54500 Vandœuvre, France

Ray Vijaylaxmi, National Plasma Fractionation Centre, K.E.M. Hospital Complex, Parel, Bombay 400012, Inde

Regnault V., INSERM, Plateau de Brabois, C.O. 10, 54500 Vandœuvre, France

Rempeters Gerold, Armour Pharma, Grüberstrasse 46A, 8011 München, Allemagne

Rentsch Markus, 2LB Wankdorfstrasse 10, 3000 Berne, Suisse

Rivat C., INSERM, Plateau de Brabois, C.O. 10, 54500 Vandœuvre, France

Roberth Irawati, Pharmacia, 751 82 Uppsala, Suède

Rocton Christian, Filtron Technologie, 42 R.N. 10, 78180 Coignères, France

Rothstein Fred, Middlesex Sciences, P.O. Box 347, Mansfield, 02048, États-Unis

Rouger Philippe, INTS, 6, rue Alexandre-Cabanel, 75015 Paris, France

Ryan Jack, Miles Inc., P.O. Box 1986, Berkeley, CA 94701, États-Unis

Sanchez José, Instituto Grifols S.A., C/Con Guash s/n, Poligono Levante, 08150 Barcelona, Espagne

Schmitthaeusler Roland, CNTS, 3, avenue des Tropiques, B.P. 100, 91943 Les Ulis Cedex, France

Schooneman François, CRTS, avenue de Bourgogne, 54500 Vandœuvre, France

Schroeder Duane, Miles Inc., 4th Parker Street, P.O. Box 1986, Berkeley, CA 94701, États-Unis

Schuurmans Renno Peter, NPBI/Biotrans, Runde ZZ 41, 7881 HM Emmer-Compascuum, Pays-Bas

Sengfelder Hermann, Fa Menck, 6100 Darmstadt, Allemagne

Setter Jurgen, Blutspendedienst, Feithstrasse 182-184, D-5800 Hagen, Allemagne

Shepherd Ailsa, Inversek Research International Ltd, Tranent EH33 2NE, Royaume-Uni

Sikorova Jana, Institute Sera and Vaccines, Korunni 108, 101 09 Prague, République Tchèque

Smeds Anne-Lisa, Kabi Pharmacia, Plasma Products, S-11287 Stockholm, Suède

Stewart David J., Affinity Chromatography Ltd, 307 Huntingdon Road, Cambridge CB3 0JX, Royaume-Uni

Stocker Ulrich, Blutspendezentrale, Gunzenbachstrasse 35, D-7570 Baden-Baden, Allemagne

Stoltz J.F., INSERM, Plateau de Brabois, C.O. 10, 54511 Vandœuvre Cedex, France

Stoltz M., 1, rue du Gué, 54180 Heillecourt, France

Stucki Martin, Zentrallaboratorium, Wankdorfstrasse 10, 3000 Bern, Suisse

Sumi Akinori, The Green Cross C.O., Central Research Laboratory, 2-25-1 Shodai-Ohtani, Hirakata, Osaka 573, Japon

Suomela Hannu, Blood Transfusion Service, Kivihaantie 7, 00310 Helsinki, Finlande

Teisner Borge, Statens Seruminstitut, 5, Artillerivej, 2300 Copenhague, Danemark

Thill Werner, 850 Stonewall Drive, Bourbonnais, IL 60914, États-Unis

Thomas Janette, Institute of Biotechnology, University of Cambridge, Tennis Court Road, Cambridge CB2 1QT, Royaume-Uni

Tideman Olaf, Pharmacia Bioprocess Tech., Box 17, 3440 AA Woerden, Pays-Bas

Tschammer Thomas, Behringwerke AG, Postfach 11 40, 3550 Marburg, Allemagne

Turecek Peter, Immuno AG, Industriestrasse 72, A-1220 Wien, Autriche

Ubrich N., INSERM, Plateau de Brabois, C.O. 10, 54500 Vandœuvre Cedex, France

Vallar L., INSERM, Plateau de Brabois, C.O. 10, 54500 Vandœuvre Cedex, France

Van Aken Willen, Red Cross Blood Transfusion, Central Laboratory, P.B. 9190, 1006 Amsterdam, Pays-Bas

Van der Zwalhen M., rue J.-Stallaert 5, 1060 Bruxelles, Belgique

Van Wyngaarden Leen, Rankestraat 42-44, 9713 Groningen, Pays-Bas

Varga Ilona, Serobacteriological Research Institute, H-2100 Gogollo, Hongrie

Vatkovsky Petko, Street Shandor petiofy 2, Sofia, Bulgarie

Véron Jean-Luc, Pasteur Mérieux, 1541, avenue Marcel-Mérieux, 69280 Marcy-l'Etoile, France

Vigneron C., Faculté de Pharmacie, 5, rue Albert-Lebrun, 54000 Nancy, France

Vijayalakshmi Mookambe A., Université de Technologie de Compiège, Laboratoire de Technologie des Séparations, 60206 Compiègne Cedex, France

Virkajarvi Timo, Blood Transfusion Service, Kivihaantie 7, 00310 Helsinki, Finlande

Voute Nicolas, Sepracor/IBF, 35, avenue Jean-Jaurès, 92390 Villeneuve-la-Garenne, France

Wallevik Knut, University Hospital, Department of Clinical Immunology, 8200 Aarhus, Danemark

Wenng Andréas, Baxter Diagnostics AG, Bonnstrasse 9, 3186 Duedingen, Suisse

Wibb Paul, Wrexham Industrial Estate, Porton Speywood Ash Road, Wrexham LL1 39UF, Royaume-Uni

Winge Stefan, Kabi Pharmacia, Linjhagensgatan 133, 112 87 Stockholm, Suède

Wyoro Robert, Berlex Biosciences, 213 East Grand Avenue, San Francisco, CA 94080, États-Unis

Yap H. Boon, CSL Limited, 45 Poplar Road, Parkville, Victoria 3052, Australie

Zuber Thomas, Serum and Vaccine Institue, P.O. Box 3001, Berne, Suisse

Opening remarks

Ladies and Gentlemen, dear Colleagues,

On behalf of C. Rivat and in my own name it is an honour and a great pleasure to open today here in Nancy the 2nd International Symposium on Blood Protein Biotechnology.

May I first extend grateful thanks to INSERM' Symposia Department, the Lorraine Regional Council, the Nancy Urban District and City Council, Nancy 1 University, the Lorraine National Polytechnic Institute as well as to all the firms taking part in the exhibition, for their invaluable assistance.

Since the first symposium, which was held here in this conference centre just over four years ago, there have been very few meetings devoted specifically to the problems of preparing blood fractions and the restrictions involved in the procedure.

Five major proteins are still the basis of all plasma fractionation activity to-day : albumin, IgG, FVIII, FIX and fibrinogen. More recently other proteins have been added to the list : ATIII, α-1-AT and biological glues. Other fractions could, in the near future, be used as therapeutic agents (activated or non-activated protein C, protein S, ceruloplasmin, transferrin, etc.).

Further, can we anticipate the possibility of using the proteins for non-therapeutic applications ? For example, would it be worthwhile to produce human culture media with a defined protein composition for biotechnology applications ?

Finally, one very important question calls for an answer: in the age of cell engineering and genetic engineering is there still a place for extraction therapeutic proteins ? We cannot, unfortunately, examine all these problems during the five half-day sessions of the conference. We do, however, hope that the wide range of papers presented will provide a general view of the present situation regarding the recent developments in industrial technology for blood protein separation. We hope too that during your stay you will have the opportunity of visiting our city and the sourrounding countryside in spite of the weather.

J.-F. Stoltz

Allocution d'ouverture

Madame, Monsieur et chers Collègues,

C'est un plaisir et un honneur pour moi que d'ouvrir aujourd'hui à Nancy, au nom de C. Rivat et en mon nom, ce 2e Symposium International consacré à la Biotechnologie des Protéines du Sang.

Je voudrais tout d'abord remercier le bureau des Colloques de l'INSERM, la Région de Lorraine, le District Urbain de l'Agglomération de Nancy, l'Université de Nancy I, l'Institut National Polytechnique de Lorraine, ainsi que les industriels qui participent à l'exposition, de l'aide qu'ils nous ont apportée.

Depuis le 1er symposium qui s'est tenu dans cette salle, voici un peu plus de quatre ans, peu de réunions spécifiques ont été consacrées aux problèmes de la préparation de fractions du sang et aux contraintes qui en découlent.

Aujourd'hui, cinq grandes protéines sont toujours à la base de l'activité du fractionnement plasmatique : albumine, IgG, FVIII, FIX et fibrinogène, auxquelles il faut ajouter plus récemment l'ATIII, l'alpha-1AT ainsi que les colles biologiques. D'autres fractions pourraient devenir, dans un proche avenir, des agents thérapeutiques (la protéine C et S : activée ou non; céruloplasmine, facteur XIII, transferrine...).

Par ailleurs, des applications non thérapeutiques sont-elles envisageables ? Ainsi, par exemple, y-a-t-il intérêt à produire des milieux de culture humains à composition définie pour les biotechnologies ?

Cependant, une question essentielle se pose : à l'heure du génie cellulaire et du génie génétique, y-a-t-il encore une place pour les protéines thérapeutiques d'extraction ? Tous ces problèmes ne seront malheureusement pas traités au cours de ces cinq demi-journées. Nous espérons, cependant, que la diversité des communications permettra de faire le point sur les évolutions récentes dans les technologies industrielles de séparation des protéines du sang et que vous aurez également l'opportunité de visiter notre ville et notre région malgré le temps.

J.-F. Stoltz

Contents
Sommaire

V   Aknowledgments
       Remerciements
VII   List of participants
       Liste des participants

       J.-F. Stoltz
XVII   Opening remarks
XVIII Allocution d'ouverture

       I. SEPARATION TECHNIQUES USED IN PLASMA FRACTIONATION
       I. TECHNIQUES DE SÉPARATION UTILISÉES DANS LE FRACTIONNEMENT DU PLASMA

3   **E. Boschetti, P. Girot, L. Guerrier, N. Voute**
      Chromatography packing design matching human plasma protein separation requirements
      Définition de supports chromatographiques adaptés à la séparation des protéines plasmatiques

13   **M. Bailly, R.M. Nicoud**
      The simulated moving bed: a powerfull process for purification
      Le lit mouvant simulé : un procédé puissant pour la purification

19   **S.J. Burton**
      Considerations in the use of synthetic dye-ligand affinity adsorbents for the manufacture of blood proteins
      Considérations sur l'utilisation d'adsorbants d'affinité à base de colorants synthétiques pour la production

25 **J.A. Thomas, C.R. Lowe**
Design of novel affinity ligands for the purification of proteases and protease inhibitors
Préparation de nouveaux ligands d'affinité pour la purification de protéases et d'inhibiteurs de protéases

31 **J.H. Berglöf**
Validation aspects relating to the use of chromatographic media
Les aspects de la validation en relation avec l'utilisation des supports chromatographiques

37 **D.J. Stewart**
Evaluation of current methods for antibody immobilization in the preparation of immunoaffinity adsorbents
Evaluation de méthodes destinées à l'immobilisation d'anticorps dans la préparation d'immuno-adsorbants

43 **N. Ubrich, P. Hubert, V. Regnault, E. Dellacherie, C. Rivat**
Immunopurification of proteins. Comparison of the stability of various activated beaded-agarose matrices
Immunopurification des protéines. Comparaison de la stabilité de matrices d'agarose activées par différentes méthodes

49 **E. de Jonge, M.A.W. van Leeuwen, H. Radema, P.H.J.M. Linssen, J. Over**
Filtration processes in the Cohn-fractionation
Procédés de filtration dans le fractionnement de Cohn

II. COAGULATION FACTORS
II. FACTEURS DE COAGULATION

57 **D. Boyeldieu, Y. Sultan**
Clinical evaluation of coagulation factor concentrate
Evaluation clinique des concentrés de facteurs de coagulation

63 **P.A. Feldman, L. Harris, D.R. Evans, H.E. Evans**
Preparation of a high purity factor IX concentrate using metal chelate affinity chromatography
Préparation d'un concentré de facteur IX de haute pureté par chromatographie d'affinité sur métal chélaté

69 A.L. Löf, E. Berntorp, B. Eriksson, C. Mattson,
   L. Svinhufvud, S. Winge, A. Östlin
   Characterization of a highly purified factor IX concentrate
   Caractérisation d'un concentré de facteur IX de haute pureté

75 C. Lutsch, P. Gattel, B. Fanget, J.-L. Véron, K. Smith,
   J. Armand, M. Grandgeorge
   Immunoaffinity purified, solvent-detergent treated factor IX
   Facteur IX immunopurifié, traité au solvant-détergent

81 A.H.L. Koenderman, H.G.J. ter Hart, C.T. Hakkennes,
   E.J. Muller, L. Brands, N. van Duren, H. Hiemstra, J. Over
   Development and preclinical evaluation of a high-purity factor IX concentrate (Factor IX-HP)
   Développement et évaluation préclinique d'un concentré de facteur IX de haute pureté

87 I. MacGregor, L. MacLaughlin, O. Drummond, J. Ferguson,
   C. Prowse
   Limitations of *in vitro* thrombogenicity tests applied to high purity factor IX
   Limitations des tests de thrombogénicité in vitro *appliqués aux concentrés de facteur IX de haute pureté*

91 C. Michalski, T. Burnouf, J.-J. Huart
   Five years of experience in the production and quality control of a highly purified factor IX concentrate
   Expérience de cinq années dans la production et le contrôle de qualité d'un concentré de facteur IX de haute pureté

97 V. Regnault, C. Geschier, M.-E. Briquel, C. Rivat,
   P. Alexandre, J.-F. Stoltz
   Preparation by immunoaffinity chromatography of therapeutic human protein C concentrates
   Préparation par chromatographie d'immuno-affinité de concentrés de protéine C à usage thérapeutique

103 K. Wallevik, S. Glavind, E. Hansen, J. Ingerslev,
    J. Jørgensen
    Method for manufacturing chemically virus-inactivated, high purity FVIII concentrate with an overall yield of 35%, feasible for small pool production in developing countries
    Méthode de production d'un concentré de facteur VIII de haute pureté, viralement inactivé, avec un rendement de 35 %, réalisable pour une petite production dans les pays en voie de développement

109 L. van Wijngaarden, H.S. Hoff, K. Koops, J.J. van Weperen, P.C. Das, C.T. Smit Sibinga
Pilot immunoaffinity purification of factor VIII/vWF complex (preliminary results)
Immunopurification à l'échelle pilote du complexe VIII/vWF (résultats préliminaires)

115 M. Ezzedine, F. Lawny, M.A. Vijayalakshmi
Purification and depyrogenation of antihemophilic FVIII:C from human plasma
Purification et dépyrogénéisation de facteur VIII:C à partir de plasma humain

125 A. Knevelman, J.H.C. de Wit
The effect of monosaccharides glucose and fructose during 80°C heat treatment of a factor VIII concentrate
Effet du glucose et du fructose pendant le traitement par chauffage à 80°C d'un concentré de facteur VIII

131 F. Verroust, Y. Laurian, J. Chabbat, M.-J. Larrieu
Three year experience with plasma derived factor VIIa concentrate
Expérience de trois années avec un concentré de facteur VIIa

III. PURIFICATION OF IgG AND ALBUMIN
III. PURIFICATION DES IgG ET DE L'ALBUMINE

137 Zhao Shuliang, Zhong Lu, Zhou Quing, Luo Liang, Li Shujin, Chen Chunsheng
Application of chromatography system in plasma protein fractionation on pilot scale
Application de la chromatographie dans le fractionnement des protéines du plasma à l'échelle pilote

143 H.B. Yap, I.F. Young, V. Micucci, R.W. Herrington, P.J. Turner, J.R. Davies
Development of a process for the preparation of human serum albumin using chromatographic methods
Développement d'un procédé pour la préparation de l'albumine sérique humaine par des méthodes chromatographiques

151 **V. Ray, M.V. Kamath**
Our initial experience with large scale chromatography for plasma fractionation
Notre expérience initiale avec la chromatographie à grande échelle pour le fractionnement du plasma

155 **V. Micucci, I.F. Young, H.B. Yap, J.R. Davies, R.W. Herrington, B.R. White, G. Naylor, P.J. Turner**
Design of a large scale chromatographic plant for the purification of human albumin
Conception d'une installation de chromatographie à grande échelle pour la purification de l'albumine humaine

163 **I. Stefas, M. Rucheton, H. Graafland**
Chromatographic purification of plasmatic human albumin
Purification chromatographique de l'albumine plasmatique humaine

169 **S.B. Marrs**
Large scale albumin fractionation by chromatography
Fractionnement de l'albumine par chromatographie à grande échelle

175 **J.-F. Stoltz, C. Geschier, L. Dumont, C. Rivat, M. Grandgeorge, J. Ribeyron, E. Boschetti, J. Liautaud, F. Streiff**
Description and assessment of an industrial chromatography unit for preparing human plasma albumin
Description et évaluation d'une installation industrielle de chromatographie pour préparer de l'albumine humaine

183 **J.-L. Véron, P. Gattel, J. Pla, P. Fournier, M. Grandgeorge**
Combined Cohn/chromatography purification process for the manufacturing of high purity human albumin from plasma
Un procédé combinant la méthode de Cohn et la chromatographie pour la production d'albumine humaine de haute pureté

189 **S. Mandjiny, M.A. Vijayalakshmi**
Membrane based pseudobioaffinity chromatography of placental IgG using immobilized L-histidine
Chromatographie de pseudo-affinité sur membrane des IgG placentaires en utilisant la L-histidine immobilisée

201 G. Birkenmeier, H. Dietze
Separation of immunoglobulins from human plasma by affinity membrane filtration
Séparation des immunoglobulines du plasma humain par filtration sur membranes d'affinité

207 N. Nourichafi, C. Geschier, J.-F. Stoltz
Comparison of various chromatographic supports for purifying human plasmatic immunoglobulins for Cohn II+III fraction
Comparaison de différents supports chromatographiques pour la purification des immunoglobulines humaines à partir de la fraction II+III de Cohn

IV. VIRUS SAFETY
IV. SÉCURITÉ VIRALE

215 P. Brunko
The regulation of medicinal products derived from human blood or plasma in the European Community
Réglementation communautaire des médicaments dérivés du sang ou du plasma humain

221 J.-J. Morgenthaler
Methods for inactivation of viruses in plasma products
Méthodes d'inactivation des virus dans des produits dérivés du plasma

229 F. Horaud
Biological products and viral safety
Produits biologiques et sécurité virale

237 B. Horowitz, A.M. Prince, M.S. Horowitz, C. Watklevicz
Viral safety of solvent/detergent treated blood products
Sécurité virale des produits du sang traités au solvant-détergent

249 M. Burnouf-Radosevich, T. Burnouf, J.-J. Huart
Development and experience of a pasteurization process for pooled fresh frozen plasma
Développement et expérience d'un procédé de pasteurisation de mélange de plasma frais congelé

255 **H. Mohr, B. Lambrecht**
Optimization of parameters for photodynamic virus inactivation of human fresh plasma
Optimisation des paramètres pour l'inactivation photodynamique des virus de plasma frais congelé

261 **H. Suomela, E. Hämäläinen**
Intravenous immunoglobulin of high purity when production includes solvent-detergent treatment
Immunoglobulines intraveineuses de haute pureté dont la production inclut un traitement par solvant-détergent

267 **J.-F. Stoltz, C. Rivat, M. Grandgeorge, C. Geschier, P. Sertillanges, J.-L. Véron, J. Liautaud, L. Dumont**
Study of the virus inactivation or elimination capacity of a chromatographic procedure for purifying human plasma albumin
Etude de l'inactivation ou de la capacité d'élimination des virus d'un procédé chromatographique de purification de l'albumine humaine

V. RECOMBINANT PROTEINS
V. PROTÉINES RECOMBINANTES

275 **C.V. Prowse**
Comparison between proteins from plasma fractionation and recombinant proteins
Comparaison entre les protéines obtenues par fractionnement du plasma et les protéines recombinantes

283 **J. Montreuil**
Recombinant glycoproteins: pitfalls and strategy
Glycoprotéines recombinantes : pièges et stratégie

293 **A. Sumi, W. Ohtani, K. Kobayashi, T. Ohmura, K. Yokoyama, M. Nishida, T. Suyama**
Purification and physicochemical properties of recombinant human serum albumin
Purification et propriétés physicochimiques de l'albumine humaine recombinante

VI. OTHER PLASMATIC PROTEINS
VI. AUTRES PROTÉINES PLASMATIQUES

301 V. Regnault, L. Vallar, C. Geschier, C. Rivat, J.-F. Stoltz
Dye-affinity purification and assessment of the biosafety of human plasma transthyretin destined to clinical uses
Purification par affinité sur colorant et évaluation de la biosécurité de la transthyrétine destinée à une utilisation thérapeutique

307 C. Chao, X. Wang, S. Chen, T. Zhang
Preparation of fibrin glue and its clinical application (summary)
Préparation de colle à base de fibrine et ses applications cliniques (résumé)

309 R. Bouguerne, J.-L. Guéant, C. Masson, F. Bois, P. Guimelly, J.-C. Michalski, J.P. Nicolas
Identification by HPLC of a hyperglycemic peptide induced by temperature in rat and human serum
Identification par HPLC d'un peptide hyperglycémique induit par chauffage du sérum humain ou de rat

315 Author index
Index des auteurs

I. Separation techniques used in plasma fractionation

I. Techniques de séparation utilisées dans le fractionnement du plasma

Chromatography packing design matching human plasma protein separation requirements

Egisto Boschetti, Pierre Girot, Luc Guerrier and Nicolas Voute

SEPRACOR S.A., 35, avenue Jean-Jaurès, 92395 Villeneuve-la-Garenne Cedex, France

SUMMARY

Chromatographic fractionation techniques are increasingly popular in isolating proteins from human plasma.

Considering that plasma is very rich in protein content, and that large quantities are treated to isolate proteins of medium value in very high safety level, special chromatographic sorbents may be desirable.

In this paper, productivity and safety aspects are discussed first with special emphasis on the sterilization and pyrogen removal from contaminated sorbents.

In a second part, a review of existing and potentially adapted media for human plasma separation is given.

INTRODUCTION

Human plasma is a very complex biological fluid where proteins are present at high total concentration and in large number. Only few of them are today separated for therapeutic applications in pure form. Contrary to most of the feedstocks used in downstream processing of proteins, human plasma implies separation schemes designed in such a way to purify simultaneously several entities to ensure the economics of the process.

In this context and considering the very large number of proteins present, specificities linked to human plasma can be listed permitting to define what should be the most adapted sorbents and the separation conditions.

Human plasma is a quite unclear viscous liquid where the concentration of proteins reaches more than 50 mg/ml.

The most represented proteins are albumin and immunoglobulins which are characterized on economic level by low value and are produced in large quantities.

Like many biological liquids, human plasma can contain virus particles that must be inactivated and/or eliminated in validated processes.

Consequently it seems important to consider two key issues when purifiying human plasma proteins by chromatography : high level of productivity for most low value proteins and total security in respect of viral sterility, apyrogenicity and absence of leached material from chromatographic packings.

In this paper, we analyze these two parameters and give specific recommendations in order to avoid inconsistent work on non adapted sorbents. A situation between the real needs and the main characteristics of existing sorbents will also be discussed.

CHROMATOGRAPHIC PRODUCTIVITY ANALYSIS

Productivity in chromatography can be defined as the amount of purified proteins in a given time for a given amount of sorbent. This definition should be completed then by the cost of the packing material.

It is known that the mathematical parameters governing the productivity are the dynamic capacity at a given flow rate *(Janson and Hedman, 1987)*, the column geometry and the cycle length. *(Boschetti, 1992)*.

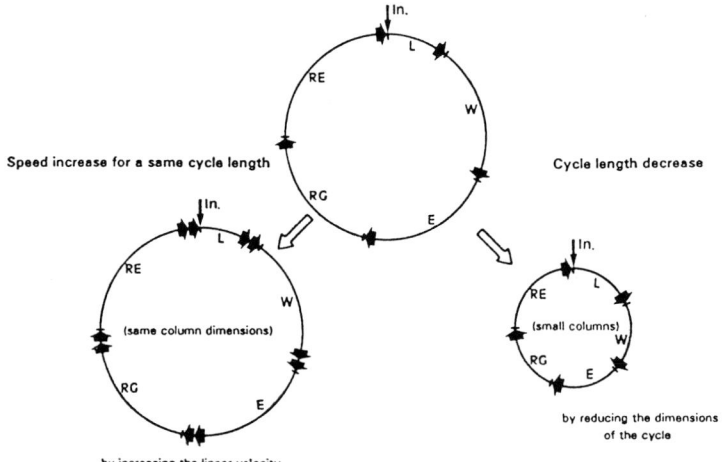

Fig.1 : Schematic representation of the modification of cycle duration by decreasing the column size using a sorbent with higher capacity (right) (loading time "L" is unchanged.), or by decreasing the time spent to cover the same cycle by speeding up the flow rate (left). In all cases loading duration was the same.

L = loading ; W = washing ; E = elution ; RG = regeneration ; **RE** : reequilibration

In non isocratic chromatography that represents most of the solid phase processes, a cycle is constituted of five main steps : loading, washing (collection of proteins in the flowthrough), elution (it can be decomposed of several substeps), regeneration and reequilibration (see Fig. 1). To improve the productivity of such a cycle considering that the loading remains constant, two ways can be followed : the diminution of the cycle length or the increase of the speed for the same cycle length (both could also be associated). In the first case, the solution consists in choosing more capacitive packings permitting, for an unchanged loading per cycle, to work with smaller columns.

In this situation the loading time remains the same while all other four steps are proportional to the column volume : total cycle will be much smaller.

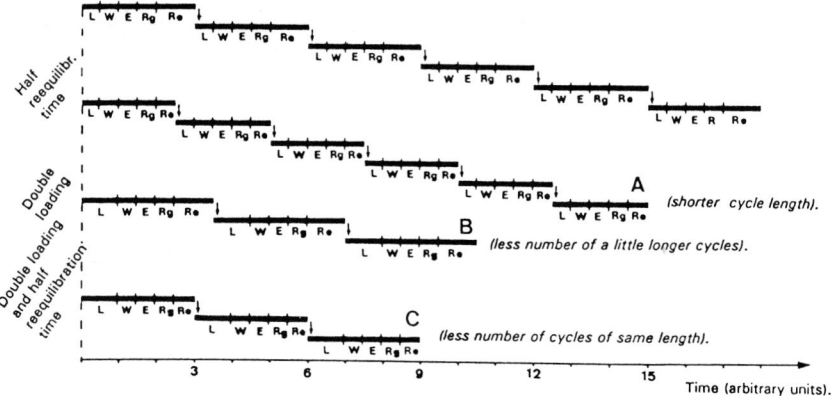

Fig.2 : Schematic representation of productivity improvement in a multicycle chromatographic separation. Total duration can be decreased choosing a sorbent with shorter reequilibration step (A) or diminishing the number of cycles with a more capacitive sorbent (B). Both improvements are illustrated in (C).

L = loading ; W = washing ; E = elution ; RG = regeneration ; RE : reequilibration

In the second case when speeding up the cycle velocity for the same column the time needed to cover the total distance could be much shorter. As for the first case here an appropriate sorbent must also be chosen because dynamic capacity decreases when the flow rate increases and for some sorbents, this parameter is dramatically modified. *(Boschetti, in preparation)*.

When considering the production of a given amount if proteins in a multicycle configuration (Fig. 2) it is clear that the impact of loading and column reequilibration are of importance to reduce the production time.

Here the key parameters when keeping constant the flow rate and the column size are the loading capacity and the time spent to reequilibrate the column with a shorter reequilibration time (this parameter is an intrinsic characteristics of chromatographic sorbent *(Boschetti, 1988)* ; the six cycles are covered in a shorter time. With a higher loading capacity, the number of cycles needed is lower and consequently the overall separation time shorter. Both parameters could be associated resulting in an even better situation.

As stated above, human plasma fractionation industry is characterized by large volumes of plasma to be treated involving large chromatographic columns. In this situation flow rate is not only limited due to the decrease of dynamic capacity, but also as a result of non rigid packings.

All considered, and independently on recovery and resolution theoretical solution is to use the smallest columns possible filled with uncompressible sorbents which show high dynamic capacities at very high flow rates.

SAFETY CONSIDERATIONS

Among the safety concerns we analyze here biological sterility, apyrogenicity and safety against chemical compounds coming from unperfectly washed sorbents or from degraded sorbents subsequent to too strong regeneration treatments. All safety concerns are of importance and should comply with validation procedures ; some of them depend on operating conditions (contaminations due to viruses, bacteria, DNA, pyrogens, and proteases) others depend on the chromatographic packing like leaching.

a) Sterilization :

It has been demonstrated that there are several solutions to sterilize a chromatographic column in acceptable conditions.*(Girot et al., 1990 ; Boschetti et al., 1990 ; 1992 ; Adams and Agarwal, 1989 ; Joyce et al., 1989).* Sodium hydroxide alone is a good solution for eliminating most of strains except spores (e.g. *Bacillus subtilis).* Acidic solutions are also behaving as sodium hydroxide as far as the degradation of spores is concerned even in the presence of ethanol. However when alternating acidic ethanol solutions in water with diluted sodium hydroxide, total sterility has been reached even in the presence of very large amount of spores. Alkaline solutions of ethanol are also very effective depending on the concentration of each component. For instance when sodium hydroxide is 0.2 M, concentration of ethanol must be close to 40-45 %, however it decreases down to 30-35 % in the presence of 0.5 M sodium hydroxide.

Additionally, sterilization using alternative washings or alkaline ethanolic solutions are also very useful to remove components very tightly adsorbed on the sorbent like lipidic material, non covalent aggregates and pigments.

b) Pyrogen removal :

Above mentioned solutions contribute also to destroy or remove pyrogenic material. Endotoxins, constituted of saccharidic sequences and of a terminal hydrophobic part called "lipid A", are present in large aggregates stabilized by divalent ions and hydrophobic associations *(Weary and Pearson, 1988).* Ethanol-containing solutions (as well as detergents) desorganize the aggregates while acidic solutions remove first metal ions and hydrolyze partially the endotoxin molecule. More specifically, acids cleave ketosidic linkage between lipid A and the core-polysccharide resulting in a dramatic decrease of the pyrogenic activity *(Weary and Pearson, 1988).*

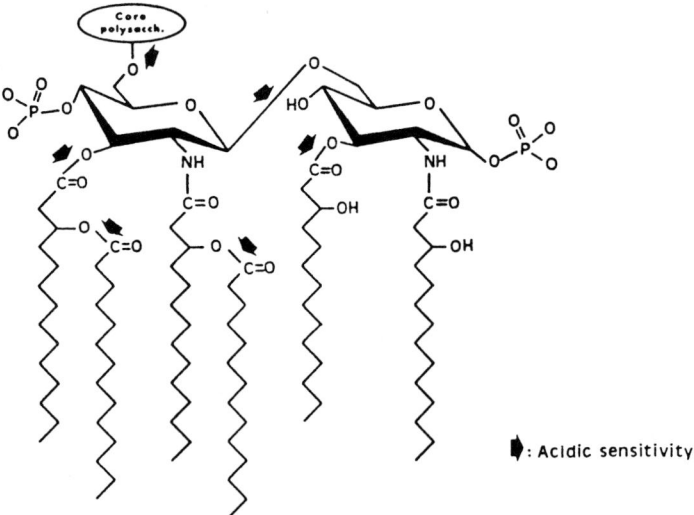

Fig.3 : Possible schematic structure of a Lipid A molecule. Substitution of the sugars with other molecules is possible according to origin of lipopolysaccharide. Hydroxylated and non hydroxylated fatty acids represent a major constituent of the structure.

Arrows indicate possible clivage sites in acidic conditions.

Acids contribute also to hydrolyse the lipid A at the level of ester linkages between the disaccharide and the fatty acids. Alkaline solutions which are uneffective for osidic hydrolysis permit the saponification of the lipid A releasing sodium salts of fatty acids (see Fig. 3)

c) Removal of leachables :

Strong washing procedures for regenerating and sanitizing can unfortunately degrade partially the macromolecular structure of the chromatographic sorbent *(Boschetti, 1988 ; Ahrgren et al., 1979 ; Johanson et al. 1987)*. Released molecules must be identified, assayed and eliminated. More importantly when dealing with affinity chromatography, toxicity of ligands that can be leached as a result of a labile linkage must be known.

Before considering these specific aspects it is important to determine in the virgin sorbent the presence of chemicals and reagents used during the synthesis of the chromatographic sorbent. Here attention have to be focused essentially on toxic or reactive organic molecules that may be present as a consequence of uncomplete reactions or uncomplete washing process. General examples are the determination of the presence of cross-linkers widely used when making gels. Most of them are very reactive toxic molecules.

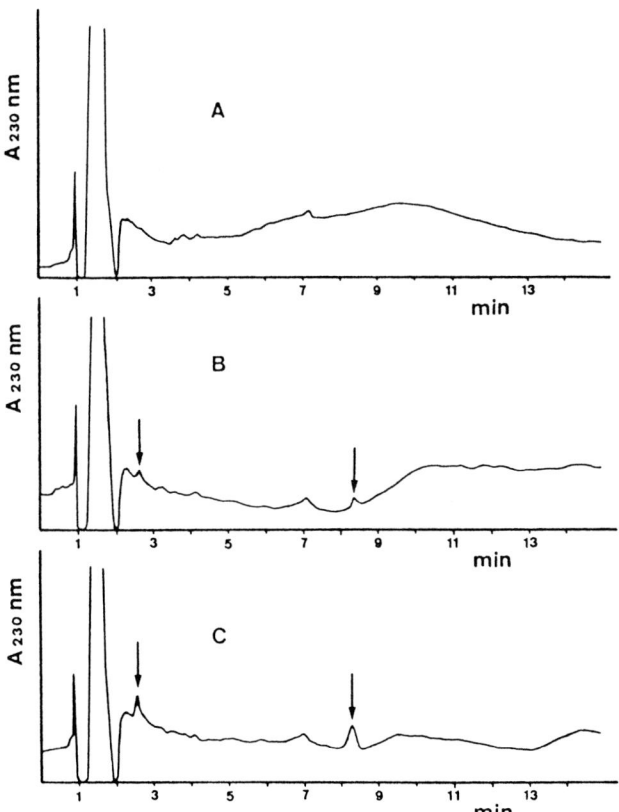

Fig.4 : HPLC analysis of virgin (A) and doped supernatant (B and C) of DEAE-Spherodex. Doping was realized by adding traces of cross-linking agent BDDGE (butanedioldiglycidyl ether) used in sorbent synthesis.
Arrows in B and C indicate the localization of BDDGE peaks which are absent in the original supernatant (A). Supernatants of B and C were respectively added with 25 µg and 50 µg/ml. For separation conditions see text.

An example is given here by HPLC quantification of butanedioldiglycidylether used as cross linking agent for polysaccharides. This component is utilized during the manufacturing of DEAE-Spherodex to stabilize the gel network. Excess of this reagent is eliminated by repeated washings with alkaline and acidic aqueous solutions. Fig.4 illustrates the quantification of BDDGE in a sample of supernatant of DEAE- Spherodex. Separation was effected by HPLC on a column (4.6 I.D x 150 mm) filled with nucleosil C-8 of 5 μm particle size. Elution was effected with 60 % distilled water and 40 % acetonitrile (v/v) at 1 ml/min.

Localisation of BDDGE peaks and method sensitivity were realized easily by adding increasing amount of fresh BDDGE in the DEAE-Spherodex supernatant. As demonstrated, no traces of reagent have been found as far as the sensitivity of the method is considered.

Only few published papers describe mechanisms of leakage and give recommendations for identification methods *(Ahrgren et al. 1979 ; Johanson et al., 1987 ; Boschetti et al., 1992)*. Here an example is proposed describing first a sensitive and reliable method for the quantification of dye traces and then a determination of toxicity in vitro. Reactive Blue 2 used extensively as immobilized dye for pseudo affinity chromatography has been recently investigated in order to establish an immunoenzymatic sensitive method to detect small traces that can be released from solid phases *(Santambien et al., 1992)*.

Additionally preliminary toxicity studies of native dye as well as modified dye that mimic the possible released material (carboxylic derivative) have been performed.

Table I : TOXICITY DATA ON REACTIVE BLUE 2

	Without dye	Native dye (average)	Carboxylic derivative (average)
In vitro cell proliferation (3rd pass.) (5μg/ml of dye)	100 %	90 %	92 %
Cell morphology and behaviour	normal	normal	normal
Polyploidia level	7/521	10/517	6-13/520
LD-50 (mouse)	-	>2000g/K	>2000 g/K

Table I summarizes some of the numerous data and shows that the behaviour of human cell in culture was not modified by adding 5 μg/ml of dye in the medium over three passages. Growth was at normal levels, morphology of the cells was also unchanged. After six passages and according to W.H.O. recommendations, chromosome polyploïdia level determination was in any cases significantly below the limits of acceptance (17/520).

All determinations were effected over 2500 metaphases per assay. The same dyes administrated to a population of 20 mices (male and female) in unique doses of 2000 mg per kilo of body did not evidence any trouble ; no mouse died.

Beyond the demonstration that this dye can be used safely and can be very specifically quantified by antibody-antigen reaction in all column effluent included in the presence of protein *(Santambien et al., 1992)*, this study is a good model to validate separation processes whatever the packing mateiral can be. These determinations should be naturally effected after regeneration and sanitization protocols that are mostly at the origin of sorbent deterioration.

PACKING MATERIAL REVIEW

The most used chromatographic sorbents are macromolecules constituted of polysaccharides (agarose, dextran, cellulose), synthetic polymers (polyacrylamide, poly-HEMA, Trisacryl, polystyrene), mineral (silica) and organo-mineral composite material. They are conceptually based on different principles like perfusivity *(Afeyan et al., 1991)*, tentacular trapping *(Muller., 1990)* macroporosity *(Girot and Boschetti., 1981)* or more classically based on homogeneous networks. Each of existing sorbents brings special features but none of them is really associating all advantages in an unique sorbent.

Though perfusive sorbents are of a good performance at high flow rates (quite constant capacity at medium-high linear velocities) their sorption capacity is generally quite low. Tentacular sorbents show very good adsorption efficiency (ratio between sorption capacity and amount of ion exchange groups) however, the sorption capacity is not very high and additionally tentacles are sensitive to strong acidic and alkaline treatments *(Boschetti., 1992)*. Macroporous sorbents are attractive by their wide pores and their synthetic nature but ionic accessibility is limited and some time they are sensitive to strong alkaline treatments. Finally, in spite of their high capacity, homogeneous networks suffer generally of a limited mass transfer (particularly in large beads), prohibiting very high flow rates.

Very recently *(Boschetti., 1992)*, new introduced packing material called HyperD showed a firtst tentative to associate the most important chromatographic features like high protein sorption capacity and sorption efficiency, low decrease of dynamic capacity versus linear velocity, total uncompresibility up to 1000 psi and a high degree of robustness in alkaline, acidic and oxydative environments.

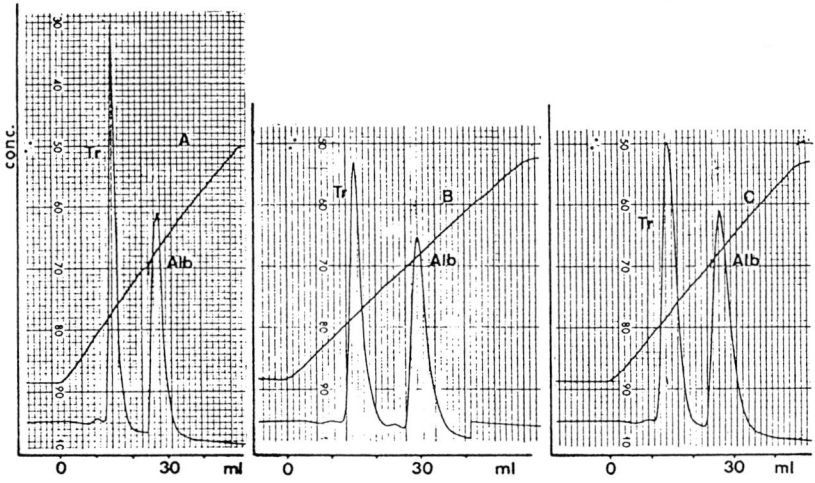

Fig.5 : Ion exchange separation of human transferrin (Tr) and albumin (Alb) on Q-Hyper D "F" grade at different flow rates. Linear velocities were 10 cm/h (A), 200 cm/h (B) and 500 cm/h (C).

Columns : 1.0 cm I.D. x 4 cm ; Buffer : 50 mM tris-HCl pH 8.6 ; Elution gradient : NaCl from zero to 0.4 M ; Loading : 10 mg of proteins in 200 μl buffer.

Table II : MAIN CHARACTERISTICS OF Hyper-D IEX "F" GRADE

	Q-Hyper D	S-Hyper D
Paricle size (μm)	25-60	25-60
Sorption capacity (mg/ml)	125 (BSA)*	100 (LP)**
Ionic groups (μeq/ml)	150	90
Sorption efficiency (mg/μeq)	0.85	11
pH stability	< 1-14	< 1-14
pk ionic groups	11	1
Pressure resistance (psi)	1000	1000
Volume changes	uncompressible	uncompressible

*   BSA : Bovine serum albumin in 0.05 M Tris-HCl pH 8.6
**   LP : Lactoperoxydase in 0.05 M acetate, pH 4.5

Table II assemblies the most important available data and Fig.5 shows separation performances as a function of flow rate. Resolution decrease was very low from a linear velocity of 10 cm/h (very classical flow rate : 1 column volume per hour) to 700 cm/h corresponding at 70 column volumes per hour.

Dynamic capacity at linear velocities up to 700 cm/hour was also decreasing very moderately from 112 mg/ml to 65 mg/ml (42 % loss) when compared to more than 80 % loss for more classical chromatographic ion exchangers.

Taking into consideration the specific needs of human plasma protein purification as discussed above, Hyper D material should represent a significant step in the direction of an optimized sorbent for these applications. It associates major feature for a real high productivity while permitting a high degree of safety as a result of its stability in extreme conditions necessary to perfect a very pushed cleaning (see prevoius chapters).

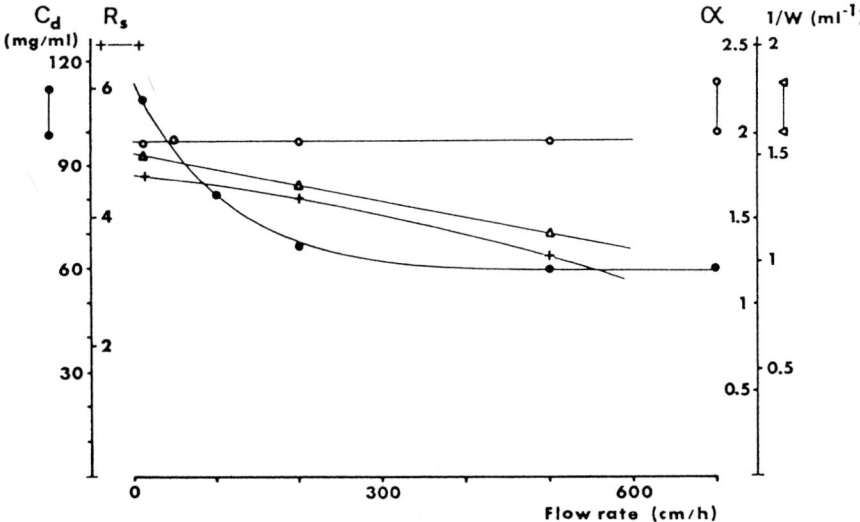

Fig.6 : Chromatographic parameters behaviour versus linear flow rate of Q-Hyper D column "F" grade.

Dynamic capacity Cd was determined using 10 mg/ml BSA in 50 mM tris-HCl buffer pH 8.6. Resolution (Rs) and selectivity (α) were calculated from results presented on figure 5. Efficiency in expressed here by the inverse of peak width (1/w) and measured on the second peak (albumin).

REFERENCES

Adams D.G., Agarwal D., (1989), Clean in place system design. *Biopharm.* 2(6), 48-57.

Afeyan N.B., Fulton S.P. et al. (1991), Perfusion chromatography packing materials for proteins and peptides., *J. Chromatogr.* 544, 267-279.

Ahrgen L,, Belder A. et al., (1979), Decomposition of diethyl aminoethyl derivatives of polysaccharides. In *Polymeric amines and ammonium salts*, ed. E.J. Goethals, pp 293-294. Oxford : Pergamon Press.

Boschetti E. (1988), Theoretical and practical approaches for liquid chromatography scale-up. *Proc. Inst. Conf. Biotech USA*, pp. 236-243.

Boschetti E., (1988), Design de supports : une notion importante dans la chromatographie liquide des protéines. *Protein Purification Technology*, vol.3, 23-31.

Boschetti E., Girot P. et al., (1990), Silica-dextran sorbent composites and their cleaning in place. *J. Chromatogr.*, 523, 35-42.

Boschetti E., (1992) Designing protein separation sorbents in the 90's., Personal communication.

Boschetti E., Bertrand O. et al., (1992), Produits de relargage de colorants immobilisés : identification et dosage. In *Technologies on protein studies and purification.*, ed. Y. Briand, C.Doinel, J.Gagnan, A.Faure, pp 91-103. Paris : G.R.B.P. press.

Boschetti E., Pouradier Duteil X. et al., (1992), Concerns and solutions for a proper decontamination of chromatographic packings. *Chemistry today*, submitted.

Boschetti E., (1993), Advanced sorbents for preparative purposes . *J. Chromatogr.*, in preparation.

Girot P., Boschetti E., (1981), Physico-chemical properties of new ion exchangers. *J. Chromatogr.* 213, 389-396.

Girot P., Moroux Y. et al., (1990), Composite affinity sorbents and their cleaning in place. *J.Chromatogr.* 510, 213-223.

Johansson B.L., Hellberg U. et al., (1987). Determination of the leakage from Phenyl-Sepharose CL-4B, Phenyl-Sepharose FF and Phenyl-Sepharose in bulk and column experiements. *J. Chromatogr.* 403, 85-98.

Janson J.C. and Hedman P., (1987) : On the optimization of process chromatography of proteins. *Biotechnol. Prog.* 3, 9-13.

Joyce W.G., Gaudet G.G. et al., (1989), Safe process scale chromatographs : standards and options. *Biotechnology*, 7, 721-722.

Muller W., (1990)., New ion exchangers for the chromatography of biopolymers. *J. Chromatogr.* 510, 133-140.

Santambien P., Hulak I. et al., (1992), Elisa-based quantification of Cibacron Blue F3GA used as ligand in affinity chromatography. *Bioseparation* 2, 327-334.

Santambien P., Girot P. *et al.*, (1992), Immunochemical quantification of Procion Red HE-3B as ligand in affinity chromatography. *J. Biochem.Biophys. Meth.* 24, 285-295.

Weary M, Pearson F., (1988), A manufacturer's guide to depyrogenation. *Biopharm.* 1(4), 22-29.

Résumé

La séparation des protéines par chromatographie liquide trouve des applications croissantes dans le domaine du plasma humain. Ce milieu biologique complexe est caractérisé par un fort contenu protéique dont les constituants essentiels sont d'une valeur ajoutée moyenne. De plus le danger potentiel de contamination (virus, microorganismes, pyrogènes) lié à sa manipulation massive limite l'utilisation de techniques comme la chromatographie en l'absence de méthodes de décontamination validées.

Dans ce rapport , deux aspects essentiels sont pris en considération, la productivité et la sécurité sur le plan biologique et pyrogénique. La deuxième partie du rapport est consacrée à l'analyse générale de la situation en matière de supports chromatographiques industriels dans le contexte de la séparation des protéines plasmatiques avec comme exemple la présentation d'un nouveau support aux caractéristiques cohérentes.

The simulated moving bed: a powerful process for purification

Michel Bailly and Roger-Marc Nicoud*

LSGC-ENSIC, 1, rue Grandville, 54001 Nancy, France, and *SEPAREX, 5, rue J. Monod, 54250 Champigneulles, France

ABSTRACT

An original chromatographic concept for bioseparation : the Simulated Moving Bed (SMB) is presented. The principle of the system is explained and applications for biotechnology are described. Using the example of a complex enantioseparation, respective performance of SMB and usual chromatography are compared.

INTRODUCTION

Chromatography is now widely used for bio-separation purposes. For instance, a lot of proteins are yet purified using ion exchange or size exclusion chromatography. However, these purifications are almost always performed through elution chromatography : a given amount of feed is periodically injected at the inlet of the column, pure fractions are collected at the outlet, after elution with constant (isocratic mode) or variable solvent composition (gradient mode). This mode is recognized as powerful because it allows an efficient purification of various compounds, but on the other hand, it is eluent consuming : the pure fractions are often recovered in tremendous amount of liquid. Moreover, this mode is discontinuous. The aim of this paper is to describe an other chromatographic mode : the Simulated Moving Bed, which is continuous and generally allows to get concentrated fractions.

THE SIMULATED MOVING BED : PRINCIPLE

In contrast to elution chromatography which is a batch process, in the Simulated Moving Bed system feed injection and fraction recovery are simultaneous and continuous. The principle of a true moving bed is schematically illustrated in figure 1.

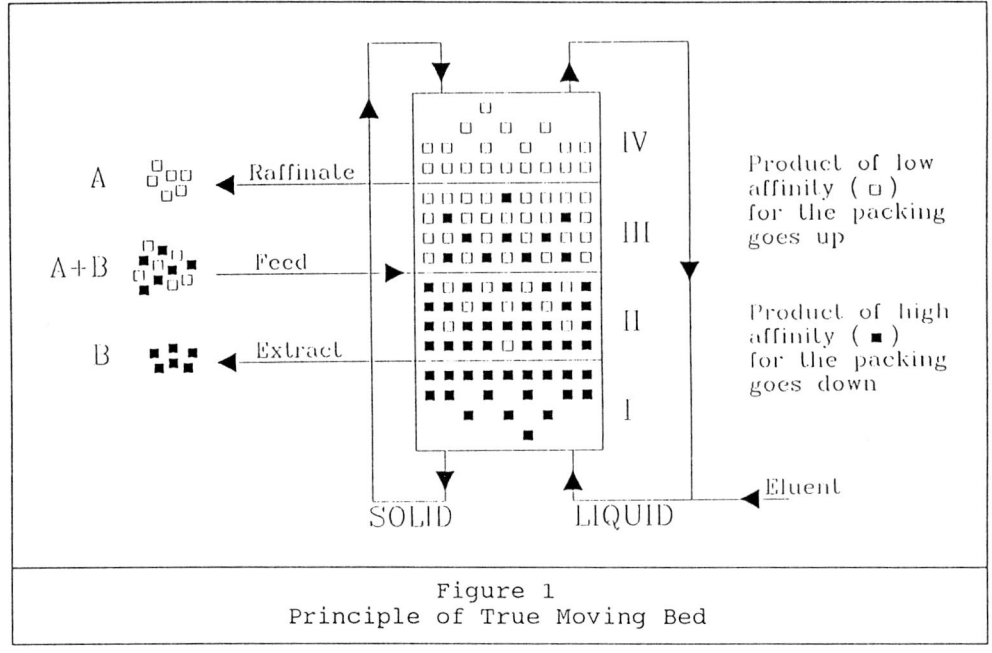

Figure 1
Principle of True Moving Bed

There is countercurrent contact between the solid phase and the eluent which move in opposite directions. Feed, containing components A and B, is injected in the middle of the column. Provided that the affinity of A and B for the solid are different (B being more retained than A), appropriate choice of the solid and liquid flow rates will split the feed into two fractions. The less retained component (A) goes up in the direction of the fluid, and is collected in the raffinate stream, whereas B moves in the direction of the solid, and is collected in the extract stream. Countercurrent systems are attractive because they are usually more efficient than batch processes.

The true moving bed adsorption process cannot be implemented directly because of lack of control over the solid flow. Thus the Simulated Moving Bed concept was developed. The basis idea is the following : rather than moving the solid in a system with inlet and outlet lines at fixed positions, it is equivalent, simply to move the inlet and outlet lines with respect to a fixed solid bed in the direction opposite to the desired solid flow. It is impractical to have continuously moving lines, and therefore a discrete implementation is preferred. One possible SMB scheme is illustrated in figure 2. There are several columns (at least four, but up to twenty four have been used in petrochemical applications) in which the solid is fixed, inlet and outlet lines being shifted step by step between these columns.

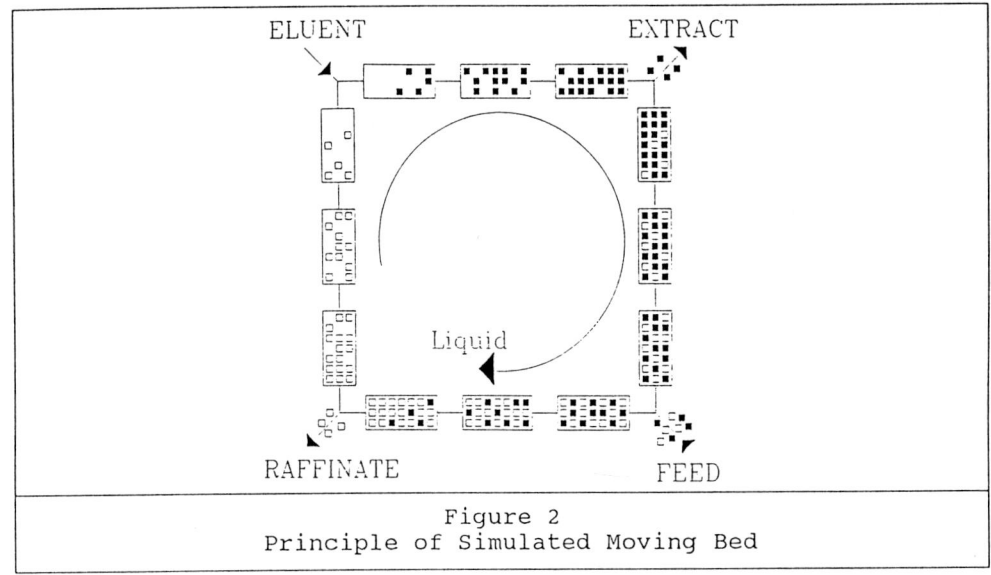

Figure 2
Principle of Simulated Moving Bed

Moving fronts appear in the system owing to elution, these fronts being followed by shifting injection and collection points. Consequently, the internal profiles are continuously moving in the system, but the outlet concentrations are almost constant.

The complete design of an SMB unit requires the choice of five flow rates (feed, extract, raffinate, eluent make-up and recycle flows), one rotation period, the column number and the column size.

The key is the proper selection of flow rates : they must be chosen in order to stabilize the B front between zones I and II, the A front between zones III and IV and to allow separation between zones II and III. The flowrate estimation relies on the knowledge of the adsorption isotherms of the components. Some simple expressions for flow rate selection are available in the case where the isotherms are linear [1]. However, in the more usual case where the isotherms are non linear, the situation is significantly more complex, and requires process simulation.

MAIN APPLICATIONS AND DEVELOPMENTS

The SMB was basically developed by UOP [2-5] : a single vertical column made up of several stages is used. The use of a master valve allows the inlet and outlet lines to be moved between the compartments. The Sorbex processes are usually named according to the application [6] : Parex, for the production of pure p-xylene ; Ebex, for ethylbenzene recovery ; Olex for the separation of n-paraffin-olefin mixtures ; Molex for the recovery of n-paraffins from light naphthas ; and Sarex for the recovery of fructose from fructose-glucose mixtures. Since 1963, more than 60 Sorbex units have been licensed, representing a total capacity of 5 million tons per year [7].

Rather than using a unique column with several compartments and a unique complex rotary valve, a combination of commonly used chromatography columns and commercial valves can be used. This type of technology has been developed by SEPAREX (Champigneulles,

France) and the Institut Français du Pétrole (IFP, Rueil-Malmaison, France) for their commercial plants (LICOSEP). The main industrial applications are in the petrochemical industry and in fructose-glucose separations [8-9].
However some development work is done in the following areas.

Chemistry and fine chemicals :

Different fractionations have been studied on a pilot scale. For example, Ching [10] reported the monoethanolamine-methanol separation, Liappis [11] the 2-butanol-ter-amylalcohol separation, and Storti [12] has worked on xylenes, ethylbenzene, toluene, and isopropylbenzene mixtures.

Biotechnology and pharmaceutical applications :

Until now, the most important and well-described application is the fructose-glucose separation using ion-exchange resins [13-16]. This application involves large-scale equipment, with productivity being higher than 100 tonnes/day. Different applications are also under development leading to more high-value sugars such as xylose-arabinose [17] or palatinose-trehalulose [18]. Barker has worked extensively with the purification of dextrans [19]. Research on the purification of enzymes [20-21], proteins [22], amino acid or sugar desalting [23-24], and fatty acid methyl esters [25] has also been carried out. Moreover, separation between glutamic acid and glutathione [26] has been recently described.

Optical isomers :

Complex enantioseparations appear to lead to promizing applications for SMB [27-28]. An example is given below.

A CASE STUDY : COMPARISON BETWEEN USUAL CHROMATOGRAPHY AND SMB

The enantio-separation of the chiral epoxyde 1a, 2, 7, 7a-tetrahydro-3-methoxinapht (2, 3b)-oxyrene is highly desirable, this compound being an important intermediate for asymetric synthesis [29].
This separation has been performed using methanol as eluent and cellulose triacetate as stationary phase.

Optimization of LC and estimation of productivity has been performed with a fully automated Gilson HPLC system in conjunction with a Metrohm column (2 cm I.D. x 25 cm length) containing 42 g CTA (15-25 µm, Merck n° 16362). Methanol has been used as mobile phase with a flow rate of 12.5 ml/min.

The Simulated Moving Bed pilot plant (LICOSEP plant at SEPAREX, Champigneulles, France) can deal with systems having from 4 up to 24 columns. In order to separate our epoxide enatiomers, 10 and 12 column configurations were investigated.

The columns were Superformance columns (Merck) of 2.6 cm I.D. and 11 cm length, packed with 25-40 µm cellulose triacetate (Merck) which was first carefully settled to remove the finest particles. in order to achieve good column stability, each column was packed with 26 g CTA.

As stated in the first paragraph, the estimation of the operating parameters for SMB must be carefully achieved. After determination of the isotherms, the operating parameters have been determined

using the HELP simulation software (proprietary software of SEPAREX). The obtained results are given below.
Starting from a feed containing 50 % of both enantiomers, usual LC as well as SMB allow to get 98 % pure fractions. The obtained experimental internal profiles for SMB are given on figure 3.

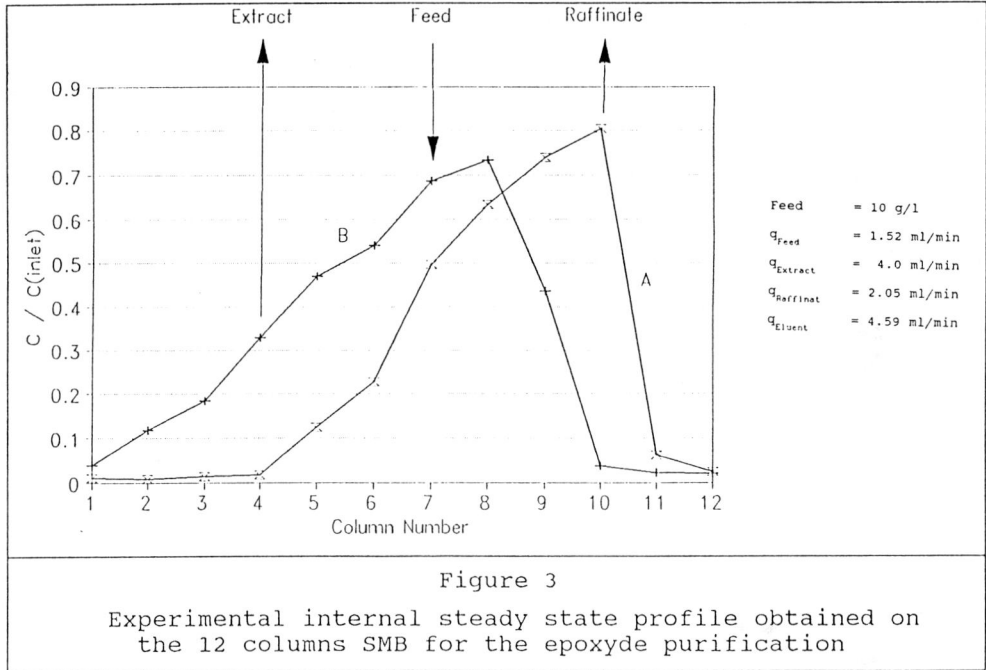

Figure 3
Experimental internal steady state profile obtained on the 12 columns SMB for the epoxyde purification

The comparison between SMB and results LC is given below.

Eluent consumption :

Compared with LC, eluent consumption in SMB is lower by a factor of 8. It should be pointed out that the LC system has been carefully optimized under overloaded conditions. The more conventionally used LC mode with baseline separation would require about 100 times more solvent than the SMB unit.

Specific productivity :

Based on the available results, the productivity obtained for SMB is two times lower than for LC. However, a larger particle size sorbent was used in SMB : 25-40 μm as opposed to 15-25 μm in LC. Since efficiency usually scales up with the square of the particle diameter, we expect that we can improve productivity in SMB by a factor of 4 using particles of half the diameter, leading to a specific productivity two times greater for SMB than for LC.

Recovery ratio :

Due to the intrinsic behavior of SMB units, the recovery is 100 %, as compared with only 70 % in LC. This could be a significant factor, depending on the feed cost.

REFERENCES

[1] R.M. NICOUD LC-GC Int. 5 (5) : 43-47, 1992.
[2] D.B. BROUGHTON, Chem. Eng. Prog. 64 (8), 6 (1968).
[3] D.P. THORNTON, Hydrocarbon Process. 49 (11), 151 (1970).
[4] D.B. BROUGHTON et al., Chem. Eng. Prog. 66 (9), 70 (1970).
[5] R.de ROSSET, R.NEUZIL, D.B.BROUGHTON, Percolation Processes : Theory and Applications, A.E. RODRIGUES and D. TONDEUR, Eds. (Sijthoff and Noordhoff, Dordrecht, The Netherlands 1981).
[6] D.B.BROUGHTON, Sep. Sci. Technol. 19(11/12), 723 (1984).
[7] D.B.BROUGHTON and S.A.GEMBICKI, AIChE Symp.Ser.80, 233 (1962)
[8] H. HEIKKILÄ, Chem. Eng. 24 January (1983).
[9] P.E.BARKER and G.GANETSOS, NATO ASI, Ser. E471-490 (1989).
[10] C.B. CHING, C. HO and D.M. RUTHVEN, Chem. Eng. Sci. 43(3), 703-711 (1988).
[11] A.I. LIAPPIS, AIChE J. 25(3), 455 (1979).
[12] G. STORTI, M. MASI and S. CARRA, Chem. Eng. Sci. 44(6), 1329-1345 (1989).
[13] C.B. CHING, J. Chem. Eng. Jpn. 16(1), 49 (1985).
[14] C.B.CHING and D.M.RUTHVEN, Chem.Eng.Sci.40(6), 877-885 (1985)
[15] P.E. BARKER and G. GANETSOS, J. Chem. Technol. Biotechnol. 35B, 217-228 (1985).
[16] P.E. BARKER and G. GANETSOS, Sep. Sci. Technol. 22(8-10), 2011-2035 (1987).
[17] G. HOTIER, Revue Française de l'IFP, in press.
[18] S. KISHIHARA et al., J. Chem. Eng. Jpn. 22(4), 434 (1989).
[19] P.E. BARKER, B.W. HART and A.N. WILLIAMS, Chromatographia 11(9), 487 (1989).
[20] S.Y. HUANG, C.K. LIN, W.H. CHANG and W.S. LEE, Chem. Eng. Commun. 45, 291-309 (1986).
[21] S.Y HUANG et al., Chem. Eng. Commun, 45, 291-309.
[22] K. HASHIMOTO, S. ADACHI, and Y. SHIRAI, Agric. Biol. Chem. 52(9), 2161-2167 (1988).
[23] K. HASHIMOTO, S. ADACHI, and Y. SHIRAI, J. Chem. Eng. Jpn, 22(4), 432 (1989).
[24] HASHIMOTO et al., Preparative and Production scale chromatography p. 273, Edited by G. GANETSOS and P.E. BARKER, Marcel Dekker Inc., New-York. Basel, Hong-Kong.
[25] L.SZEPY, Zs. Sebestyén ; I. Fehér and Z. NAGY, J. Chromatogr. 108, 285-297 (1975).
[26] HARUHIKO MAKI, Preparative and Production scale chromatography, p. 359.
[27] G. FUCHS, R.M. NICOUD and M. BAILLY, Optical isomers purification with the S.M.B. technology : experimental and theoritical approaches. Proceedings of the 9th Int. Symposium on Preparative and Industrial Chromat. "Prep 92", Nancy, France, April 1992, Edited by Société Française de Chimie, 395, 1992.
[28] M. NEGAWE, F. SHOJI, Optical resolution by simulated moving bed adsorption techn., J. of Chromatogr., 590, 113-117, 1992.
[29] Common work SEPAREX-SANDOZ PHARMA, to be published in Chirality.

Résumé

Un procédé chromatographique original pour les bioséparations est présenté : le Lit Mobile Simulé (LMS). Le principe du système est expliqué et des applications en biotechnologie sont décrites.
A partir d'un exemple d'une difficile séparation d'énantiomères, les performances du Lit Mobile Simulé sont comparées avec celles de la chromatographie classique.

Considerations in the use of synthetic dye-ligand affinity adsorbents for the manufacture of blood proteins

Steven J. Burton

Affinity Chromatography Ltd, 307 Huntingdon Road, Cambridge CB3 OJX, United Kingdom

Affinity chromatography is an attractive method for the isolation of blood proteins since it provides very high degrees of purification and is applicable to use on a large-scale. The requirements of affinity adsorbents for use in protein purification are well documented (Lowe., 1979). In particular, the immobilised ligand must exhibit selective and reversible binding and it should be possible to elute the bound protein without loss of biological activity. The adsorbent should also offer good protein binding capacities and recoveries, and for large scale applications, the support matrix should be sufficiently rigid to withstand high linear flow rates. However, there are a number of additional requirements demanded of affinity adsorbents which are to be used in the manufacture of therapeutic protein products.

First and foremost, the adsorbent must be chemically and biologically stable so that ligand leakage (and subsequent loss of column capacity) is reduced to a minimum. Current legislation requires that any compounds which leach from the adsorbent during chromatography must be identified and proven to be non-toxic, non-carcinogenic etc. at the levels which are encountered (Johansson, 1992). This means that in addition to availability of sensitive detection assays, any ligands used must be inherently non-toxic, and the adsorbent must be highly defined to enable the identification of leakage products. These requirements can only really be met by immobilisation of pure ligands under good manufacturing practice (GMP) conditions.

In addition to low ligand leakage, the adsorbent must be stable in order that rigorous column sanitisation methods can be employed. Sodium hydroxide is a particularly favoured cleaning agent since it is highly effective in destroying bacteria, viruses and endotoxin. Sodium hydroxide is also essentially non-toxic yielding sodium chloride and water after neutralisation. Consequently, it is highly desirable if an affinity adsorbent is alkali resistant. For this to be achieved, the ligand, the coupling chemistry and the support matrix must all be equally resistant to high pH's. The inadvertent introduction of biological contaminants (particularly viruses and endotoxin) into a process by way of contaminated adsorbent must also be considered. Synthetic ligands have obvious advantages compared to biologically derived ligands such as antibodies and protein A. A further degree of protection is afforded by manufacturing the adsorbent in a clean room environment where microbial contamination can be strictly controlled. Such attention to manufacturing detail facilitates the registration of chromatography adsorbents with the various pharmaceutical regulatory bodies (eg. FDA Drug Master Files).

REACTIVE TEXTILE DYES AS AFFINITY LIGANDS

Synthetic textile dyes, particularly reactive dyes containing a chlorotriazine group, have proved to be very successful for the purification of a variety of blood proteins, including serum albumin (Travis et al., 1976; More et al., 1984) plasminogen (Harris & Byfield, 1979), interferon (Jankowski et al., 1976), transferrin (Werner et al., 1983) and many others (Miribel et al., 1988). The most commonly used dye is C.I. Reactive Blue 2 (Cibacron Blue 3GA), a blue anthraquinone dye containing a monochlorotriazine reactive system (Fig. 1). In addition to selective and reversible binding to many blood proteins, reactive dyes also have the advantage of being easy to immobilise and inexpensive to produce. Hydroxylic support matrices are simply dyed in the same way as cellulosic cloth (Lowe, 1984). Furthermore, since the ligands are synthetic, the presence of biological contaminants is minimised. The dyes in question are also very stable, non-toxic and, theoretically, can be produced to high purities. These features make dye ligand adsorbents ideally suited to use in blood protein manufacture.

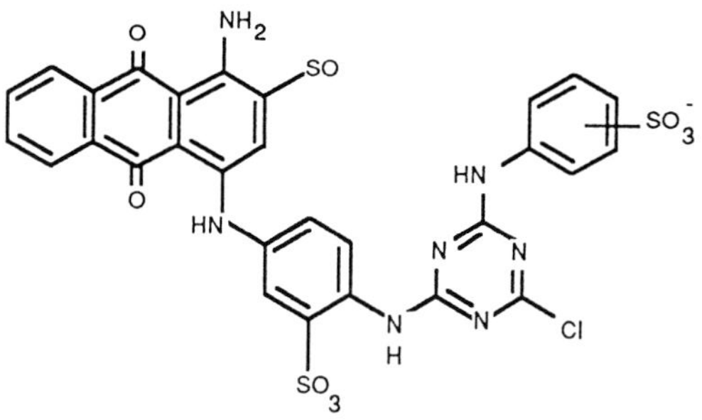

Fig.1. Structure of C. I. Reactive Blue 2

Unfortunately, most reactive dyes available on the open market are manufactured to meet the demands of the textile industry and do not meet the rigorous standards now required by the biopharmaceutical industry. In particular, commercial textile dye preparations are often highly heterogeneous and contain a number of unwanted contaminants, including isomeric species, reaction intermediates and by-products, antidusting agents and buffer salts (Burton et al., 1988). Thus the purity of a typical commercial dye preparation is normally in the region of 50 per cent and it is difficult, if not impossible, to identify the components of these crude mixtures which immobilise to (and subsequently leach from) a support matrix. A further problem is created by the widespread immobilisation of these dyes via the chlorotriazine moiety. Reaction of chlorotriazine groups with hydroxyl containing compounds yields alkoxytriazine derivatives which are known to be unstable, particularly at extremes of pH (Lowe, 1984). As the alkoxytriazine group constitutes the linkage between the dye and the support matrix, it is not surprising that dyes immobilised in this manner exhibit appreciable ligand leakage, particularly at alkaline pH. Ligand leakage may also occur by degradation of the support matrix and desorption of species which are non-specifically adsorbed during ligand immobilisation.

Because of the problems of heterogeneity and ligand leakage, reactive textile dyes would not appear to meet the requirements of the blood fractionation industry. However, all of the problems encountered relate to the nature of commercial textile dye preparations and associated bonding chemistries. By synthesising dye ligands specifically for use in the isolation of therapeutic protein products, these problems can be overcome.

BENEFITS OF SPECIFICALLY ENGINEERED DYE LIGANDS

Several advantages are obtained by manufacturing dye ligands specifically for affinity applications. Firstly, once the decision to adopt the synthesis route is made, then the problematic chlorotriazine bonding method can be abandoned in favour of more appropriate bonding chemsitries which may be engineered into the ligand itself. An example is the Mimetic^{TM} range of synthetic dye ligands manufactured by Affinity Chromatography Ltd which incorporate a highly stable spacer-arm bonding chemistry. During the course of ligand synthesis emphasis can be placed upon product purity, rather than product yield, with the result that very high purity dye ligands can be manufactured without having to resort to difficult and expensive post-synthesis purification methods such as preparative HPLC. Thus, for example, single isomer preparations of C.I. Reactive Blue 2 can be produced economically with purities in excess of 99 per cent. As both ligand and adsorbent synthesis can be accurately controlled, highly defined and reproducible adsorbents may be obtained. This is of great assistance, particularly for the identification and detection of potential leakage products.

An increasing volume of data is now being generated on the toxicology of reactive dyes. Most of the information has been obtained using standard, or partially purified preparations of commercial textile dyes, particularly C.I. Reactive Blue 2. This compound and related dyes have been shown to be essentially non-toxic, non-mitogenic and non-carcinogenic (Hulak et al., 1991; MacGregor et al., 1980). Consequently, purely on toxicity grounds there would appear to be no barrier to the use of C.I. Reactive Blue 2 and related poly-sulphonated dyes for the purification of therapeutic protein products. One would expect highly purified dye ligands to have an even greater safety margin. However, it is important that users establish that any dye leakage products are non-hazardous at the levels that may be encountered in the final protein product.

Dramatic improvements in dye leakage can be achieved by using alternative bonding chemistries. For example, whereas conventional C.I. Reactive Blue 2 agarose exhibits significant dye leakage at both acid and alkaline pH's, improved dye ligands with more stable bonding chemistries exhibit a remarkable increase in resistance to ligand leakage (Fig. 2). These findings have been substantiated by recent studies where ligand leakage has been monitored by sensitive ELISA detection assays capable of detecting dye concentrations down to the low nanomolar range (Stewart et al., 1992). The levels of ligand leakage observed for Mimetic Blue 1 adsorbent, even at extremes of pH, were barely detectable by ELISA assay and represented a dramatic improvement on conventionally immobilised dye media.

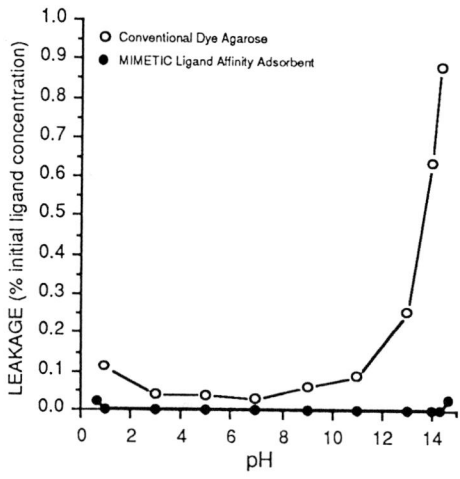

Fig. 2. Comparison of ligand leakage from conventional textile dye agarose and MIMETIC ligand affinity adsorbent

The robustness of purpose designed dye-ligand media such as Mimetic Blue 1 A6XL means that these materials can be subjected to repeated cleaning and sterilisation cycles with concentrated sodium hydroxide. This feature is very important when plasma, or various plasma fractions are applied to chromatography columns, since non-specifically adsorbed protein and lipid can stripped from the column after every cycle if required. Again sodium hydroxide is very effective at removing plasma components from chromatographic media, and in the absence of thorough cleaning, column performance deteriorates rapidly to the point where the media is no longer useable. Thus in a repetitive purification experiment where human serum albumin (HSA) is purified from diluted plasma in a single step, no decrease in column performance was observed over 300 cycles (Fig. 3). This reuseability was facilitated by a 1M NaOH cleaning step every fifth cycle. It is also notable that this approach can provide virtually pure HSA (approximately 98 per cent purity) with albumin recoveries of approximately 95 per cent. Given that the capacity of the Mimetic Blue 1 A6XL media for HSA approaches 50mg/ml (Stewart et al., 1992) one can see that this method is eminently suitable for the large scale purification of this important plasma protein.

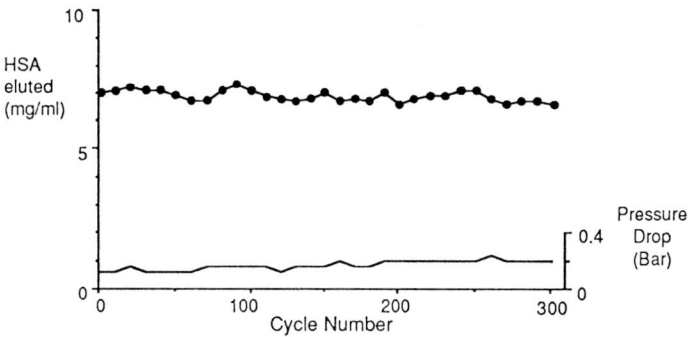

Fig. 3. Purification of HSA from Human Plasma on Mimetic Blue 1 A6XL: Column Capacity and Pressure Drop as a Function of Cycle Number

Human plasma was diluted 1:1 with 25mM MOPS buffer, pH 6.0, readjusted to pH 6.0 with 1M HCl and filtered. At the beginning of each cycle the column (0.5 cm dia. x 9.5 cm) was equilibrated with 6ml of 25mM MOPS buffer, pH 6.0 and the column loaded with 1ml of diluted plasma. After washing with 5ml of equilibration buffer, bound HSA was eluted with 5ml of 50 mM sodium phosphate buffer, pH 8.0 containing 1M KCl (NaCl could also be used). Every fith cycle the column was regenerated by flushing with 1M NaOH. Eluted HSA was collected every 10th cycle and quantified by absorbance at 280 nm. Column back pressure was also recorded every 10th cycle. The experiment was run continuously for 300 cycles at a flow rate of 1 ml/min (300 cm/h).

THE FUTURE OF DYE-LIGAND AFFINITY CHROMATOGRAPHY

A further extension to the concept of synthesising dye ligands specifically for affinity separations is the design of novel synthetic ligands which are targetted toward specific proteins. Such "biomimetic" ligands would have similar properties to the new generation of dye ligands described above, but possess increased binding selectivity. A substantial amount of work has already been directed towards increasing the selectivity of dye ligands (Burton et al., 1990; Lindner et al., 1989). More recently, de-novo design and synthesis of novel dye-like ligands has been attempted. In one of the first reported examples, a synthetic ligand for the purification of kallikrein was developed (Burton & Lowe, 1992).

Thus, in the future, it is possible to envisage a range of totally synthetic affinity ligands which are specific for most commercially important plasma proteins. In common with current state-of-the-art materials, these new adsorbents are likely to be highly stable, non-toxic, free of contaminants and produced to high quality standards. Such materials would offer tremendous advantages to the blood fractionation industry.

REFERENCES

Burton, S.J., McLoughlin, S.B., Stead, C.V., and Lowe, C.R. (1988). J. Chromatogr. 435: 127-137.
Burton, S.J., Stead, C.V., and Lowe, C.R. (1990). J. Chromatog. 508: 109-125.
Burton, N.P., and Lowe, C.R. (1992). J. Mol. Recog. 5: 55-68.
Harris, N.D., and Byfield, P.G.H. (1979). FEBS Lett. 103: 162-164.
Hulak, I., Nguyel, C., Girot, P., and Boschetti, E. (1991). J. Chromatogr. 539: 355-362.
Johansson, B.-L. (1992). Pharmaceut. Technol. Internat. 4: 24-29.
Lindner, N.M., Jeffcoat, R., and Lowe, C.R. (1989). J. Chromatogr. 473: 227-240.
Lowe, C.R. (1979). In Laboratory Techniques in Biochemistry and Molecular Biology. Vol. 7, eds T.S. Work and E. Work, pp. 267-522. Amsterdam: North Holland.
Lowe, C.R. (1984). In Topics in Enzyme and Fermentation Biotechnology. Vol. 9, ed A. Wiseman, pp. 78-161. Chichester: Ellis Horwood.
MacGregor, J.T., Diamond, M.J., Mazzeno, L.W., and Friedman, M. (1980). Mutagenesis 2: 405-418.
Miribel, L., Gianazza, E., and Arnaud, P. (1983). Arch. Biochem. Biophys. 226: 393-398.
More, J.E., Hitchcock, A.G., Price, S., Rott, J., and Harvey, M.J. (1989). In Protein-Dye Interactions: Developments and Applications, eds M.A. Vijayalakshmi and O. Bertrand, pp. 265-274. London: Elsevier.
Stewart, D.J., Purvis, D.R., Pitts, J.M., and Lowe, C.R. (1992). J. Chromatogr. 623: 1-14.
Travis, J., Bowen, J., Tewksbury, D., Johnson, D., and Pannell, R. (1976). Biochem. J. 157: 301-306.
Werner, P.A.M., Galbraith, R.M., and Arnaud, P. (1983). Arch. Biochem. Biophys. 226: 393-398.

Design of novel affinity ligands for the purification of proteases and protease inhibitors

Janette A. Thomas and Christopher R. Lowe

Institute of Biotechnology, University of Cambridge, Tennis Court Road, Cambridge, CB2 1QT, United Kingdom

Affinity chromatography harnesses the specific interaction that occurs between biological macromolecules and their ligands such as enzyme substrates, inhibitors, coenzymes, effectors, antigens, nucleic acids, hormones and sugars. The fundamental feature of affinity purification is the predictive and rational character, since the ligand selected is designed to interact specifically with the molecule to be purified. As a result, the use of affinity chromatographic techniques should simplify process design and make the selective adsorption step much less sensitive to the composition of the feedstock.

Biological compounds such as proteins tend to be expensive to use as ligands for affinity adsorbents since the ligands themselves are chemically and biologically labile and are difficult to immobilise in high yield with retention of activity. However, to circumvent many of these difficulties, biomimetic ligands can be designed and used in place of their natural counterparts as ligands for affinity chromatography. By far the most universal class of biomimetic ligand is the reactive textile dyes. For example, many proteins have been purified on immobilised Cibacron Blue F3G-A affinity adsorbents, including albumin and other blood proteins. The use of immobilised textile dyes offers significant advantages over conventional affinity adsorbents (Table 1). Thus they are inexpensive, commodity chemicals which are readily coupled to a variety of support matrices via their reactive groups and are resistant to biological and chemical degradation.

Table 1. Comparison of immobilised 'biomimetic' dyes with conventional affinity adsorbents

Criterion	Conventional biospecific ligands	Biomimetic ligands
Cost	Can be expensive	Inexpensive, commodity chemicals
Stability	Tend to be labile	Chemically and biologically stable
Specificity	High to moderate	Moderate
Synthesis of adsorbents	Often lengthy, synthetic route and/or by use of toxic activation agents	Facile, often one step reaction
Capacity	Low	High (>10% ligand utilisation)
Scale-up potential	Limited	Large scale potential
Sterilisability	Often low	High
Re-usability	Limited	Very high

To date, however, almost all studies have been performed with commercially available dyes which have fortuitously been found to mimic natural biological compounds in their specificity of binding. The selectivity of these affinity ligands can be improved by designing dyestuffs which mimic the structure and binding of natural biological ligands much more than the commercial dyes.

This paper describes the design of novel affinity ligands for the purification of alkaline phosphatase and kallikrein as examples of the approach to be taken in the design of affinity ligands to purify other proteins such as alpha1-proteinase inhibitor.

Immobilised commercial dyes were screened for the binding of alkaline phosphatase from calf intestinal mucosa. The results revealed an average 8.4-fold purification with enzyme recoveries >90%. The specific activity achieved (~25.2 u/mg) fell far short of the specific activity of commercial 'high purity' preparations (850-1250 u/mg). The inability of commercial dyes to purify alkaline phosphatase may be ameliorated by using specifically designed and synthesised triazine dyes as ligands (Lindner et al., 1989). Carboxylate, phosphonate and boronate are known to be potent competitive inhibitors of alkaline phosphatase and the enzyme prefers aromatic rather than aliphatic phosphate esters. Substitution of these groups on dye chromophores would be expected to yield more effective adsorbents and so several dyes were synthesised with these substituents on the terminal ring of Cibacron Blue F3G-A (Fig. 1). Preliminary evidence showed that the p-aminobenzyl phosphonate analogue proved superior for the purification of alkaline phosphatase, with up to 200 fold increase in specific activity.

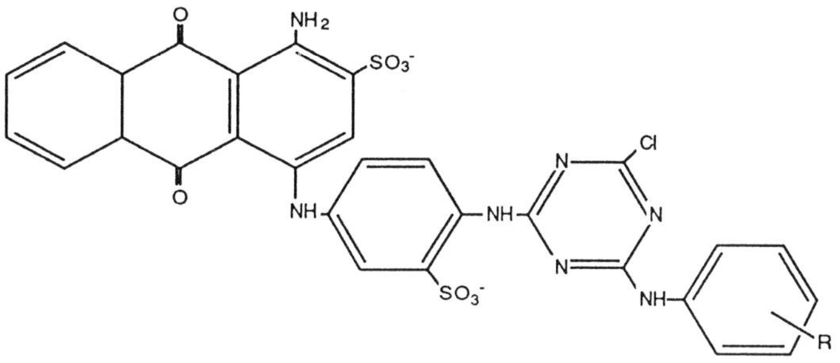

Terminal ring analogue	R
I aniline	-H
II p-aminobenzoic acid	-COOH
III m/p-aminobenzenesulphonic acid	-SO$_3$H
IV p-aminobenzyl phosphonic acid	-CH$_2$PO$_3$H$_2$
V m-aminobenzeneboronic acid	-B(OH)$_2$

Fig. 1. The structure of Cibacron Blue F3G-A and the terminal ring substituents.

With optimisation of adsorption and elution protocols, a 330-fold one-step purification of the enzyme from crude calf intestinal extract was achieved using specific elution with inorganic phosphate (5mM). The major contaminant in purified alkaline phosphatase is phosphodiesterase but using this methodology the purified enzyme contained <0.05U phosphodiesterase/mg protein. The final alkaline phosphatase product displayed a specific activity in excess of 1000 u/mg and was of equivalent purity to commercial 'high purity' preparations (Lindner *et al.*, 1989).

The effectiveness of specifically designed dye molecules as ligands for affinity chromatography prompted consideration of the possibilities of *de novo* design and synthesis of biomimetic ligands targeted at an individual protein, in this way an affinity ligand for the proteolytic enzyme, kallikrein, was designed.

The trypsin-like family of enzymes forms one of the the largest groups of enzymes requiring cationic substrates and includes enzymes involved in digestion (trypsin), blood clotting (kallikrein, thrombin, factor Xa), fibrinolysis, (urokinase, tissue plasminogen activator), and complement fixation. These enzymes possess similar catalytic machinery and bind the side chains of lysine or arginine in a binding pocket (the primary binding pocket, denoted S1) proximal to the reactive serine (Ser-195). Substrate specificity is determined partly by the side chain of Asp-189 lying at the bottom of the pocket interacting with the cationic side chain, and partly by secondary interactions with the side chains of other amino acids nearby in the substrate. For example, the binding specificity of tissue kallikrein differs from pancreatic trypsin in that it displays a marked preference for phenylalanine in the secondary site. This specificity arises because the phenyl ring of the phenylalanine residue neatly slips in a hydrophobic wedge shaped pocket between the aromatic side chains of residues Trp-215 and Tyr-99 whereas trypsin does not have this hydrophobic pocket. Consequently, designing a ligand specific for kallikrein should be achieved by designing and synthesising a mimic for the Phe-Arg dipeptide (Burton and Lowe, 1992). Figure 2 shows the structure of the analogue designed to mimic the Phe-Arg dipeptide comprising of p-aminobenzamidine and phenethylamine functions substituted on a monochlorotriazine moiety.

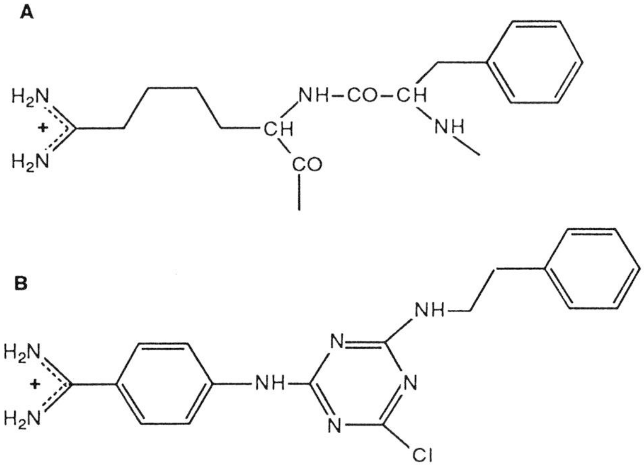

Fig. 2. Comparison of the structures of: (A) the Phe-Arg dipeptide, and (B) the "biomimetic" ligand designed to bind at the active site of the porcine pancreatic kallikrein.

The ligand was designed using the crystal structure of kallikrein bound with BPTI (Bode et al., 1983) and the known position of benzamidine, which binds to kallikrein with the triazine ring projecting partly into solution. Using computer modeling to examine the binding site, replacement of one of the chlorines on the triazine ring with the phenethylamine group made it possible to place the terminal phenyl group of this substitution in the hydrophobic secondary binding pocket between the side chains of residues 99 and 215: this arrangement leaves the third chlorine available for immobilisation of the ligand to the matrix. However, the active site of of kallikrein lies in a depression in the surface of the enzyme and direct immobilisation of the ligand to the matrix causes problems of steric hindrance. Insertion of a hexamethylene spacer arm between the ligand and the matrix circumvented this problem and generated a highly effective adsorbent for the purification of pancreatic kallikrein. Experiments showed that kallikrein bound strongly to the immobilised 6-aminohexyl analogue of the biomimetic ligand with over 90% of activity being recovered on elution with 4-aminobenzamidine. In contrast, other proteinases, such as trypsin, did not bind to the column showing the ligand is specific for kallikrein and yet not for broad specificity proteinases.

These studies clearly show the value of designing ligands which mimic natural biological molecules and the effectiveness of using a combination of structural knowledge with computer aided design for producing novel 'biomimetic' ligands for affinity chromatography.

REFERENCES

Bode, W., Chen, Z., Bartels, K., Kutzbach, C., Schmidt-Kastner, G., Bartunik, H. (1983): Refined 2A X-ray crystal structure of porcine pancreatic kallikrein A, a specific trypsin-like serine proteinase. *J. Mol. Biol.* 164, 237-282.

Burton, N.P. & Lowe, C.R. (1992): Design of novel affinity adsorbents for the purification of trypsin-like proteases. *J. Mol. Recognit* 5, 55-68.

Lindner, N. M., Jeffcoat, R. & Lowe, C.R. (1989): Design and applications of Biomimetic anthraquinone dyes. *J. Chromatogr.* 473, 227-240.

Lowe, C.R., Burton, S.J., Burton, N.P., Alderton, W.K., Pitts, J.M., & Thomas, J.A. (1992): Designer dyes: "Biomimetic" ligands for the purification of pharmaceutical proteins by affinity chromatography. *Trends in Biotech.* 10, 442-448.

Validation aspects relating to the use of chromatographic media

J.H. Berglöf

Fast Trak Consulting, Pharmacia BioProcess Technology AB, 751 82 Uppsala, Sweden

Production and purification processes for all biological products intended for medical use need to be validated. This is one of requirements of the Good Manufacturing Practice (GMP) regulations in both the USA and Europe, and it applies irrespective of whether the source material is recombinant or human plasma.

Validation is defined by the Federal Drug Administration (FDA) in their "Guidelines on general principles of process validation" May 1987, as: "Establishing documented evidence which provides a high degree of assurance that a specific process will consistently produce a product meeting its pre-determined specifications and quality attributes".

Chromatographic media play an important role in most modern purification processes due to their high selectivity, as a result, their function as a specific unit operation needs to be established and qualified. This paper covers some of the aspects that concern the use of chromatographic media when validating a process.

COLUMN QUALIFICATION

To give assurance that a chromatographic medium will perform as expected, its packing into a column has to be qualified. Column qualification is an important aspect that must be considered at process development in small columns, during scale up and also when verifying scale down in spiking experiments.

A packed column is relatively easy to qualify by using a test sample, for example 2% acetone, or a salt solution that can be detected by UV- or conductivity monitoring. From the results, Height Equivalent to a Theoretical Plate (HETP) and/or peak asymmetry values can then be calculated as shown in Fig. 1.

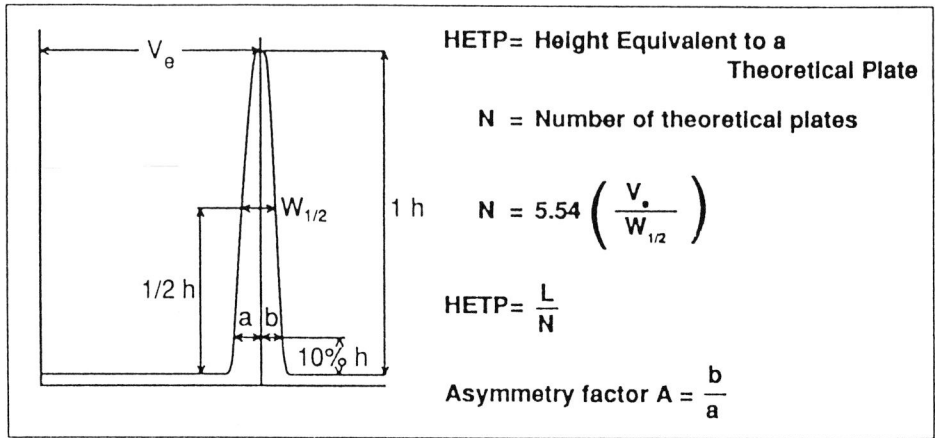

Fig. 1. Determination of HETP and peak asymmetry.

When using HETP and peak asymmetry it is important that the parameters are set at the maximum acceptable values for a given step. These values should then be used for all work, regardless of column size. There are a few rules of thumb that may be followed when setting these values. Firstly, the best HETP that can be achieved is 2 dp (dp = mean particle diameter). In practice, values of 3-5 dp are acceptable in situations where demands on resolution are high. However, values of 5-10 dp are normal where there is less demand on resolution. Peak asymmetry values usually lie between 0.7-1.3. If values for HETP and peak asymmetry fall within the above limits, it is possible to prove that packed columns perform identically regardless of size.

Secondly, when performing spiking experiments, for example with viruses in a scaled down process, it is important to consider the materials in use and the design of the small scale column. This is to ensure that the small scale column really mimics the column intended for use in the production process. If the large scale column has stainless steel or polyamide nets, the small scale column should have the same. Sintered frits could cause artefacts.

Thirdly, scale up and down will be linear and well controlled if linear flow rates are kept within the same range and sample loadings with proteins are proportional. As long as these two parameters are controlled during virus spiking experiments, the magnitude of the scale down is not as important as the ability to scale down to a level which suits the virus testing requirements. These require that maximum log reduction be demonstrated.

REMOVAL OF CRITICAL CONTAMINANTS

To demonstrate some of aspects of column qualification and scale down, the example below was developed. The process that was validated is a chromatographic procedure for the fractionation of plasma into albumin and IgG; it has been reported previously (2). An simple overview of the ion exchange steps is shown in Fig. 2. For the requirements of this demonstration, however, we shall focus on the last step in the IgG purification procedure.

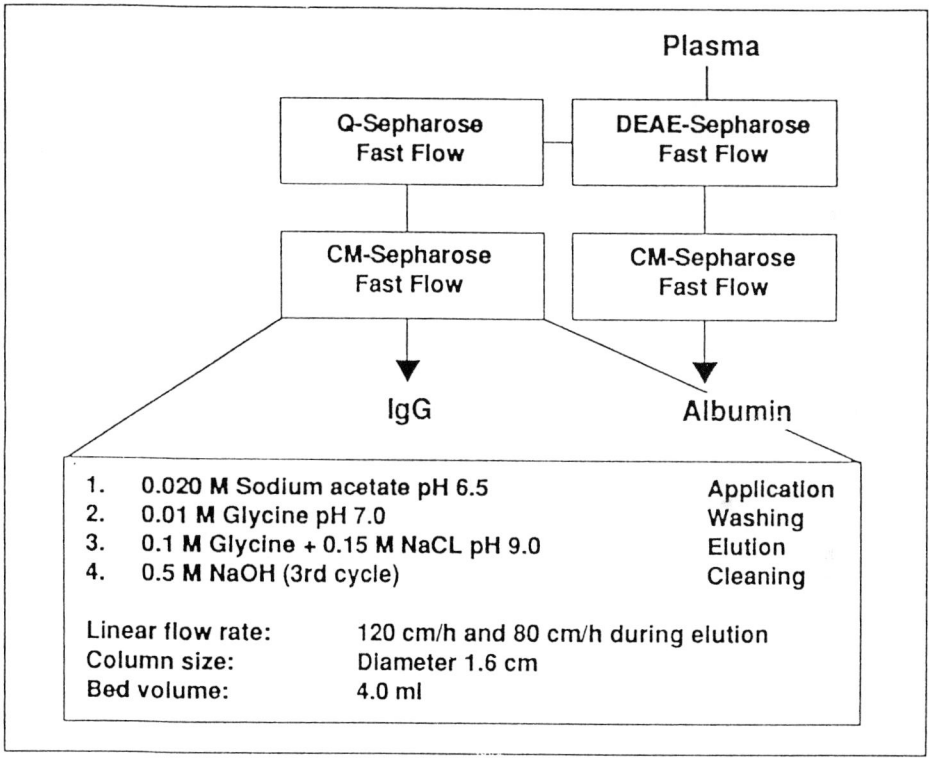

Fig. 2. Fractionation of plasma

Strictly speaking, several viruses should be used in order to reflect a variety of characteristics. In our example, however, only one virus was used, Bovine Herpes Virus (BHV). BHV was chosen as there are no neutralising antibodies present in plasma. Acceptable HETP and peak asymmetry values were then set. For HETP it was decided that columns should give values below
0.05 cm and for peak asymmetry, values between 0.7-1.3.

The design of this step involved three applications from one batch without any intermediate wash. Product quality is demonstrated in Fig. 3 where the chromatogram from one of the cycles performed on a 4 ml column used for spiking is shown together with an analytical gel filtration run of the product.

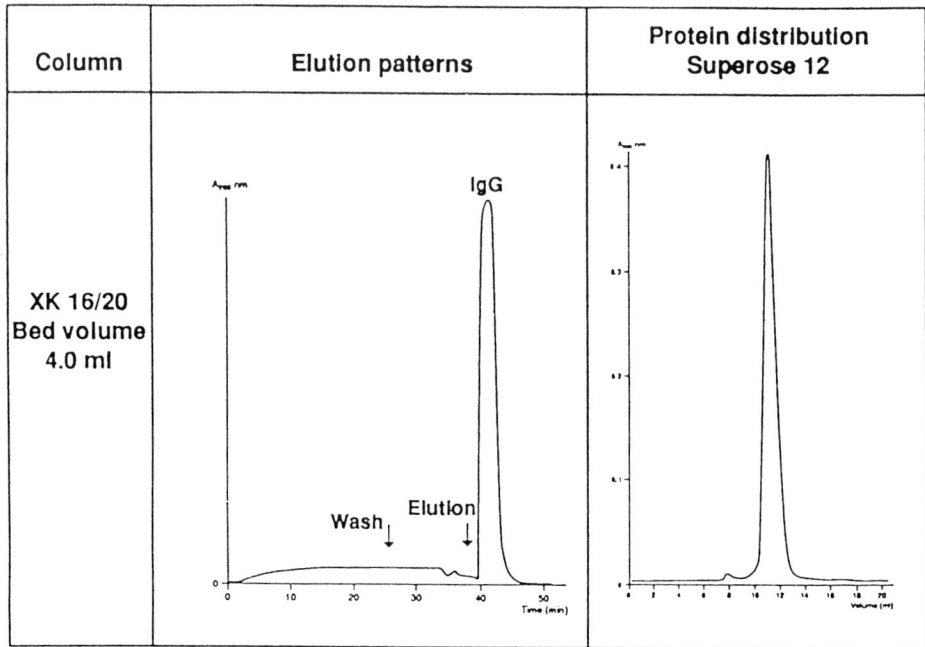

Fig. 3. Elution of IgG from CM Sepharose® Fast Flow in 4.0 ml column and analytical gel filtration of the product on Superose® 12.

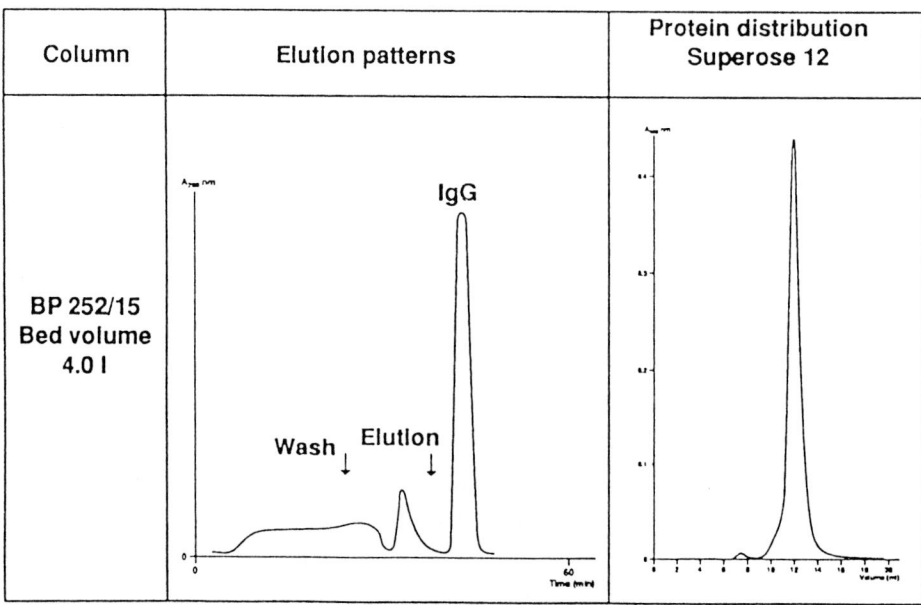

Fig. 4. Elution of IgG from CM Sepharose® Fast Flow in a 4 litre column and analytical gel filtration of the product on Superose® 12.

The large scale run shown in Fig. 4. was performed in a column with a volume of 4 litres, the scale down was thus 1000-fold. Note that the UV monitor used at large scale is not linear due to the large flow cell. This means that measurements within the protein peaks are not linear either. As a result, the protein peaks have to be verified by an analytical technique, in this case by checking the product by analytical gel filtration. By using this method, scale down could thus be demonstrated.

Two virus spiking experiments were also performed. In the first experiment, spiking was carried out in the first cycle and in the second experiment from the third cycle. The products from the first and third cycles were then tested for the virus to check carry over. In the first cycle the virus was below detection limit, in the third cycle it was slightly above detection limit. This indicates that viruses adsorb easily, but can just as easily leak in later cycles. Consequently cleaning must be performed between cycles in order to avoid accumulation of the virus on a column and carry over between batches. The experiments are outlined in Fig. 5.

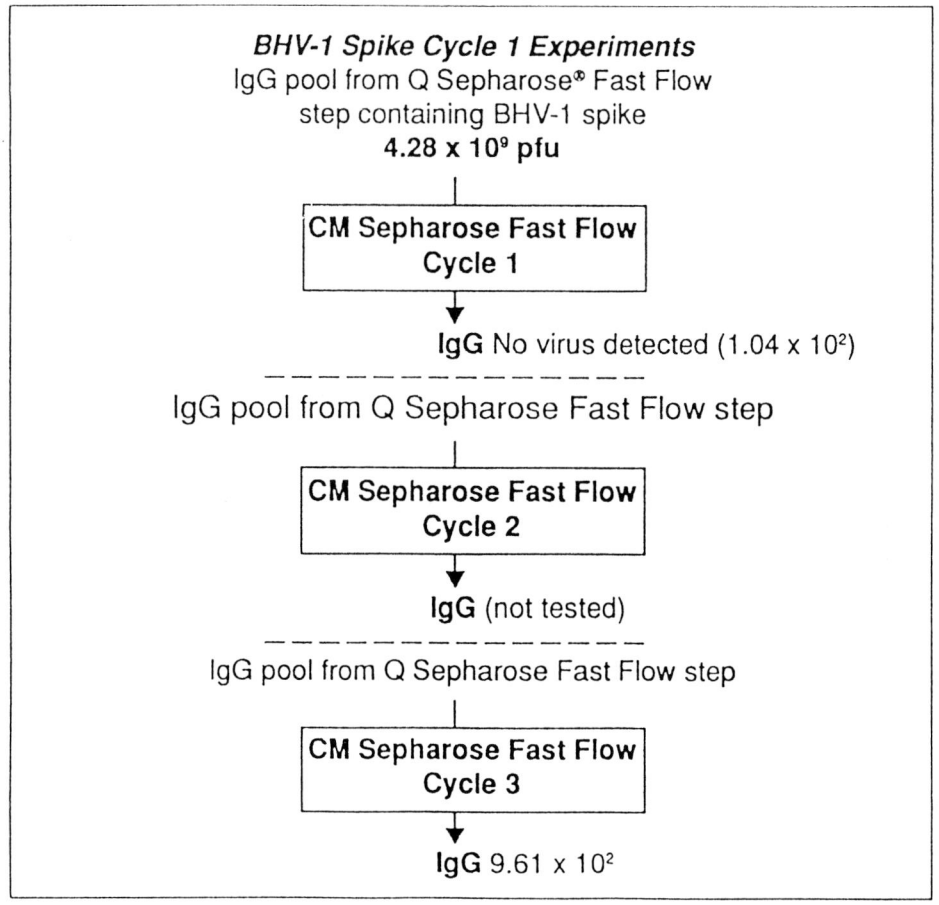

Fig. 5. Virus spiking experiments.

CLEANING

Cleaning of columns is vital in order to stop carry over between batches. One cleaning agent that is recognised for its effectiveness in inactivating viruses and other substances such as endotoxins is sodium hydroxide. Indeed our own data (1) show that viruses are effectively inactivated by sodium hydroxide. Since viruses can accumulate on a column, there is a risk of cross contamination between cycles and batches; columns should therefore be cleaned with sodium hydroxide after every cycle. Cleaning will also contribute to the life time of the chromatographic media.

CONCLUSION

Aspects of process validation that concern chromatographic media are very straightforward to deal with. Column qualification is an effective way to assess scale down and scale up. Validation of cleaning procedures will assess their effectiveness in removing/ inactivating potentially harmful agents such as viruses.

ACKNOWLEDGEMENTS

The experimental work behind this paper has been prepared by A. J. Darling, Quality Biotech Ltd., Glasgow, United Kingdom and I. Andersson, Pharmacia BioProcess Technology AB, Uppsala, Sweden

REFERENCES

Berglöf, J.H. et al., (1992): Validation of Chromatographic Procedures used in Fractionation of Plasma Derivatives presented at Virological Safety Aspects of Plasma Derivatives, Cannes, France Nov. 3-6.
Berglöf, J.H. & Eriksson, S. (1989): Plasma fractionation by chromatography of albumin and IgG. In *Biotechnology of plasma proteins,* eds. J.F. Stoltz, C. Rivat, pp 201-206. Colloque INSERM, Vol. 175. Paris: INSERM.
Janson, J.C. & Pettersson, T. (1992): Large-Scale Chromatography of Proteins. In *Preparative and Production Scale Chromatography,* eds. G. Ganetsos, P.E. Barker, pp. 559-590. New York: Marcell Dekker Inc.
Sofer, G.K. & Nyström, L.E. eds. (1991) Process Chromatography: A Guide to Validation. London: Academic Press.

Evaluation of current methods for antibody immobilization in the preparation of immunoaffinity adsorbents

David J. Stewart

Affinity Chromatography Ltd., 307 Huntingdon Road, Cambridge, CB3 OJX, United Kingdom

ABSTRACT

Trichloro-s-triazine activation may be applied to the immobilisation of proteins and antibodies to agarose in the preparation of adsorbents for immunoaffinity chromatography and related techniques. Triazine activation chemistry offers a non-hazardous and stable alternative to CNBr-activated agarose, and allows rapid immobilisation of antibody via surface imidazole, amino, hydroxyl and thiol groups under mildly acidic conditions to yield stable and neutral linkages. Under non-saturating conditions more than 95% of antibody is immobilised in 1 hour at 4°C. Immobilised antibody is functionally active with up to 52% of the theoretical maximal capacity available for antigen binding. Monitoring of antibody leakage by enzyme-linked immuoassay clearly demonstrates the greater stability of triazine linkages over isourea bonds. The activated support is stable on storage as wet slurry and upon lyophilisation.

INTRODUCTION

Applications of immobilised proteins include bioreactors, biosensors, *in vitro* and *in vivo* diagnostics, medical devices and downstream processing. The preparation of most affinity adsorbents relies on the use of activating agents to facilitate coupling of the affinity ligand. Cyanogen bromide has been used extensively for the immobilisation of proteins and other ligands containing primary amino groups to polyhydroxylic supports (Axen & Ernback, 1971; Porath, 1974). Bonding is performed under relatively mild conditions so that biological integrity of the immobilised ligand is preserved. However, the isourea linkage is charged at neutral pH (which can promote nonspecific binding interactions) and the stability the bond is limited (Tesser et al., 1974; Wilchek et al., 1975). Despite these acknowledged disadvantages of CNBr activation, alternative coupling reagents (eg. epoxides, divinylsulphone) are often less efficient, more costly, or, more importantly, require conditions for immobilisation to which biological ligands are not suited. With the growth in importance of immunoaffinity chromatography on both the laboratory and process scales, secure and efficient coupling of intact immunoglobulin molecules remains a primary application of any activated matrix.

Trichloro-s-triazine (cyanuric chloride) is a commonly available precursor used in many branches of organic chemistry. It contains three labile chlorines which can be displaced sequentially by nuleophiles. Reaction of substituted triazines with cellulosic fibres plays a central role in the modern textile dye industry. Trichloro-s-triazine has been used to couple enzymes to cellulosic fibres (Smith & Lenhoff, 1974) and to couple small affinity ligands to agarose (Laing et al., 1977). We describe the application of triazine activation to the immobilisation of proteins on agarose. The results suggest that triazine provides a non-hazardous and stable alternative to CNBr-activated agarose, and allows rapid immobilisation of proteins via surface imidazole, amine, hydroxyl and thiol groups under mildly acidic conditions to yield stable and neutral linkages.

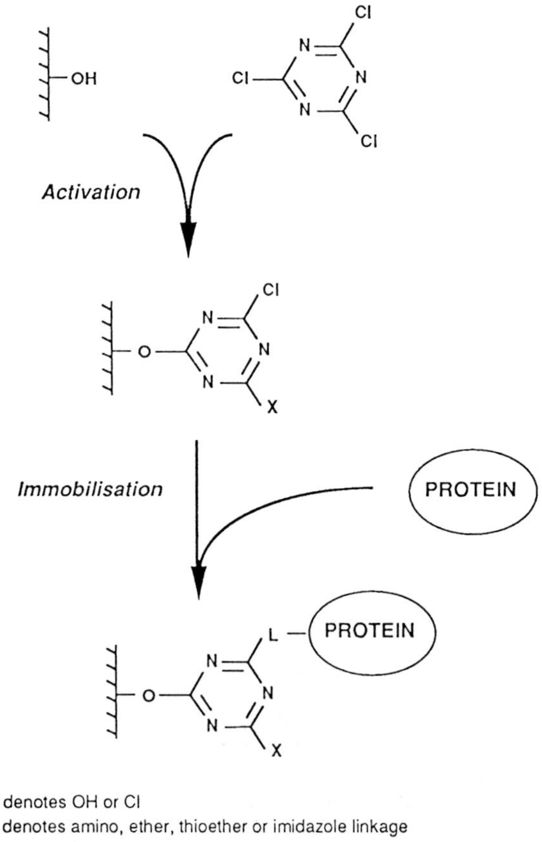

X denotes OH or Cl
L denotes amino, ether, thioether or imidazole linkage

Figure 1. Schematic of the immobilisation of protein on agarose via activation with trichloro-s-triazine.

TRIAZINE ACTIVATION OF AGAROSE

Activation of polyhydroxylic supports such as agarose may be carried out in organic solvents such as dioxane in the presence of sterically hindered base (Hodgkins & Levy, 1980). Alternatively, biphasic mixtures between strong aqueous alkali and certain organic solvents can be used. Typically, activation (Fig. 1) is carried out at below 4°C to prevent overhydrolysis of the triazine to cyanuric acid. Triazine content of the activated gel is determined using Konig's assay (Kohn & Wilchek, 1982) and can be carefully controlled by varying the initial concentration of triazine present (Fig. 2). Activated agarose may be used immediately, freeze-dried in the presence of stabilisers such as lactose or dextran, or stored in preservative. Maximal levels of activation (~50 µmol/g for 4% cross-linked agarose) are similar to those found with other activation chemistries.

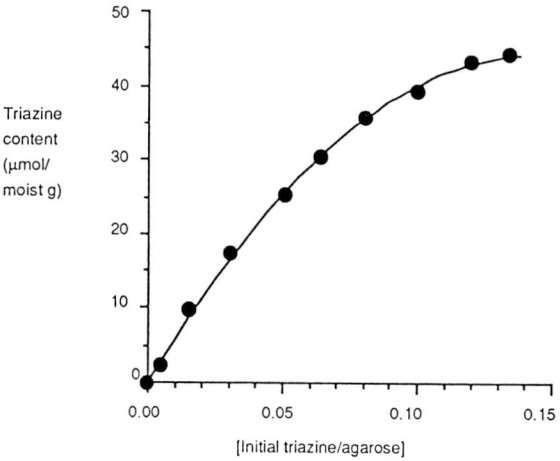

Fig. 2. The concentration of reactive triazine groups as a function of initial trichloro-s-triazine: agarose ratio in the activation reaction

PROTEIN IMMOBILISATION

Figure 3(A) shows the pH dependency of protein immobilisation on triazine and CNBr-activated agarose. Coupling of proteins to triazine-activated agarose is unusual in being favourable in mildly acidic conditions and is very efficient (the gels contain similar levels of respective reactive group), typically binding >95% of protein, while low molecular weight ligands are preferentially bound between pH 9 and 10. Figure 3(B) shows the immobilisation with time of human IgG to the two activated supports, indicating that coupling is almost complete within two hours. In the case of triazine activation, the level of bound protein attained is largely independent of protein type.

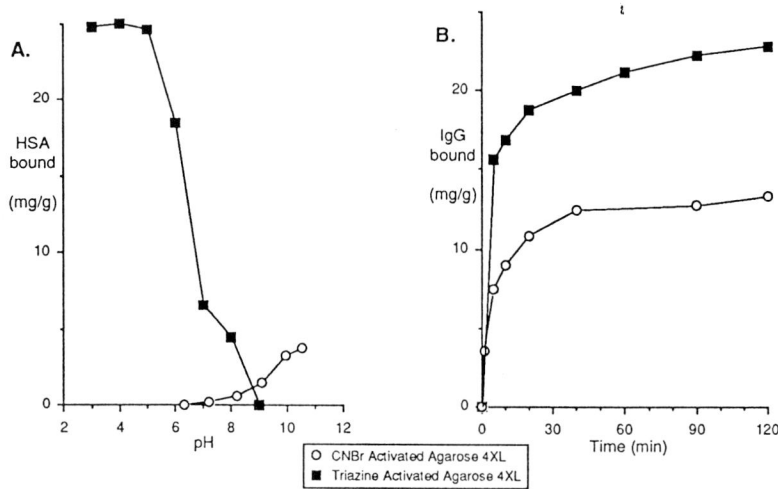

Fig. 3. Immobilisation of protein to CNBr and TST activated agaroses as a function of A) pH (Human serum albumin); and B) Time (Human IgG)

A. 100 mg moist washed, rehydrated activated gels were mixed with 1ml 25 mM buffer solution (sodium acetate, MES, MOPS, Tricine, pyrophosphate, sodium carbonate etc.) at appropriate pH containing 2.5 mg HSA. Coupling mixtures were tumbled overnight at room temperature, allowed to settle and unbound protein was measured using the Bradford assay against an HSA standard curve, from which the concentration of bound protein was deduced.

B. 100 mg moist washed, rehydrated activated gels were mixed with 1ml optimal coupling solution containing 2.5 mg human IgG [Triazine-activated gel: 25 mM sodium acetate, pH 4.0; CNBr-activated gel: 50 mM carbonate, pH 9.9] and incubated by rotary tumbling at 4°C (coupling solutions were pre-cooled prior to incubation). At various intevals, coupling mixtures were rapidly centrifuged, small aliquots (5µl) removed and unbound protein measured as above.

APPLICATIONS

Affinity adsorbents prepared with immobilised proteins are typically capable of achieving high degrees of purification because of their complex biological recognition of the target molecule. Thus antibodies will bind their complementary antigens, lectins their complementary sugar moieties and proteins A and G, various subclasses of immunoglobulin. The advantages of using such complex, labile and costly ligands are lost if the immobilisation procedure damages or inactivates the biological functioning of the ligand. Figure 4 shows the application of an anti-human serumn albumin immunosorbent prepared via triazine activation to the purification of serum albumin from human plasma showing the retention of function after coupling.

The capacity of such adsorbents is typically in the range 1 - 5 mg/ml which represents good protein binding efficiency (ligand useage), and purity of the eluted peak is usually high. We have found that, after optimisation, Protein A coupled via triazine activation to cross-linked agarose binds immunoglobulin molecules quantitatively, routinely giving ligand useage values in excess of 75% (1 molecule of Protein A will bind 2 molecules of IgG in free solution). In separate studies, immobilised enzymes prepared via triazine activation chemistry, retained up to 70% of soluble activity upon coupling.

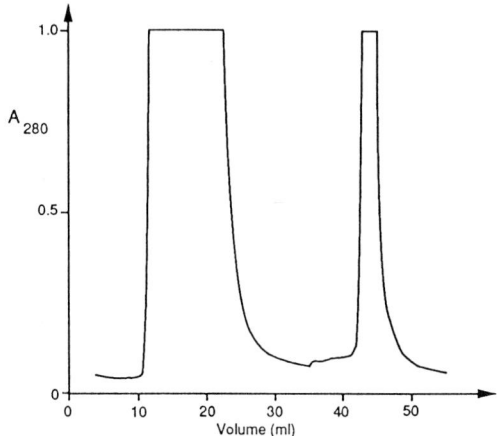

Fig. 4. Purification of serum albumin from human plasma by chromatography on ovine anti- human serum albumin immobilised via trichloro-s-triazine on 4% cross-linked agarose.

Column dimensions: 10 mm (I.D.) x 13 mm; bed volume: 1 ml; flow rate: 76.4 cm/h. Packing: ovine α-HSA immobilised via trichloro-s-triazine activation on 4% cross-linked agarose; 5 mg/moist g agarose. Equilibration buffer: 50 mM potassium phosphate, pH 7.7. Load: Human plasma, diluted 1/10 in equilibration buffer. Eluent: 20 mM glycine, pH 2.0. Peaks: 1) unbound contaminants; 2) human serum albumin. Capacity: 1.1 mg/g moist gel. Ligand useage: 52%.

LIGAND LEAKAGE

A crucial aspect of immunosorbents and other immobilised proteins is the leaching of ligand or ligand fragments from the support during the chromatographic operation, and in particular during elution of the target protein. Figure 5 compares the level of protein leaching from CNBr- and triazine-activated supports using an ELISA-based detection method to measure nanomolar concentrations of free immunoglobulin. Leakage was detectable from the cyanogen bromide-coupled material at pH 7 and 10, and from the traizine-coupled material at pH 10 at a concentraton approximately one order of manitude lower. An earlier comparative analysis (Laing et al., 1977) of leakage of radio-labelled small molecular weight ligands found that in 30 days at pH 9, the CNBr-coupled gel lost 50% of immobilised ligand while the triazine-linked gel lost approximately 0.6%. Multi-point attachment of immobilised protein should significantly reduce these leakage rates but it remains clear that triazine coupling produces a substantially more stable (immuno)affinity adsorbent.

SUMMARY

Trichloro-s-triazine activation ofers a superior alternative to cyanogen bromide for the immobilisation of biological macromolecules to polyhydroxylic supports. Levels of activation are reproducible and the activated support is stable at neutral pH. Furthermore, the coupling efficiency of triazine activated agarose in mildly acidic conditions is very high, which minimises wastage of valuable ligand during the bonding process. The immobilisation procedure ensures that the biological specificity of the immobilised antibody is retained while the

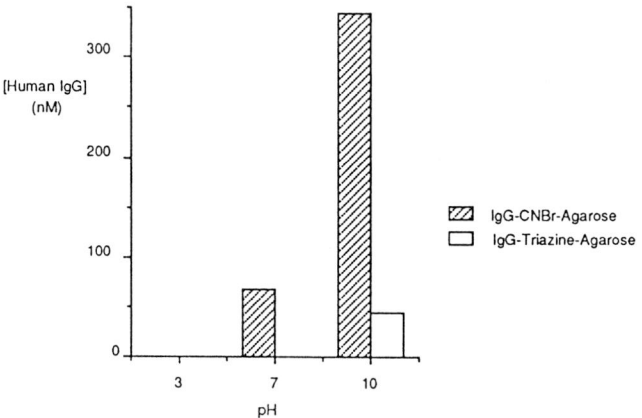

Figure 5. Comparison of leakage for immobilised human immunoglobulin G from triazine- and CNBr-coupled agaroses at various pH values.

(100nM IgG is equivalent to 15.5µg/ml)

CNBr-activated and triazine-activated agaroses (3g) were incubated with human IgG (5 mg/ml) in 3 ml either 50 mM sodium carbonate, pH 9.5, and 50 mM sodium acetate, pH 4.0, respectively, by rotary tumbling for 1h at 20°C. Bradford assays of supernatants revealed both gels contained 5 mg IgG/moist g agarose. Residual reactive sites were blocked overnight with 2 M ethanolamine, pH 9.5. Gels were then thoroughly washed with distilled water prior to determination of leakage.

Gels (0.5 g) were mixed with 0.5 ml of either 50 mM glycine, pH 3.0, 50 mM phosphate, pH 7.0, or 50 mM carbonate, pH 10.0, by rotary tumbling for 16 h at 20°C. Supernatants were assayed for human IgG using a competitive enzyme-linked immunosorbent assay (ELISA), in which serial dilutions of known and unknown IgG samples were incubated with anti-human IgG-peroxidase conjugate in microtitre plates pre-coated with human IgG. Bound peroxidase activity was measured using tetramethylbenzidine as enzyme substrate. Sample concentrations were deduced from the known standard curve. Assay detection limit = 10 nM IgG.

considerably enhanced stability of the triazinyl linkage allows more rigorous cleaning of the immunosorbent *in situ* and guarantees longer column lifetimes. The growing requirements for ultra-pure proteins for therapeutic and *in vivo* diagnostic applications, coupled with more sensitive methods for detection of contaminants, will ensure that novel coupling chemistries such as triazine activation will rapidly replace current immobilisation procedures based on CNBr activation.

REFERENCES

Axen, R. & Ernback, S. (1971): *Eur. J. Biochem.*, **18**, 351-356.
Hodgkins, L. T. & Levy, M. (1980): *J. Chromatogr.*, **202**, 381-390.
Kohn, J. & Wilchek, M. (1982): In <u>Affinity Chromatography and Related Techniques</u>, eds. Gribnau, T. C. V., Visser, J. & Nivard, R. J. F., pp.235-244, Amsterdam: Elsevier.
Lang, T., Suckling, C.J. & Wood, H. C. S. (1977): *J. C. S. Perkin 1*, 2189-2194.
Porath, J. (1974): *Methods Enzymol.*, **34**, 13-30.
Smith, N. L. & Lenhoff, H. M. (1974): *Anal. Biochem.*, **61**, 392-415.
Tesser, I. G., Fisch, H. U. & Schwyzer, R. (1974): *Helv. Chim. Acta*, **57**, 1718-1725.
Wilchek, M., Oka, T. & Topper, Y. J. (1975): *Proc. Natl. Acad. Sci. (USA)*, **72**, 1055-1058.

Immunopurification of proteins. Comparison of the stability of various activated beaded-agarose matrices

N. Ubrich[1,2], P. Hubert[2], V. Regnault[1], E. Dellacherie[2] and C. Rivat[1]

[1]INSERM, Plateau de Brabois, C.O. 10, 54511 Vandœuvre-lès-Nancy Cedex, France. [2]Laboratoire de Chimie-Physique Macromoléculaire, URA CNRS 494, ENSIC, BP 451, 54001 Nancy Cedex, France

INTRODUCTION

Immunoadsorption is becoming an attractive method and affords a high degree of purification owing to the specific recognition between antigens and antibodies. However, besides its cost, the leakage of small amounts of antibodies from the support hampers the practical use of this method (Sato et al., 1987, Bessos et al., 1991). In fact, these released antibodies contaminate the purified media, and when a clinical use is concerned, may lead to side effects to patients, especially if these antibodies are of animal nature. As the products thus purified could still pose a potentiel threat to patients, it is of prime importance that the immunoadsorbents exhibit a satisfactory stability over the whole range of chemical and biochemical conditions involved during their clinical handling.

One reason of such leakage involves the chemistry of immobilization of antibodies to the support. Therefore, the purpose of this study was to prepare immunoadsorbents by covalent coupling of goat anti apolipoprotein B polyclonal antibodies on Sepharose CL-4B previously activated by various chemical reagents (carbonyldiimidazole, 1,4-butanediol diglycidylether, divinyl sulfone, tresyl chloride and trichloro-s-triazine). The resulting immunoadsorbents aimed to remove the excess of apolipoproteins B of patients affected by familial hypercholesterolemia (Stoffel and Demant, 1981) were compared in terms of yield of coupling, adsorption capacity and stability, with that obtained earlier by activation of Sepharose CL-4B with cyanogen bromide (Regnault et al., 1990).

This approach will serve as a model system to compare the stability of the immunoadsorbents according to the various activation methods used, and will be possibly applied to other immobilized proteins.

EXPERIMENTAL

Materials

The matrix used was Sepharose CL-4B from Pharmacia (Uppsala, Sweden). Carbonyldiimidazole (CDI), 1,4-butanediol diglycidylether (BDGE), divinyl sulphone (DVS), tresyl chloride (TC) and trichloro-s-triazine (TsT) were purchased from Aldrich (Milwaukee, WI, USA). Goat immune serum was purchased from Sebia (Issy-les-Moulineaux, France). Goat anti apolipoprotein B polyclonal antibodies (anti apo B) were obtained by affinity chromatography of goat plasma on Sepharose-immobilized human apolipoproteins B (apo B). Fresh blood plasma from healthy donors was provided by the Centre Régional de Transfusion Sanguine de Nancy (France). All other chemical reagents were obtained from Merck (Darmstadt, Germany) and Prolabo (Strasbourg, France) and were of analytical grade.

Methods

Carbonyldiimidazole activation

This activation was carried out according to Bethell et al. (1979). Decanted Sepharose CL-4B (5ml) was washed on a glass filter successively with water (100 ml), water-dioxane (7:3, 5:5, 3:7, v:v, 100 ml of each) and finally anhydrous dioxane (100 ml). The gel was suspended in 2.5 ml of anhydrous dioxane and CDI (20, 30 or 50 mg/ml of gel) was added. The suspension was rotated at 40°C for 2 h, then washed with 100 ml of anhydrous dioxane, dioxane-water (7:3, 5:5, 3:7, v:v), distilled water and used immediately.

The amount of imidazole and carbonyl groups was determined according to a procedure previously described by Bethell et al. (1981).

1,4-butanediol diglycidylether activation

This activation was performed according to the procedure described by Sundberg and Porath (1974). Decanted Sepharose CL-4B (5 ml) was washed on a glass filter with water (100 ml) and stirred by rotation at room temperature for 8 h with 5 ml (or 10 ml) of BDGE, in the presence of 5 ml (or 10 ml) of 0.6 M NaOH containing 10 mg (or 20 mg) of sodium borohydride. The activation reaction was stopped by washing the gel on a glass filter with 1 l of distilled water.

The amount of oxirane groups immobilized on the support was determined after treatment of the activated matrix with sodium thiosulfate (Sundberg and Porath, 1974).

Divinyl sulphone activation

This activation was carried out according to the procedure described by Porath et al. (1975). Decanted Sepharose CL-4B (5 ml) was washed on a glass filter with 25 ml of water, then with 15 ml of 0.5 M sodium carbonate buffer NaOH pH 11. The gel was suspended in 5 ml of the same buffer and reacted under stirring with DVS (0.01, 0.10 or 0.15 ml/ml of gel) at room temperature. The resulting matrix was then washed with water (2 l) in order to remove the excess of DVS.

The content in linked vinyl groups was determined after preliminary treatment of the activated matrix by sodium thiosulfate (Porath et al., 1975). The content in total sulphur was measured according to the procedure described by Belcher (1962).

Tresyl chloride activation

This activation was performed according to Nilsson and Mosbach (1981). Typically, decanted Sepharose CL-4B (5 ml) was washed on a glass filter successively with water (500 ml), water-acetone (7:3, 5:5, 3:7, v:v), and finally with dry acetone (100 ml). The gel was suspended in 3 ml of dry acetone containing 20, 40 or 60 ml of pyridine, according to the amount of tresyl chloride (10, 20 or 30 ml/ml of gel) subsequently added dropwise to the suspension. After the mixture was shaken for 15 min, the gel was washed with dry acetone (100 ml), acetone-HCl 1 mM (7:3, 5:5, 3:7, v:v) and finally HCl 1 mM (100 ml).

The content in total sulphur was determined according to the procedure described by Belcher (1962).

Trichloro-s-triazine activation

This activation was adapted from Finlay et al. (1978). Decanted Sepharose CL-4B (5 ml) was washed on a glass filter with water (500 ml), water-acetone (7:3, 5:5, 3:7, v:v) and finally with dry acetone (200 ml). The gel was suspended in 7 ml of dry acetone containing 50, 80 or 100 mg/ml of gel and stirred at room temperature for 30 min. The activation was stopped by washing the gel on a glass filter with dry acetone (200 ml), acetone-PBS pH 5 (7:3, 5:5, 3:7, v:v) and finally PBS pH 5 (100 ml).

The content in chlorine was determined according to the procedure described by Kirsten (1976).

Typical coupling procedure

Each activated support (5 ml) was washed on a glass filter with 0.5 M NaCl, 0.1 M sodium bicarbonate buffer and mixed under gentle stirring at room temperature with the goat anti apo B solution (6 mg/ml) in the same buffer, volume to volume. This concentration was previously determined as the one affording an optimal adsorption capacity (Regnault et al., 1990). The reaction time was 22 h for the gels activated by CDI, TC or TsT, 48 h for the BDGE-activated supports and 24 h for the DVS-activated matrices. The resulting immunoadsorbents were then washed successively with sodium bicarbonate buffer, 1 M ethanolamine pH 8.5 for 2 h to block the unreacted active groups, then with 0.3 M glycine-HCl pH 2.8 in order to disrupt possible antibody-antibody interactions. After final washings with phosphate buffered saline (PBS : 0.01M Na_2HPO_4, 0.15M NaCl, pH 7.3), each immunoadsorbent was stored at 4°C in 25% aqueous ethanol.

Adsorption capacity

Each immunoadsorbent (5 ml) was packed in a column (1.1 cm x 5.3 cm) and washed successively with PBS pH 7.3, glycine-HCl pH 2.8 and again PBS. Blood plasma (60 ml) was pumped into the column containing each immunoadsorbent (30 ml/h). Elution with PBS pH 7.3 was then carried out until 60 ml of plasma thus purified were recovered. Adsorbed apo B were desorbed thereafter with glycine-HCl pH 2.8. Each immunoadsorbent was then washed with PBS and stored again in 25% aqueous ethanol. The amount of apo B in the initial plasma and in the eluted plasma was measured by Laurell immunoelectrophoresis rockets (Laurell, 1966), and the adsorption capacity was determined as the difference between these two values.

Assay of released antibodies

The amount of released antibodies was measured by an enzyme linked immunosorbent assay (ELISA), both in the eluted plasma at pH 7.3 and in the apo B solution desorbed. Microtiter plates (Costar) were coated with 100 µl of rabbit anti goat IgG antibodies in 50 mM sodium carbonate buffer, pH 9.6 (2.5 µg/ml), overnight at 4°C. After washing with PBS-Tween (130 mM NaCl, 5 mM Na_2HPO_4, 1 mM KH_2PO_4, pH 7.2 containing 0.05% Tween 20), 125 µl of 0.5% cold water fish skin gelatin were added in each well, and the plates were incubated at 37°C for 3 h. A 100 µl aliquot of samples diluted in the initial plasma or PBS-Tween was added in the wells, and the plates were incubated at 37°C for 2 h. Goat purified IgG were used as a standard. After washing with PBS-Tween, 100 µl of biotinylated rabbit anti goat IgG antibodies were added to each well. The plates were incubated at 37°C for 2 h and washed with PBS-Tween. A 100 µl volume of peroxidase-streptavidine (Zymed) (1/1000) was then dispensed into each well and the plates were incubated at 37°C for 10 min. Finally, after washing with PBS-Tween, then with 0.14 M acetate-citrate buffer pH 6, 0.1 mg/ml of 3,3'-5,5'-tetramethylbenzidine and 0.01% H_2O_2 in the acetate-citrate buffer were placed in each well. The reaction was stopped by addition of 25 ml of 2 M H_2SO_4 and the absorbance was measured at 450 nm in a Titertek plus micro ELISA reader (Flow Laboratories, Middlesex, UK).

RESULTS and DISCUSSION

Purification of proteins requires preparation of immunoadsorbents exhibiting both a high yield of coupling, a good adsorption capacity and especially an extensive stability over the whole range of chemical and biochemical conditions to which they are submitted. To optimize these caracteristics, the matrix, Sepharose CL-4B, was activated by 5 chemical reagents, and for each of them, various amounts were allowed to react with the gel. For each resulting activated support, the coupling with the goat anti apo B solution was performed at various pH values, and the results obtained for an optimal coupling yield are collected in Fig. 1. CDI- and moreover BDGE-activated matrices afford rather low coupling yields. Therefore, for this latter matrix, no further investigations was done. In opposition, DVS-, TC- and TsT-activated supports lead to highly substituted-immunoadsorbents exhibiting an adsorption capacity similar to that obtained with the previously described CNBr activated gel (Regnault et al., 1990) (Fig. 2).

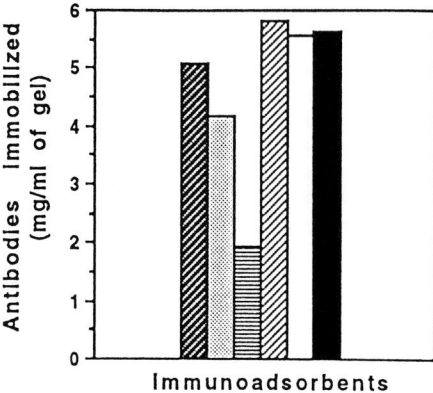

Fig. 1. Optimal coupling yields of the immunoadsorbents prepared by reaction of 5 ml of goat anti apo B polyclonal antibodies (6 mg/ml) with Sepharose CL-4B (5 ml) previously activated with various chemical reagents : (▨) CDI (30 mg/ml of gel), (▤) BDGE (2 ml/ml of gel), (▧) DVS (0.15 ml/ml of gel), (☐) TC (20 ml/ml of gel) (■) TsT (100 mg/ml of gel) and (▨) CNBr (100 mg/ml of gel). The coupling was performed at pH 9 for CDI-, BDGE- and DVS-activated supports, pH 7.5 for the TC-activated matrix, pH 5 for the TsT-activated gel and pH 8.5 for the CNBr-activated one.

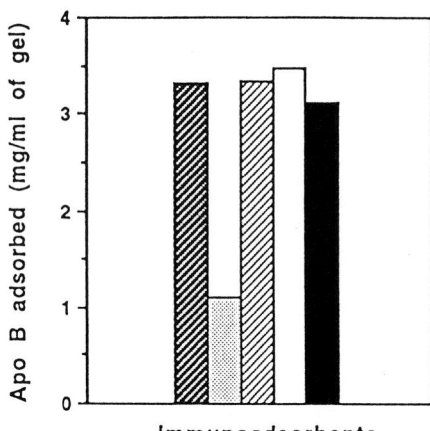

Fig. 2. Optimal adsorption capacities of the various immunoadsorbents (5 ml) obtained by activation of Sepharose CL-4B with (▨) CDI (4.20 mg of antibodies/ml of gel), (▧) DVS (5.80 mg of antibodies/ml of gel), (☐) TC (5.55 mg of antibodies/ml of gel), (■) TsT (5.65 mg of antibodies/ml of gel) and (▨) CNBr (5.10 mg of antibodies/ml of gel), when loaded with blood plasma (60 ml).

Fig. 3 shows the antibodies released at pH 7.3 in the eluted plasma, for each activated support, and Fig. 4 those released from the various immunoadsorbents, during the elution of adsorbed apo B at acidic pH (2.8). This leakage can be explained by the cumulative unstabilities of the spacer arm and the matrix itself. The most striking evidence is that the extent of release depends on pH.

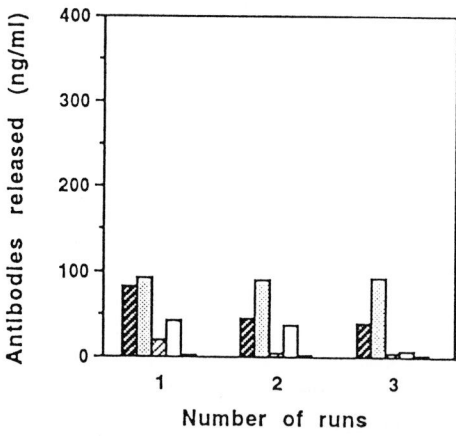

Fig. 3. Stability of the various immunoadsorbents at pH 7.3. Antibodies released in the eluted plasma at pH 7.3 vs the number of runs for each immunoadsorbent previously activated by (▨) CDI, (▧) DVS, (☐) TC, (■) TsT and (▨) CNBr.

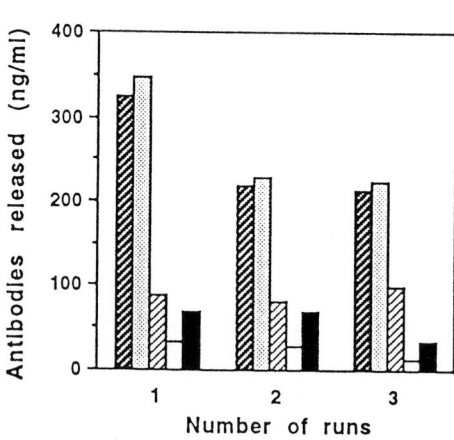

Fig. 4. Stability of the various immunoadsorbents at pH 2.8. Amounts of antibodies released at pH 2.8 in the apo B solution vs the number of runs for (▨) CDI-, (▧) DVS-, (☐) TC-, (■) TsT- and (▨) CNBr-activated immunoadsorbents.

At neutral pH, a very limited leakage is observed for the DVS-, TC- and TsT-activated immunoadsorbents. As around neutrality, the nature of the chemical bonds between the matrix and the antibody (Fig. 5) makes them unlikely to be broken, this leakage is probably due to the matrix disruption. An enhanced stability is obtained for DVS- and TsT-activated supports (compared to the TC-activated one), presumably because of the extra cross-linking of the gel, resulting respectively of the bi- and trifunctional character of these activation reagents.

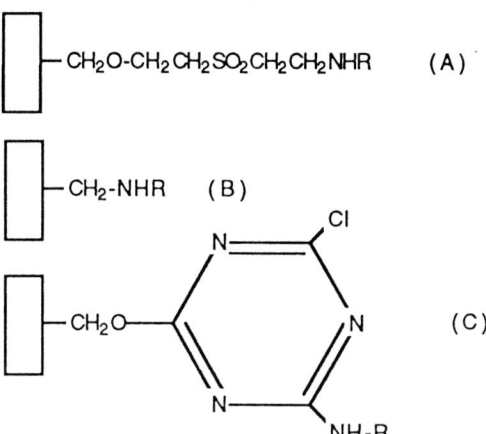

Fig. 5. Chemical structure of immunoadsorbents prepared by activation of Sepharose CL-4B with DVS (A), TC (B) and TsT (C) followed by coupling to goat anti apo B polyclonal antibodies (R-NH_2).

At acidic pH, the DVS-, TC- and TsT-activated supports behave quite differently from each other. Since the same matrix was used for their preparation, the degradation of the matrix cannot be the only reason of the leakage, and a breaking of the bond between the matrix and the ligand or the degradation of the ligand itself must be therefore considered.
In fact, it is expected that the secondary amino groups involved in the TC-activated support would be insensitive to acidic conditions, unlikely to the ether functions involved in the DVS- and TsT-activated supports.

From these results, it appears that an optimal stability can be anticipated for immunoadsorbents obtained by TC-activation and the use of highly cross-linked matrices such as Sepharose Fast Flow for the preparation of higher performance immunoadsorbents is presently in progress in our laboratory.

REFERENCES

Belcher, R., Campbell, A.D., Gouverneur, P., Macdonald, A.M.G. (1962) : Submicro-methods of organic analysis. Part XV. Determination of sulphur by the oxygen-flask method. *J. Chem. Soc.* 585, 3033-3037.
Bethell, G.S., Ayers, J.S., Hancock, W.S. Hearn, M.T.W. (1979) : A novel method of activation of cross-linked agaroses with 1,1-carbonyldiimidazole which gives a matrix for affinity chromatography devoid of additional charged groups. *J. Biol. Chem.* 254, 2572-2574.
Bethell, G.S., Ayers, J.S., Hearn, M.T.W. Hancock, W. S. (1981) : Investigation of the activation of cross-linked agarose with carbonylating reagents and the preparation of matrices for affinity chromatography purifications. *J. Chromatogr.* 219, 353-359.
Bessos, H., Appleyard, C., Micklem, L.R., Pepper, D.C. (1991) : Monoclonal antibody leakage from gel: effect of support, activation and eluant composition. *Prep. Chromat.* 1, 207-220.
Finlay, T.H., Troll, V., Levy, M., Johnson, A.J. and Hodgins, L.T. (1978): New methods for the preparation of biospecific adsorbents and immobilized enzymes utilizing trichloro-s-triazine. *Anal. Biochem.* 87, 77-90.

Kirsten, W.J.(1976) : Ultramicro and trace determination of chlorine, bromine, and iodine. *Mikrochimica Acta* II, 299-310.

Laurell, C.B. (1966) : Quantitative estimation of protein by electrophoresis in agarose gel containing antibodies. *Anal. Biochem.* 15, 45-52.

Nilsson, K. and Mosbach, K. (1981) : Immobilization of enzymes and affinity ligands to various hydroxyl group carrying supports using highly reactive sulfonyl chlorides. *Biochem. Biophys. Res. Commun.* 102, 449-457.

Porath, J., Laas, T., Janson, J.C. (1975) : Agar derivatives for chromatography, electrophoresis and bound enzymes. Rigid agarose gels cross-linked with divinyl sulfone. *J. Chromatogr.* 103, 49-62.

Regnault, V., Rivat, C., Marcillier, P., Pfister, M., Michaely, J.P., Didelon, J., Schooneman, F., Stoltz, J.F. and Siadat, M. (1990) : Study of parameters involved in specific immunoadsorption of apolipoprotein B. *Int. J. Artif. Organs* 13, 760-767.

Sato, H., Kidaka, T., Hori, M. (1987) : Leakage of immobilized IgG from therapeutic immunoadsorbents. *Appl. Biochem. Biotech.* 15, 141-158.

Stoffel, W. and Demant, T. (1981) : Selective removal of apolipoprotein B containing serum lipoproteins from blood plasma. *Proc. Natl. Acad. Sci.* 78, 611-615.

Sundberg L., Porath J. (1974) : Preparation of adsorbents for biospecific affinity chromatography. Attachment of group-containing ligands to insoluble polymers by means of bifunctional oxiranes. *J. Chromatogr.* 90, 87-98.

ACKNOWLEDGEMENTS

This work was supported in part by a grant from the Pôle Technologique Régional de Génie Biologique et Médical-Biotechnologies.

Biotechnology of Blood Proteins. Eds C. Rivat, J.-F. Stoltz. Colloque INSERM/John Libbey Eurotext Ltd.

Filtration processes in the Cohn fractionation

E. de Jonge, M.A.W. van Leeuwen, H. Radema, P.H.J.M. Linssen and J. Over

CLB, Department of Product and Process Development, PO Box 9190, 1006 AD Amsterdam, The Netherlands

Introduction

The Cohn fractionation process was developed during the second world war (Cohn, 1946). Although it has undergone many changes since then, the essentials of the process are still the same.

Figure 1 shows a block scheme of the Cohn fractionation process at the CLB. In general the raw material consists of cryoprecipitate-depleted plasma. The final products immunoglobulin and albumin are derived from precipitate II and V respectively. The total capacity of the fractionation plant, at present, is about 200.000 kg plasma per year.

Figure 1: Block scheme of the CLB fractionation process

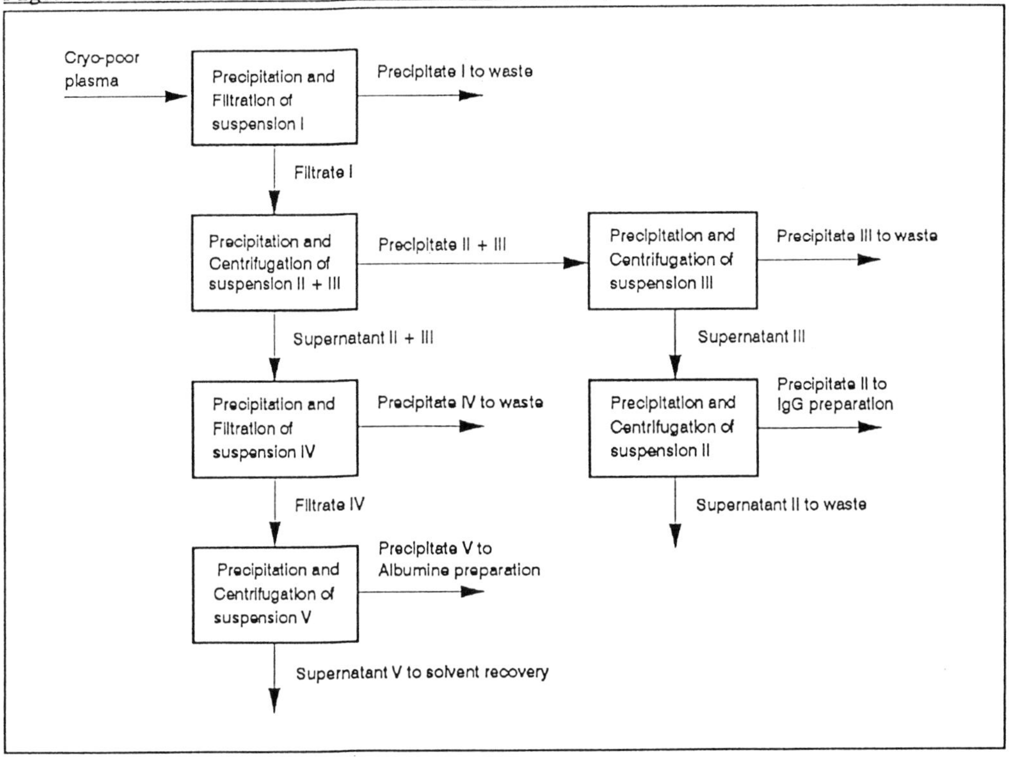

The waste fractions I and IV are separated by means of filtration, while all the other solid-liquid separations are carried out in centrifuges. The centrifuges that are used are Sharples AS 16; these are so-called vertical tubular bowl centrifuges.

At the end of the last decade it became clear that these should be replaced, mainly due to lack of compliance with current GMP requirements, but also because of the relatively high maintenance costs.

An analysis was carried out with respect to the advantages and disadvantages of filtration in comparison to centrifugation. From this analysis it was concluded that filtration has the following advantages over centrifugation:
- relative ease of recovery of mother liquor from the solid,
- faster rate of separation and thus a high capacity per unit of floor space,
- improved compliance with current GMP requirements, for instance by applying cleaning in place,
- convenience to maintenance,
- less noise disturbance,
- reduced energy costs.

The investment costs proved to be roughly comparable.

Process development

Table 1 shows the precipitation conditions that are currently used for the various fractionation steps. To make sure that the characteristics of the final products are not affected, the physico-chemical parameters of the fractionation process must remain unchanged. However, to accomplish an effective implementation of filtration over centrifugation as a separation process in the Cohn fractionation, it was necessary to investigate and improve the filtration properties of each of the various fractions. This was done by combining investigations on both laboratory and production scale.

Table 1: Current precipitation conditions (C: centrifugation; F: filtration)

Fraction	Ethanol v/v %	Temp.°C	pH	Filter aid w/w %	Separation
I	8.0	-3	7.4	0.75	F
II + III	25.0	-5	6.8	-	C
III	12.0	-3	5.10	-	C
II	25.0	-5	7.30	-	C
IV	40.0	-5	5.85	3.0	F
V	40.0	-5	4.8	-	C

The first step in these investigations was to develop a standardized method to measure the rate of filtration on laboratory scale. Figure 2 shows a scheme of the laboratory arrangement. In this arrangement, the filtrate volume is measured as a function of time, while applying a constant pressure.

Figure 2: Scheme of the laboratory arrangement

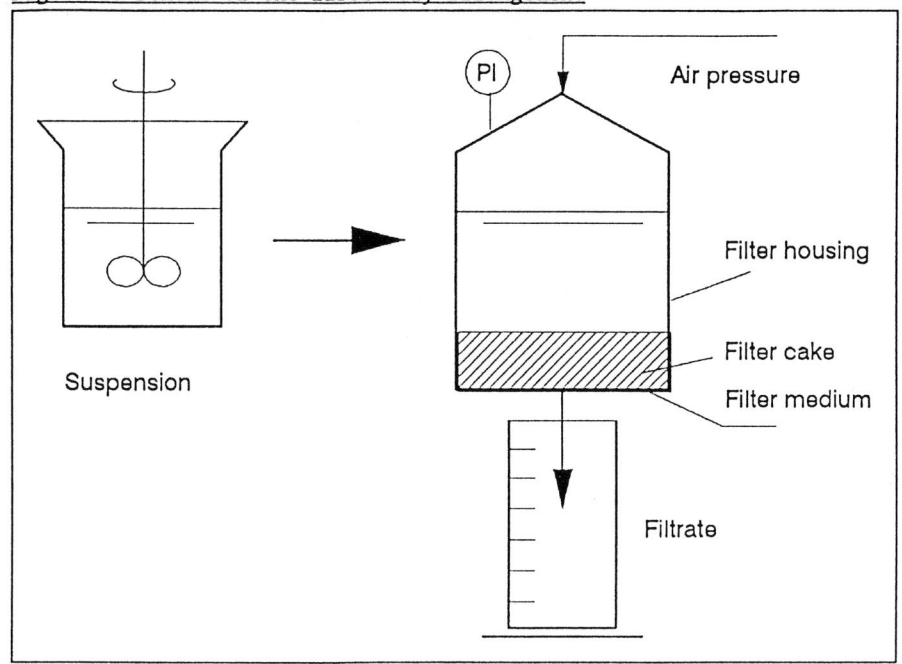

For evaluation of the results of the filtration experiments, the standard filtration theory was applied. Flow through a porous medium is governed by the law of d'Arcy (Krijgsman, 1989). Applying it to a system of cake and filter medium, one obtains equation 1:

$$\frac{1}{A} \cdot \frac{dV}{dt} = \frac{\Delta p}{\eta \cdot (\frac{V}{A} \phi_v R_c + R_m)} \tag{1}$$

Herein is:
- A : filter surface area [m²]
- V : filtrate volume [m³]
- t : filtration time [s]
- Δp : pressure difference over filter [Pa]
- η : filtrate viscosity [Pa.s]
- R_c : specific cake resistance [m⁻²]
- R_m : filter medium resistance [m⁻¹]
- ϕ_v : volume fraction of solids (as volume of cake) in suspension

Integration of equation 1 with the boundary condition $V=0$ at $t=0$, in case of constant pressure filtration and an incompressible filter cake, yields:

$$\frac{t}{(\frac{V}{A})} = \frac{\eta}{\Delta p} (\frac{1}{2} \phi_v R_c (\frac{V}{A}) + R_m) \tag{2}$$

From equation 2 it follows that a plot of $t/(V/A)$ plotted against (V/A) should yield a straight line. The slope of the line provides a measure of the resistance of the filter cake R_c, whereas the extrapolated value at the intercept of the Y-axis, $(V/A)=0$, yields a measure for the medium resistance R_m.

Figure 3 shows one of the plots that were obtained as an example. This graph shows the results of experiments with fraction IV with three different filter aid concentrations. In general it was found that for suspensions containing more than 1% filter aid, d'Arcy's law was applicable. In those instances it was possible to predict the filtration times on full production scale by scaling up from the results of laboratory experiments.

Figure 3: Filtration characteristics of suspension IV with three filter aid concentrations at 0.5 bar.

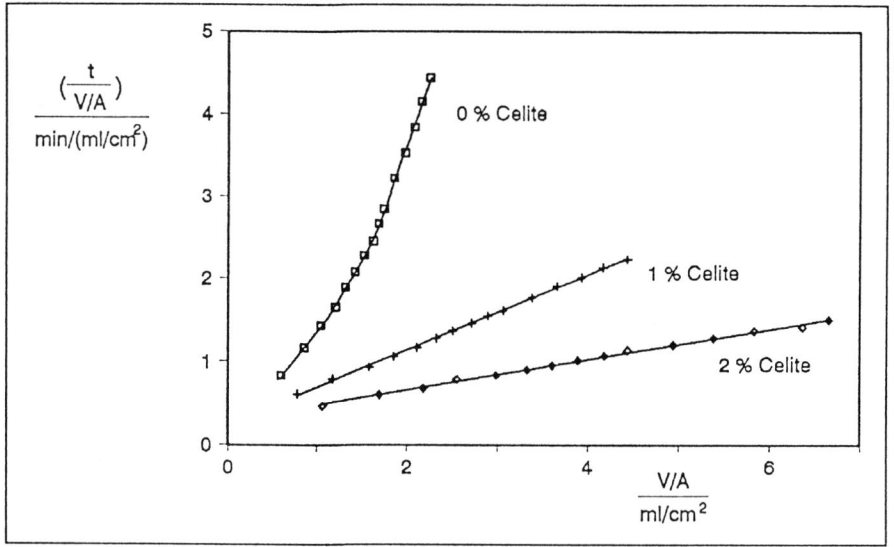

By using this standardized method it was possible to evaluate the effect of changing process parameters on filtration properties. This was done on laboratory scale as well as on full production scale. In general, improved filtration properties can be obtained, by creating a more uniform size distribution of the precipitate particles. In practice this can be achieved by:
1) avoiding the build-up of locally excessive precipitant concentrations, which may lead to a large amount of precipitate nuclei, instead of growth of precipitate particles.
2) avoiding intensive mixing, because this may lead to generation of small particles due to shear break-up.

In view of this, the following process parameters were investigated:
- rate of addition of citric acid or sodium hydroxide solution to adjust pH,
- rate of addition of ethanol,
- the way by which ethanol is added (within the fluid or by spraying over the fluid),
- concentration of added ethanol,
- mixing regime.

Results and discussion
The main findings from these investigations were that the filtration properties of fractions I, II+III, III, II and V could be improved by:
- decreasing the rate of pH adjustment (except for fraction III),
- decreasing the rate of ethanol addition,
- adding the precipitant in the fluid, just above the tip of the anchor mixer.
- creating a mildly turbulent mixing regime.
The results are summarized in table 2.

Table 2: Main results of investigation.

fraction	pH adjustment time*		ethanol addition time*		filter aid (W/W %)		filter area (m^2)	
	old	new	old	new	old	new	old	new
I	-	-	2 - 3	12 - 16	0.75	0.75	13	6
II + III	0.25	2	4 - 6	12 - 16	-	2.0	-	13
III	3	2	5 - 7	6 - 16	-	2.0	-	13
II	0.25	2	4 - 5	12 - 16	-	-**	-	4
IV	0.25	2	4 - 6	12 - 16	3.0	2.5	13	13
V	2	16	-	-	-	precoat	-	13

* time in hours   ** no filter aid necessary

Despite the improvements of filtration properties of fraction I, II+III and III the use of small amounts of filter aid still proved to be necessary. The filtration of fraction II and V could be optimized in such a way that addition of filter aid as body-feed was not needed. The filtration properties of fraction IV however, could not be improved further by the changes mentioned above. This is probably due to the complex protein composition of this fraction.

In quality control of albumin and immunoglobulin preparations, produced from fractions filtered at full production scale, revealed that the products complied with the requirements stated in the European Pharmacopoeia. Furthermore no results were obtained that differed from the routine ones. The test included for instance aluminium and PKA content.

Apparatus
The findings presented in this paper will result in the design and installation of a so-called horizontal pressure vessel, vertical leaf filter for the filtration of fractions II+III and V. The filtration process will be operated automatically, which, together with an automated cleaning-in-place procedure, will result in a higher overall capacity in the fractionation facility.
For the separation of the waste fractions I, III and IV, the CLB will continue to use horizontal plate filters. For fraction II a small plate filter will be designed.

Conclusions

The main conclusion is that for <u>all</u> fractions a filtration process could be developed. For <u>most</u> fractions it was possible to optimize the filtration characteristics. For <u>some</u> fractions the filtration characteristics could be improved in such a way that the use of filter aid is not needed.

Acknowledgement

The authors wish to express their thanks to Mr. Olschewski of the German Red Cross Plasma Fractionation Facility in Springe, for his advice and helpful suggestions in this investigation.

References

Cohn, E.J. et al. (1946): Preparation and properties of serum and plasma proteins, A system for the separation into fractions of the protein and lipoprotein components of biological tissues and fluids. J. Am. Soc. 68, 459.

Krijgsman, J et al. (1989), Advanced Course on Downstream Processing, 4-6, Delft University of Technology.

II. Coagulation factors

II. Facteurs de coagulation

Clinical evaluation of coagulation factor concentrate

D. Boyeldieu and Y. Sultan

Centre d'Accueil et de Traitement des Hémophiles, Hôpital Cochin, 27, rue du Faubourg Saint-Jacques, 75014 Paris, France

SUMMARY

Congenital and acquired coagulation factor deficiencies are associated to bleeding episodes. A substitutive therapy may be required. Clotting factors need purification and concentration from plasma to be efficacious. Clinical evaluations are needed to conclude about efficacy and safety of these concentrates. Recommandations about these trials are defined by an international consensus. Among these protocols, studies of efficacy, tolerance, safety and immunogenicity are currently conducted. The impact of purification processes of these concentrates on the immune functions of the recipients have still to be studied. Trials on a long follow up, and trials on previously untreated patients are recommanded.

Congenital and acquired coagulation factor deficiencies are associated to bleeding complications which require replacement therapy with plasma derivatives enriched in the deficient clotting factor. The most frequently observed are hemophilia due to factor VIII or IX deficiency, Von Willebrand's disease, afibrinogemia and vitamine K dependant clotting factor deficiencies. More recently thromboembolic episodes occuring in young patients have been attributed to coagulation inhibitor deficiencies and concentrate of antithrombin III and protein C have been prepared and have shown to be helpful in such circUmstances.

Replacement therapy in clotting factor deficiencies might be administred through fresh frozen plasma or "home made" preparations such as cryoprecipitate from single donor blood donation. However since many years concentrate are industrial products prepared from large pool of plasma. Several thousand liters of plasma are currently required to prepare batches of plasma derivatives. The same basic material ie human plasma is used to prepare in following processes factor VIII, Von Willebrand factor, prothrombin complex concentrate, factor IX, protein C, albumin, fibrinogen, immunoglobulins . . . Once purified and lyophilised clotting factors concentrate need clinical evaluation before marketing.

The most important qualities to be controled and established are: efficacy, recovery and half life in circulation, safety, purity, immunogenicity, control of appropriate labelling. At least, commercial presentation and easiness for patients care are also important qualities.

Efficacy of plasma derived products is difficult to establish as most of the criteria are subjectives ones. Efficacy is evaluated on the pain, the swelling of the joint or soft tissues, the stop of the bleeding if gastro intestinal or exteriorised bleedings are concerned. The criteria can be appreciated either by the patient himself or the doctor or both. Some criteria are more objective such as the measurement of the swelling, mobility of the limbs which can be appreciated in degrees of mobility. The necessity of a second or third injection to control the bleeding episode is also a mean of efficacy evaluation. However this criteria depends on the time interval between the onset of the bleeding and the injection of concentrate, it depends also on the initial dose of concentrate administered to the patients. Efficacy on single bleeding episode such as hemarthrosis or muscle bleeding is usually completed by evaluation of efficacy in surgical conditions. The control of bleeding during elective surgery or emergency surgical procedures is an important mean of evaluation providing that daily dosages of clotting factors in circulation might be compared to the dosages of concentrates administered during and after surgery.

Recovery and half life of the product after injection in coagulation factor deficient patients are the most objective criteria which can be used to evaluate the characteristics of clotting factor preparations. Standardized conditions for such studies have been established and an international consensus has been approved by a standardization committee; the rules for these evaluations have been published and manufacturers can establish protocols of studies according to comparative evaluation from one center to another. Patients with hemophilia A and hemophilia B, eligible for recovery studies must have not been treated with any blood or blood product for a delay of 8-15 days, be severe patients with no detectable plasma FVIII or FIX and without neutralizing antibodies towards these coagulation factors. It is also recommended that high doses of concentrate be administered per kilogramme body weight, not less than 40U/kg as a bollus or a short period of infusion not more than 10 to 15 minutes. Blood samples must be multiple and at critical times: before injection, 15 or 30 minutes after, and during 48 hours samples are collected at hours 1, 2, 4, 8, 24, 36 and 48.

Recovery is appreciated as a percentage of what is expected to be in circulation at the peak of activity. It is theorically expected that 1 U/kg rises the FVIII level of 2U/dl. Half life of the product is the time between the peak level and half of the clotting factor concentration at the peak.

Tolerance must be evaluated. General tolerance is appreciated by clinical examination, pulse, blood pressure, temperature, respiration frequency and any side effect. Local tolerance is appraised by redness, hematoma, pain, stinging or burning on the injection site. Biological tolerance is analysed on tests of hemostasis, cytology and biochemistry.

Safety studies. The risk of viral transmission is the most important concern for industrial preparations of clotting factor concentrate. Large pool of plasma from thousand of donors is a cause of viral contamination despite the control of individual plasma and donor. This is the reason why in addition to the control made on the donor, which is the single one possible for labile products (red cells and platelets), a method of viral inactivation is applied during the purification process. Inactivation procedures are multiple: heat treatment with multiple possibilities in degrees and duration, vapor treatment, solvent detergent methods. Affinity chromatography on sepharose bound antibody columns are also considered as a mean of reducing the viral content.

Evaluation of safety on virus transmission of blood products is long and difficult. Several months of follow up in populations of virgin patients is often necessary before the safety on viral transmission can be established.

If hepatitis B is now avoided by vaccination, the recommendations of the International Committee on Thrombosis Hemostatis (Mannucci & Columbo, 1989) to conduct trials about other hepatitis safety are still valid. It consist on a follow up, after the first injection, of liver enzymes every 2 weeks during 4 months and every month during the next 2 months. Non enveloped viruses are not affected by solvent detergent methods of inactivation. However they seem sensitive to heat treatment in conditions which are not fully determined yet. These viruses actually known such as non enveloped viruses concerned parvovirus and hepatitis A virus however other still unknown viruses might emerge in the following years and efficient methods of inactivation against all kind of viruses must be considered; double inactivation at different steps of the purification procedure is now proposed by some manufacturers.

Immunogenicity. Highly purified material might cause modification of the clotting factor molecules emergence of new epitopes eliciting formation of neutralizing antibodies. Evaluation of such immunologic response in the receiver patients is extremely difficult to assess: first because the prevalence of inhibitors in the population of FVIII or FIX deficient patients is not known with certainly (Ehrenforth et al, 1992) and secundly because the reason why inhibitors arise in some patients and not in others is not known either. To evaluate the response of the immune system of a new preparation of concentrate, studies on virgin patients are required using a several month follow up until a high number of injections has been reached, as well as the follow up of older patients treated for a long time with well known preparations of plasma concentrates, in whom emergence of new antibodies could be detected.

Purity is an important concern when the choice of a concentrate has been made. Several in vitro and clinical studies are available demonstrating that intermediate purity concentrate contaning large amont of proteins other than the deficient factors have deleterious effects on the immune system when compared to very high purity concentrate (Brettler et al, 1989 ; Goldsmith et al, 1991 ; Eibl et al, 1987 ; Pasi & Hill, 1990 ; Hay & McEvoy, 1992 ; Madhok et al, 1990 ; Vermot-Desroches et al, 1992 ; Faucette et al, 1992). This is a special concern for HIV positive hemophiliacs.

Purity of a concentrate is related to the specific activity (SA). The specific activity is the activity evaluated in international units (IU) per milligramme of proteins present in the preparation. Very high purity products are those with a SA > 100 IU of FVIII or FIX per mg of protein.

Clotting factor concentrate prepared using affinity chromatography or monoclonal antibody sepharose bound have a SA of 2 to 3 000 after elution. SA is reduced in the final preparation by albumin addition to stabilize clotting factor activities. Clotting factor concentrate prepared using ion exchange chromatography have currently a SA between 100 and 150 without stabilizing protein added. The choice is difficult to do in absence of long and expensive studies on the immunologic system, which are still ongoing.

Facilities and current usage must be appreciated. Dissolution of the concentrates, concentration and volume of the final product, storage, must be as easy as possible.

In conclusion, coagulation factor concentrates must be efficient, safe and without immunogenicity. The impact of purification processes on the immune function have still to be studied. Clinical evaluations are absolutly necessary, but they are difficult to carry out as they need severe deficient patients with a long, follow up. So these trials need multicentric international studies.

REFERENCES

Brettler, D.B., Forsberg, A.D., Levine, P.H., Petillo, J., Lamon, K. and Sullivan, J.L. (1989) : Factor VIII:C concentrate purified from plasma using monoclonal antibodies: human studies. Blood 73, 7, 1859-1863.

Ehrenforth, S., Kreuz, W., Scharrer, I., Linde, R., Funk, M., Gungor, T., Krackhardt, B., Kornhuber, B. (1992) : Incidence of development of factor VIII and factor IX inhibitors in haemophiliacs. The Lancet 339, 8793, 594-598.

Eibl, M.M., Ahmad, R., Wolf, H.M., Linnau, Y., Gotz, E. and Mannhalter, J.W. (1987) : A component of factor VIII preparations which can be separated from factor VIII activity down modulates human monocytes functions.Blood 69, 4, 1153-1160.

Faucette, J., Parker, C.J., McCluskey, T., Bernshaw, N.J., Rodgers, G.M. (1992) : Induction of tissue factor activity in endothelial cells and monocytes by a modified form of albumin present in normal human plasma. Blood 79, 11, 2888-2895.

Goldsmith, J.M., Deutsche, J., Tang, M., and Green, D. (1991) : CD4 Cells in HIV-1 infected hemophiliacs: effect of factor VIII concentrates. Thrombosis and Hemostasis 66, 4, 415-419.

Hay, C.R.M., and Mc Evoy, P. (1992) : Purity of factor VIII concentrates. The Lancet 339, 1613.

Madhok, R., Gracie, J.A., Smith, J., Lowe, G.D.O., and Forbes, C.D. (1990) : Capacity to produce interleukin 2 is impaired in haemophilia in the absence and presence of HIV 1 infection.

Mannucci, P.M., and Colombo, M. (1989) : Revision of the protocol recommended for studies of safety from hepatitis of clotting factor concentrates.Thrombosis and Hemostasis 61, 532-534.

Pasi, K.J., and Hill, F.G. (1990) : In vitro and in vivo inhibition of monocyte phagocytic function by factor VIII concentrates: correlation with concentrate purity. Br. J. of Haematol. 76, 88-93.

Vermot-Desroches, C., Rigal, D., Blourde, C., and Bernaud, J. (1992) : Immunosuppressive property of a very high purity antihaemophilic preparation: a low molecular weight component inhibits an early step of PHA induced cell activation. Br. J. of Haematol. 80, 370-377.

Résumé

Les deficits congenitaux et acquis en facteurs de la coagulation sont associées a des épisodes hémorragiques. Une thérapeutique substitutive peut être necessaire. Les facteurs de la coagulation doivent être purifiés et concentrés pour être efficaces. Des études cliniques doivent être menées pour conclure à l'efficacité et à l'inocuité virale de ces produits. Des recommendations au sujet de ces études sont définies par un consensus international. Parmi ces protocoles, des études de l'immunogénicité sont necessaires. L'impact des procédés de purification de ces produits sur les fonctions immunitaires des patients doit encore être étudié. Des essais au long cours, et des essais chez des patients "vierges" (patients n'ayant jamais reçu de produit sanguins ou dérivé du sang) doivent être menés.

Preparation of a high purity factor IX concentrate using metal chelate affinity chromatography

P.A. Feldman, L. Harris, D.R. Evans and H.E. Evans

Bio-Products Laboratory, Dagger Lane, Elstree, Hertshire, WD6 3BX, United Kingdom

SUMMARY

Factor IX has been purified from cryopecipitate-depleted plasma using DEAE-Sepharose anion exchange chromatography and immobilised metal ion affinity chromatography. Prothrombin complex, eluted from the anion exchange gel, was incubated with TWEEN and TnBP to inactivate viruses. This solution was applied to a column of Chelating Sepharose which had been charged with copper ions. Prothrombin did not bind to the gel. Other proteins were removed from the gel by buffer washes at low salt and low pH. Factor IX was eluted by a buffer containing glycine, at a concentration which enabled formulation and freeze-drying without further processing. The specific activity of the final Factor IX concentrate was > 150iu/mg protein.

INTRODUCTION

For more than 20 years, patients with Factor IX deficiency (Haemophilia B; Christmas Disease) have been treated by replacement therapy with Prothrombin Complex Concentrates (PCC) prepared from human plasma. These preparations are a mixture of the Vitamin K dependent proteins and other plasma proteins which co-fractionate. Depending on the method of preparation, the absolute and relative concentrations of these different proteins can vary, though Factor IX rarely exceeds 2% of the total by weight.

Sporadic incidences of thrombotic complications have been reported following the use of PCC, though it is difficult to establish the true level of risk or to attribute these events to a particular cause [1]. Various formulations in anticoagulants (e.g. ATIII and heparin) and rigorous *in vitro* testing of potential thrombogenicity have been introduced to minimise the thrombogenic risk. However, it is believed that greater purification of the Factor IX protein (or the corollary: the exclusion of unidentified thrombogenic components) may offer the best security from such untoward events.

In recent years, several processes have been developed which remove many of the unwanted proteins, producing more highly purified Factor IX concentrates. These methods are based upon affinity chromatography, using either immobilised sulphated polysaccharides [2,3] or immobilised monoclonal antibodies [4]. We have developed an alternative, novel method for the purification of Factor IX from plasma, using anion-exchange chromatography and immobilised metal ion (metal chelate) affinity chromatography. This overcomes much of the laborious processing required by other methods and yields a freeze-dried concentrate of Factor IX with a high specific activity, which is suitable for clinical use.

MATERIALS AND METHODS

Human plasma was collected using apheresis by the National Blood Transfusion Service of England and Wales. DEAE-Sepharose CL6B and Chelating Sepharose Fast Flow were from Pharmacia (Milton Keynes,

U.K.). Routine chemicals were obtained from BDH-Merck (Poole, U.K.). Antisera were obtained from Dakopatts (High Wycombe, U.K.).

Clotting factor activities were measured by one-stage clotting times in deficient plasmas (Immuno, Sevenoaks, U.K. and Diagnostic Reagents, Thame, U.K.). Factor IX activity was also measured by two-stage assay. Potencies were assigned using the 2nd British Working Standard (87/532) calibrated against the 1st International Standard for Factors II,IX and X Concentrate (84/681; NIBSC). Samples of purified Factor IX were diluted in Factor IX-deficient plasma before one-stage Factor IX assay to avoid protein denaturation and ensure equivalence with the two-stage system. Potential thrombogenicity was assessed by non-activated partial thromboplastin time (NAPTT) and Fibrinogen Clotting Time (FCT).

Antigen assays were performed by rocket immunoelectrophoresis (Laurell method) against antisera to Factors II, IX and X, Protein C and Inter-α-trypsin inhibitor, using normal pooled human plasma as the standard designated to contain an arbitrary 1 plasma equivalent unit (peu) per ml for each protein.

Protein was measured by the Biuret method and by absorbance at 280nm. Copper was measured by atomic absorption spectroscopy.

Chromatography Buffers (all citrate-phosphate except Buffer 8):

Buffer 1. 190mM NaCl, pH6.5
Buffer 2. 310mM NaCl, pH6.5
Buffer 3. 500mM NaCl, pH6.5
Buffer 4. 100mM NaCl, pH7.0
Buffer 5. 100mM NaCl, pH 4.4
Buffer 6. 100mM NaCl, pH7.0
Buffer 7. 100mM NaCl 20mM glycine, pH7.0
Buffer 8. 50mM EDTA, pH7.0

FACTOR IX PURIFICATION

200-300kg pools of cryoprecipitate-depleted plasma (CPS) were adjusted to pH7.0 and batch-adsorbed with DEAE-Sepharose at 4°C, for 1 hour. The gel was recovered in a Broadbent continuous flow basket centrifuge and washed in the centrifuge with Buffer 1. The gel was resuspended in Buffer 1 and packed into a 180mm diameter glass chromatography column (bed height 9-13cm). After further washing with Buffer 1, a fraction containing PCC was eluted by Buffer 2. Protein elution was monitored by absorbance at 280nm. The PCC eluate was collected in three fractions, of which the second contained most of the eluted Factor IX activity. These fractions were stored at -40°C.

The thawed PCC was incubated with 1% v/v polyoxyethylene (20) sorbitan monooleate (TWEEN 80) and 0.3% v/v tri-n-butyl phosphate (TnBP) at 25°C for 6 hours to inactivate lipid-enveloped viruses [5]. The solution was then prepared for metal chelate chromatography, by the addition of solid sodium chloride to achieve a final concentration of 500mM.

Chelating Sepharose Fast Flow was packed into a 70mm diameter glass chromatography column (bed height 15-21cm) and washed with copper sulphate solution (5mg/ml) to charge the chelating ligand with copper ions. The gel was then washed with the equilibration Buffer 3.

The salt-adjusted, virus-inactivated PCC was then loaded on to the column and washed with 6 bed volumes of Buffer 3 before the ionic strength was reduced by the application of Buffer 4. This was followed by the acidic Buffer 5. Each of these three buffer washes eluted proteins which were collected separately (Fractions A-C).

After re-equilibrating the gel to pH7.0 with Buffer 6, the Factor IX was eluted by Buffer 7. The eluate (Fraction D) was collected and stored at -40°C.

The copper attached to the gel, and any remaining associated protein, was then removed (as Fraction E) by washing the gel with Buffer 8.

The Factor IX fractions were subsequently thawed, pooled and diluted to a target Factor IX potency of 50iu/ml. This solution, formulated with lysine, was filtered aseptically through a 0.2μm sterilising filter, dispensed in 10ml aliquots into Type 1 glass vials (50ml capacity) and freeze-dried.

RESULTS

PCC was isolated from CPS by anion-exchange chromatography on DEAE-Sepharose. The PCC was highly concentrated (60-80iu/ml) with acceptable NAPTT (>150s) and FCT (>5h). After solvent-detergent treatment, Factor IX was isolated by metal chelate chromatography.

Figure 1a shows a typical protein elution profile during chromatography on copper-charged Chelating Sepharose Fast Flow. Figure 1b-d show the clotting activities of Factor IX, Prothrombin, and Factor X in each fraction. Only a very small proportion of the loaded Factor IX (<2%) failed to bind to the gel; in total, about 5% was eluted in Fractions A, B and C. The Factor IX eluted by Buffer 7, had high potency (60-100iu/ml) and high specific activity (120-160iu/mg). The average recovery of usable Factor IX in Fraction D was 53%. Approximately 12% of the loaded Factor IX remained bound to the gel after the glycine wash and was measured by antigen assay in Fraction E.

97 per cent of the prothrombin in the starting material failed to bind to the gel and was recovered in Fraction A. Factor X was distributed between Fractions A, B and C. Only small amounts were measured in the Factor IX-rich Fraction D (approximately 3iu Factor X per 100iu Factor IX) and this was detected mainly in the front of the protein elution peak.

Figures 1e and 1f show the antigen concentrations of Protein C and Inter-α-trypsin inhibitor respectively. All the Protein C bound to the gel and was mainly eluted by Buffer 5 and Buffer 7. In the Factor IX-rich Fraction D there were approximately 20peu Protein C per 100iu Factor IX. The Inter-α-trypsin inhibitor which bound to the gel was mainly eluted into Fraction C (40%) and Fraction E (35%). There was very little in the intervening Fraction D (0.5%), approximating to 0.4peu Inter-α-trypsin inhibitor per 100iu Factor IX.

Figure 1g shows the copper concentration, expressed in mg/L. In Fractions A, B and C the copper concentration was 8-10mg/L. The concentration in Fraction D was much lower (0.4-0.7 mg/L). Quantitation of the copper in Fraction E indicated that the final copper loading on the gel was 0.95mg per ml of gel.

Table 1 shows the mean yield and characteristics of Factor IX during the purification process. The overall yield was 178iu Factor IX per kg CPS and the Factor IX was purified ten thousand-fold from CPS. NAPTT of all Factor IX samples were >150 seconds when diluted 1/10 and the FCT at 37°C were >6 hours.

TABLE 1
Mean Yield and Characteristics of Factor IX Prepared by Metal Chelate Affinity Chromatography

Process Stage	No. batches	Factor IX:C (iu/ml)	(iu/kg CPS)	Stage Yield (%)	Sp. Act. (iu/mg)	NAPTT Range 1/10 (s)	FCT @ 37°C (h)
CPS	8	0.9	900	–	0.016	–	–
DEAE Eluate (PCC)	8	73.5	458	51	3.3	160 – 235	5 – >6
Post–virus inactivation	8	69.1	422	92	4.0	232 – 284	2½ – 5¼
Metal Chelate Eluate	8	79.7	218	53	140	150 – 230	>6
Freeze–Dried Product	4	52.8	178	82	164	175 – 217	>6

Table 2 lists some characteristics of the final product after reconstitution of the freeze-dried product.

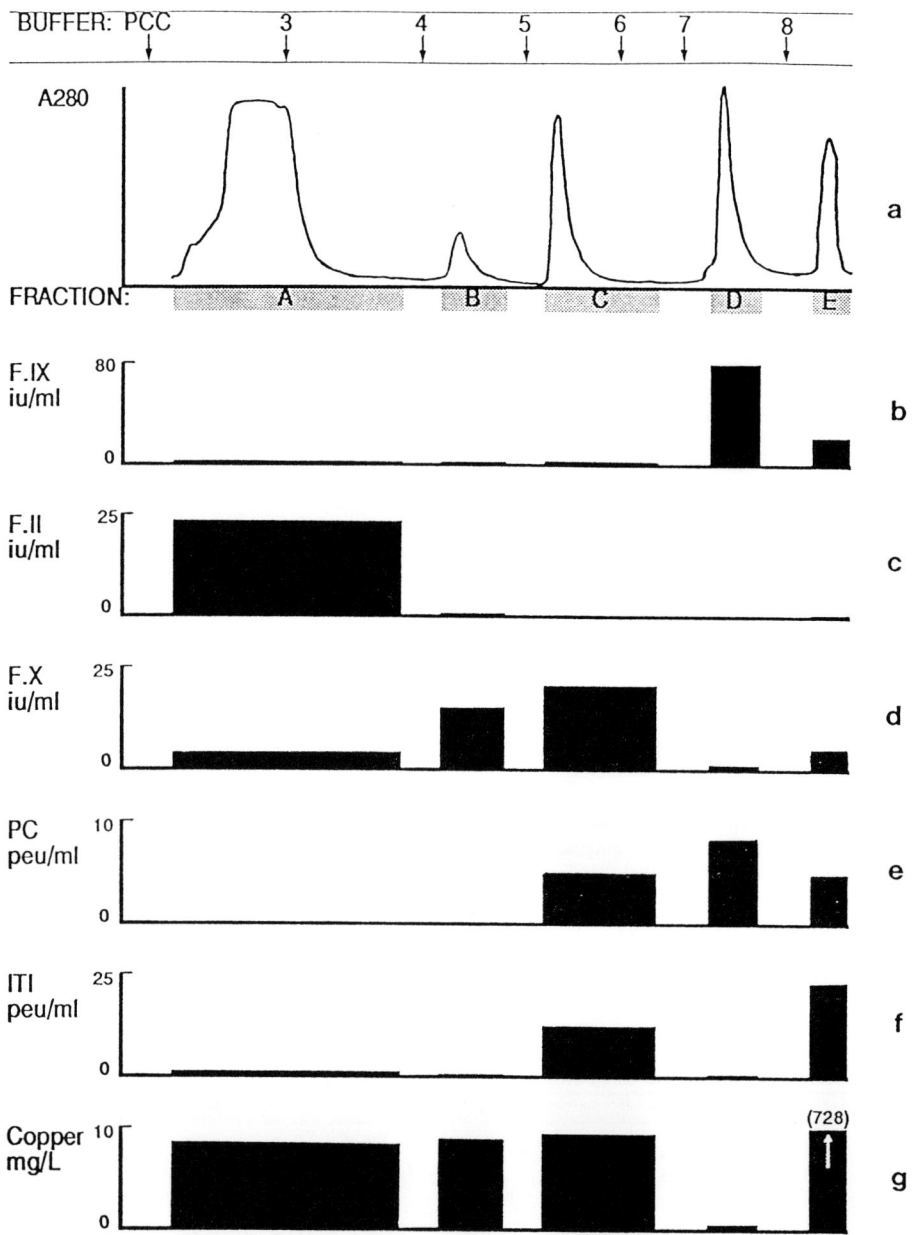

Fig. 1: Chromatography of PCC on Copper–Charged Chelating Sepharose
Solvent–detergent treated PCC was loaded on to copper–charged Chelating Sepharose Fast Flow. The gel was then washed sequentially with Buffers 3–8 (see Materials & Methods). During elution, the sensitivity of the u.v. absorbance monitor was increased ten–fold to accomodate low protein concentration of Fractions B & D. (a), typical elution profile monitored by absorbance at 280nm; other boxes show mean (n=8) elution of: (b) Factor IX; (c), Factor II (prothrombin); (d), Factor X; (e), Protein C; (f), Inter–alpha–trypsin inhibitor; (g), copper.

TABLE 2
High Purity Factor IX Final Product Characteristics
(mean of 4 batches)

Factor IX (iu/ml)	52.8
(iu/vial)	528
Protein (mg/ml)	0.32
Factor IX Sp. Act. (iu/mg)	164
NAPTT 1/10 [control] (s)	196 [285]
FCT @ 20°C, 37°C (h)	>24, >6
Factor II (iu / 100 iu Factor IX)	None Detectable
Factor X (iu/ 100 iu Factor IX)	<1.5
Copper (mg/L)	0.5

DISCUSSION

Using a combination of anion-exchange chromatography and metal chelate affinity chromatography, we have developed a highly purified Factor IX concentrate. This two-stage process has several advantages over other, more laborious methods. The plasma supernatant did not require dilution before adsorption on DEAE-Sepharose. The resulting PCC eluate had a high Factor IX potency (a function of chromatographic frontal elution using a heavily loaded, small volume of gel) and passed the NAPTT and FCT tests for *in vitro* potential thrombogenicity. This differs from our previous experience with apheresis plasma, fractionated using DEAE-cellulose, when 25% of all batches failed the NAPTT test [6]. The improvement may result from three processing modifications; (1) after adsorbing the gel at pH7.0 (to maximise Factor IX binding), it was washed with buffers at pH6.5, which reduces thrombin activity; (2) the ionic strength of the wash Buffer 1 was increased, eluting material with short NAPTT which would otherwise be retained to co-elute with the Factor IX elution peak; (3) the avoidance of CPS dilution may maintain higher functional concentrations of plasma protease inhibitors.

Inactivation of lipid-enveloped viruses was achieved by incubation with 1% TWEEN 80 and 0.3% TnBP at 25°C for 6 hours. There was greater than 90% recovery of Factor IX activity across the solvent-detergent step, and no shortening of NAPTT (Table 1). Any FCT shortening was at least partly due to distortion of the assay by the TWEEN/TnBP reagents.

The proteins in the PCC eluate were then separated by chromatography on Chelating Sepharose which had been charged with copper ions. This chromatography was not affected by the presence of 1% TWEEN and 0.3% TnBP. Factor IX binding was not critically dependent on ionic strength, so there was no need to reduce the ionic strength of the PCC before loading, as required by other chromatographic methods. Prothrombin did not bind to the gel (Fig. 1c), thus removing from the system the predominant protein by weight in the PCC. If the gel was loaded with PCC which contained thrombin (measured by FCT), the thrombin also failed to bind (data not shown). This differs from chromatography using sulphated polysaccharides, to which thrombin can bind and co-elute with the Factor IX.

Factor X bound to the gel and was eluted in Fractions B and C (Fig. 1d). After Buffer 5, very little Factor X remained bound to the gel. Protein C was virtually undetectable in both of the first two wash fractions, indicating complete and tight binding to the gel (Fig. 1e). The separation of Protein C from Prothrombin and Factor X is a further unique feature of this chromatographic method.

After exclusion of prothrombin, the most significant purification was achieved by the removal of Inter-α-trypsin inhibitor which, in PCC, constitutes 40% of the total protein by weight. Antigen to Inter-α-trypsin inhibitor was measured in Fraction C and Fraction E but only very small amounts were detected in the Factor IX-rich Fraction D (Fig. 1f). SDS polyacrylamide gel electrophoresis identified different proteins in Fractions C and E; the predominant protein in Fraction C had a molecular weight of approximately 120,000 and the protein in Fraction E had a molecular weight of approximately 230,000. These two species correspond to Pre-

and Inter-α-trypsin inhibitor moeities [7], which both react with the antiserum used for assay. Our present chromatographic method offers a novel approach to the separation of Pre-α-trypsin inhibitor from Inter-α-trypsin inhibitor and of both from Factor IX.

A potential hazard of metal chelate chromatography is that metal ions may leak from the gel. To ensure that any labile metal ions were removed before elution of Factor IX, the citrate concentration in equilibration and wash buffers was deliberately higher than in the re-equilibration and elution buffers. This strategy proved effective, causing a ten-fold reduction in eluted copper after gel washing (Fig. 1g), with only 0.5mg copper per litre in the final product (Table 2). This was the same as measured in PCC which had never been exposed to such a copper challenge and was less than the plasma copper concentration of 1 mg/L.

Factor IX was recovered in Fraction D in highly purified and concentrated form (Fig. 1b; Table 1). The eluates did not require any subsequent concentration and yielded a freeze-dried concentrate with a mean Factor IX specific activity of 164 iu/mg. Comparison with published specific activities suggests that the concentrate contained >70% pure Factor IX. *In vitro* tests for potential thrombogenicity showed no evidence of clotting factor activation. There was no detectable prothrombin activity and negligible Factor X activity. After satisfactory safety tests in animals, this product (BPL "9MC") is currently under clinical evaluation.

REFERENCES

1. Lusher JM (1991): Thrombogenicity associated with Factor IX complex concentrates. Sem Haematol 28 Suppl 6:3-5.

2. Ménaché D, Behre HE, Orthner CL, Nunez H, Anderson HD, Triantaphyllopoulos DC, Kosow DP (1984): Coagulation factor IX: method of preparation and assessment of potential in vivo thrombogenicity in animal models. Blood 64:1220-1227.

3. Burnouf T, Michalski C, Goudemand M, Huart JJ (1989): Properties of a highly purified factor IX:c therapeutic concentrate prepared by conventional chromatography. Vox Sang 57:225-232.

4. Hrinda ME, Huang C, Tarr GC, Weeks R, Feldman F, Schreiber AB (1991): Preclinical studies of a monoclonal antibody-purified factor IX, mononine. Sem Haematol 28 Suppl 6:6-14.

5. Horowitz B (1989): Investigations into the application of tri(n-butyl) phosphate/detergent mixtures to blood derivatives. In Morgenthaler J-J (ed): "Virus inactivation in plasma products." Basel, Karger, pp83-96.

6. Evans D, Walker T, Evans H (1989): Pilot scale (300kg) fractionation of plasma for factor VIII and factor IX. Transfus Sci 10:313-319.

7. Salier J-P (1990): Inter-α-trypsin inhibitor: emergence of a family within the Kunitz-type protease inhibitor superfamily. Trends Biochem Sci 15:435-439.

Characterization of a highly purified factor IX concentrate

Anna-Lena Löf, Erik Berntorp*, Bertil Eriksson, Christer Mattson, Lillemor Svinhufvud, Stefan Winge and Anna Östlin

Kabi Pharmacia AB, Plasma Products, 112 87 Stockholm, Sweden and *Department for Coagulation Disorders, Malmö General Hospital, 214 01 Malmö, Sweden

INTRODUCTION

Low purity factor IX (FIX) complex concentrates have been used for the treatment of haemophilia B since the late 1960's. Unfortunately, the use of these concentrates has been associated with severe adverse effects, such as thrombotic complications (Lusher, 1991, Kasper, 1991) and viral transmission of hepatitis and human immuno deficiency virus (HIV).
The problems with thrombogenicity have generally been attributed to the presence of activated coagulation factors and coagulant-active phospholipids in the concentrates (White et al. 1977, Giles et al. 1982) and/or the sustained elevated levels of factor II and factor X attained in the recipients (Aronson & Menache 1987). Thus, it is likely that purer products would have a lower thrombogenic potential than the cruder ones.
At Kabi Pharmacia a highly purified FIX concentrate, Nanotiv, has been developed. Viral inactivation with the solvent detergent (S/D) technique is incorporated in the manufacturing process to obtain a product with a high virus safety margin. The S/D method, initially developed at the New York Blood Center, has been demonstrated to possess a highly efficient virus-inactivating capacity against lipid-enveloped viruses (Horowitz et al. 1985, Piët et al. 1990).

MATERIAL AND METHODS

Preparation of Nanotiv 500 IU and 1000 IU
1000 l of plasma was thawed and the cryoprecipitate was separated. The cryopoor plasma was applied to a DEAE-Sepharose column for the capture of FIX. After elution FIX was subjected to SD treatment using TNBP (0.3%) as solvent and Triton X-100 (1%) as detergent. Affinity chromatography on Heparin-Sepharose was performed in order to remove the chemical agents as well as factors II, VII and X (FII, FVII, FX). Further purification of FIX was achieved by the use of a cation exchanger. The FIX solution was formulated, sterile filtered, filled and lyophilized. Before use, Nanotiv 500 IU and 1000 IU were reconstituted in 5 ml and 10 ml of water for injections, respectively, yielding a FIX potency of 100 IU/ml.

Preconativ 600 IU
Preconativ a low purity, factor II, IX and X concentrate, was obtained from the ordinary production line, Kabi Pharmacia AB, Stockholm, Sweden. Before use, Preconativ 600 IU was reconstituted in 10 ml of water for injections, yielding a FIX potency of 60 IU/ml.

Coagulation factor assays and in vitro thrombogenicity tests
FIX activity was measured by a one-stage coagulation technique using FIX-deficient plasma essentially according to Biggs, 1972. The FIX activity was expressed in International Units (IU) as defined by the first International Standard for blood coagulation factors II, IX, X concentrate (IS). The standard coded 84/681 was obtained from the National Institute for Biological Standards and Control (NIBSC), England. FII and FX activities were determined in one step using the chromogenic substrates S2238 and S2222, respectively (Axelsson et al. 1976, Aurell et al. 1977). The substrates were obtained from Chromogenix AB, Sweden. The activities were expressed in IU defined by the IS. FVII activity was measured in two steps as described by Oswaldsson et al 1985, using the chromogenic substrate S2222 and rabbit brain thromboplastin as activator. The FVII activity was expressed in IU defined by the first International Standard for factors II, VII and X in plasma. The standard coded 84/665 was obtained from NIBSC.

The thrombogenicity in vitro was evaluated by the Non Activated Partial Thromboplastin Time (NAPTT) and the thrombin assay according to the European Pharmacopoeia. Additionally, all batches were subjected to the Thrombin Generation Time (TGt50) test (Sas et al. 1975).

Protein determination
Total protein was measured as described elsewhere (Löf et al. 1992) using a modified Bradford method and Bovine Serum Albumin (BSA) as protein standard. The BSA was purchased from Bio-Rad Laboratories, Germany.

Rabbit stasis model
The in vivo thrombogenicity of Preconativ and Nanotiv batches was tested in a modified Wessler rabbit thrombus model (Wessler et al 1959).

Fourteen Preconativ batches were solubilized to a final concentration of 25 IU/ml and injected into rabbits at a dose of 25 IU/kg (1 ml/kg). Three batches of Nanotiv were reconstituted to a final concentration of 25 IU/ml, while two other batches of Nanotiv were reconstituted to a final concentration of 200, 300 and 400 IU/ml. The test compound was injected intravenously at a volume of 1 ml/kg, representing a total dose of 25, 200, 300 and 400 IU/kg, respectively. Six control animals received saline at a dose of 1 ml/kg. The thrombogenicity of each dose group is described by a "thrombogenic index" ranging from 0 (non-thrombogenic) to 1 (highly thrombogenic).

Virus safety
Several studies were performed with the objective of determining to what extent virus infectivity could be reduced and/or separated from FIX in different steps of the manufacturing process of Nanotiv. Each step was carefully adapted to a laboratory scale which as closely as possible mimicked the manufacturing procedure.

The viruses studied were human immunodeficiency virus, type 1 (HIV-1), vesicular stomatitis virus (VSV) and Sindbis virus. Virus infectivity titre was expressed in accordance with the method of Reed & Muench 1938, as tissue culture infectious dose giving an end point of 50% infected cultures (TCID$_{50}$) and normally related to a sample volume of one ml.

Clinical studies, pharmacokinetics
Six haemophilia B patients were assigned to a randomized single-blind cross-over study in which each patient served as his own control. The Factor VIII/Factor IX Scientific and Standardization Committee (SSC) of the International Society on Thrombosis and Haemostasis (ISTH) has issued recommendations for the Design and Analysis of Half-life and Recovery

studies (ISTH/SCC, Barcelona June 1990). These recommendations were followed in all essentials.

Nanotiv and Preconativ were administered intravenously in a single dose of 50 IU (FIX) per kg bodyweight. Treatment started after an initial ≥5 days wash out/run-in period. Both treatments were separated by a ≥5 days wash-out period.

Venous blood samples were drawn before injection of the FIX concentrates and at 5, 10, 15, 20, 30 and 45 minutes and 1, 2, 3, 6, 9, 12, 24, 32, 48 and 72 hours after both injections, for the determination of FIX clotting activity (FIX:C). The plasma concentration curves of FIX:C were analyzed by model-independent methods as previously described for FIX (Matucci et al 1985). Accordingly, the following pharmacokinetic parameters were estimated from each curve: total body clearence (Cl), volume of distribution at steady state (Vdss), mean residence time (MRT) adjusted to the bolus dose and half life ($t_{1/2}$).

The in vivo recovery was expressed as incremental rize IU/dl per dose IU/kg.

Clinical studies, thrombogenicity tests

Samples for the evaluation of thrombogenicity were taken before the injection and at 0.5, 1 and 24 hours after the injections. Platelet count was performed and Antithrombin III (ATIII), thrombin/antithrombin III complex (TAT), fibrin-D dimer, fibrin monomer and prothrombin fragment F_{1+2} were determined in plasma in order to evaluate possible thrombogenicity.

The platelet count was performed by visual counting under a phase contrast microscope. AT III functional activity was measured as heparin cofactor activity by an amidolytic method (Coatest, Chromogenix AB, Sweden). An ELISA technique (Enzygnost, Behringwerke, Germany) was used to determine TAT. A Latex Agglutination Slide Test (Diagnostica Stago, France) was used to assess the fibrin-D dimer level. Spectrophotometric assays with chromogenic substrate (Coaset, Chromogenix AB, Sweden) were used to determine fibrin monomer. Enzyme immunoassays (Enzygnost F 1+2, Behringwerke, Germany) were employed for the determination of human prothrombin fragment F 1+2.

RESULTS

Purity

There were no measurable amounts of FII, FVII and FX present in Nanotiv and the specific activity of FIX was about 200 IU/mg protein. Nanotiv is about 100 times purer than Preconativ, which was used as a comparative drug in this study, see Table 1.

Table 1. Purity, comparison between Preconativ and Nanotiv

	Preconativ low purity FIX concentrate	Nanotiv high purity FIX concentrate
FIX:C IU/ml	60	100
Specific activity, FIX:C IU/mg protein	2	200
FII:C IU/100 IU FIX:C	80	<0.1
FVII:C IU/100 IU FIX:C	1	<0.1
FX:C IU/100 IU FIX:C	80	<0.1
Heparin	not added	not added
NAPTT 1/10 and 1/100 dilutions sec	>150	>150
TGt50 min	>60	>60
Thrombin	approved	approved

Thrombogenicity
The in vivo thrombogenicity of Nanotiv was evaluated in a modified Wessler rabbit thrombosis model. Results obtained indicated that doses as high as 400 IU/kg can be administered to rabbits without causing severe thrombogenic problems (Fig 1). Furthermore, there was no obvious correlation between thrombogenic index and dose in the range 25-400 IU/kg. The results are in agreement with other published data for highly purified FIX concentrates (Smith 1988, Burnouf et al. 1989, Hrinda et al. 1991).

Figure 1. Assessment of thrombogenicity in vivo

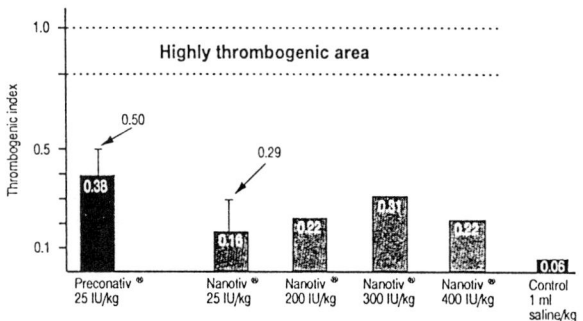

Virus safety
The major purification steps of the manufacturing process of Nanotiv were validated with respect to the inactivation and separation of viruses deliberately added to the FIX. Results from the studies performed demonstrated that the overall clearance factor for HIV-1 was ≥10.8 logs of infectivity, measured as $TCID_{50}$/ml. Corresponding overall clearance factors were ≥8.5 for VSV and ≥10.1 for Sindbis virus as shown in Table 2.

Table 2. Separation and inactivation of different viruses in the production of Nanotiv

Step investigated	Clearance factor		
	HIV-1	VSV	Sindbis
Initial separation	≥1.0	n d	n d
DEAE-Sepharose chromatography	2.1	3.0	3.1
S/D treatment	≥6.0*	≥4.0*	≥5.0*
Heparin-Sepharose chromatography	0.4	0.4	0.7
Cation exchange chromatography	1.7	1.5	2.0
Total number of accumulated clearance factor**	≥10.8	≥8.5	≥10.1

n d = not determined
* Total inactivation after <1 minute
** Any reduction factor <1.0 has not been considered in the calculation of the overall clearance factors

Clinical studies
A clinical bioequivalence trial was performed at Malmö General Hospital, Malmö, Sweden Figure 2 and Table 3 show the elimination curves and pharmacokinetic parameters after single injections of Nanotiv and Preconativ. There was no statistically or clinically-significant differences in any pharmacokinetic parameter between the two treatments.

Figure 2. FIX activities (means) after a single dose of 50 IU/kg, n=6.

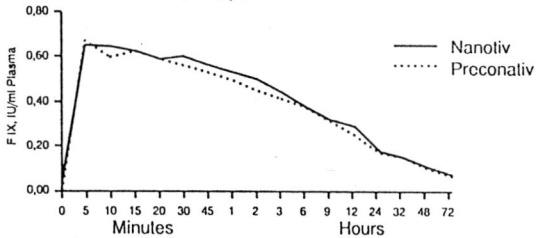

Table 3. Pharmacokinetic results (means ± SD)

	$T_{1/2}$ [h]	Cl [ml/h/kg]	Vdss [ml/kg]	MRT [h]	Incremental recovery [IU/dl per IU/kg]
Nanotiv	19 ± 8	4.9 ± 0.7	123 ± 40	26 ± 10	1.2 ± 0.2
Preconativ	20 ± 11	5.2 ± 0.6	126 ± 27	25 ± 9	1.3 ± 0.2

Safety

Nanotiv did not differ from Preconativ in its thrombotic potential, measured as platelet counts, ATIII, TAT, fibrin-D dimer, and fibrin monomer. However, the post-injection values of prothrombin fragment F_{1+2} indicated a difference. Thirty minutes after treatment with Preconativ a 2.6 fold increase in the F_{1+2} level was observed. This increase could not be ascribed to the presence F_{1+2} in the concentrate. In contrast no significant rise was observed after treatment with Nanotiv.

Efficacy

An open clinical study with the objective of assessing efficacy and safety of Nanotiv during surgical procedures in haemophilia B patients is ongoing. So far, five patients have been treated. The haemostatic effect was excellent and no adverse reactions were reported.

CONCLUSION

Nanotiv, a highly purified FIX concentrate, seems to combine an excellent haemostatic effect with a high virus safety margin and a minimal risk of thrombotic complications.

REFERENCES

Aronson, D.L., and Ménaché, D. (1987): Thrombogenicity of factor IX complex: In vivo investigation. Joint IABS CSL Symposium on Standardization in Blood Fractionation Including coagulation Factors, Melbourne 1986. Dev Biol Standard Basel, Karger 67: 149-155.

Aurell, L., Friberger, P., Karlsson, G., and Claeson, G. (1977): A new sensitive and highly specific chromogenic peptide substrate for FXa. Throm Res 11: 595-609.

Axelsson, G., Korsan-Bengtsen, K., and Waldenström J. (1976): Prothrombin determination by means of chromogenic peptide substrate. Thromb. Haemost . 36:517.

Biggs, R. (1972): Human blood coagulation haemostasis and thrombosis. ed 1. Oxford, Blackwell Scientific: p. 614.

Burnouf, T., Michalski, C., Goudemand, M., and Huart, J. J. (1989): Properties of a highly purified human plasma factor IX:C therapeutic concentrate prepared by conventional chromatography. Vox Sang 57: 225-232.

European Pharmacopoeia ed 2 (1987): Factor IX coagulations sanguinis humani cryodessiatus: Freeze-dried human coagulation factor IX. p 554.

Giles, A. R., Nesheim, M. E., Hoogendoorn, H., Tracy, P. B., and Mann, K.G. (1982): The coagulant-active phospholipid content is a major determinant of in vivo thrombogenicity of prothrombin complex (factor IX) concentrates in rabbits. Blood 59: 401-407.

Horowitz, B., Wiebe, M. E., Lippin, A., and Stryker, M. H. (1985): Inactivation of viruses in labile blood derivates I. Disruption of lipid-enveloped viruses by tri(n-butyl)phosphate detergent combinations. Transfusion 25: 516-522.

Hrinda, M. E., Chin Huang, Tarr, G. C., Weeks, R., Feldman, F., and Schreiber, A. (1991): Preclinical studies of a monoclonal antibody-purified factor IX, Mononine™. Semin Hemat 28: Suppl 6,6-14.

The International Society on Thrombosis and Haemostasis (ISTH). Morfini, M., Lee, M. (1990): The Design and Analysis of Half-life and Recovery Studies for Factor VIII and Factor IX. Scientific and Standardization Committee XXXVI Annual Meeting, Barcelona, June 20-22, .

Kasper, C. K. (1991): Hemophilia B, thrombosis and surgery. The Hemophilia Bulletin, June , p 2.

Lusher, J. M. (1991): Thrombogenicity associated with factor IX complex concentrates. Semin Hemat ; 28: Suppl 6, 3-5.

Löf , A. L., Gustafsson, G., Novak, V., Engman, L., and Mikaelsson, M. (1992): Determination of total protein in highly purified factor IX concentrates. Vox Sang 63: 172-177.

Matucci ,M., Messori, A., Donati-Cori, G., Longo, G., Vannini, S., Morfini, M., Tendi, E., and Rossi-Ferrini, P. (1985): Kinetic evaluation of four factor VIII concentrates by model-independent methods. Scand J Haematol 34: 22-28.

Oswaldsson, U., Wilson, S., and Rosen, S. (1985): A simple chromogenic assay for the determination of factor VII in microtiterplates. Thromb Haemost 54: 26.

Piët , M. P. J., Chin, S., Prince, A. M., Brotman, B., Cundell, A. M., and Horowitz, B. (1990): The use of tri(n-butyl)phosphate detergent mixtures to inactive hepatitis viruses and human immunodeficiency virus in plasma and plasma's subsequent fractionation. Transfusion 30: 591.598.

Reed, L. J., and Muench, H. (1938): A simple method of estimating fifty percent end points. Am J Hyg 27: 493-497.

Sas, G., Owens, R.E., Smith, K.J., Middleton, S. and Cash, J.D. (1975): In vitro spontaneous thrombin generation in human factor IX concentrates. Brit J Haematol 31: 25.

Smith, K. J. (1988): Immunoaffinity purification of factor IX from commercial concentrates and infusion studies in animals. Blood 72: 1269-1277.

Wessler, Reimer, S. M., and Sheps, M. C. (1959): Biological assay of a thrombosis inducing activity in human serum. J Appl Physiol 14: 934-946.

White, G. C., Roberts, H. R., Kingdon, H. S., and Lundblad, R. L. (1977): Prothrombin complex concentrates. Potentially thrombogenic materials and clues to the mechanism of thrombosis in vivo. Blood 49: 159-170.

Immunoaffinity purified, solvent-detergent treated factor IX

C. Lutsch, P. Gattel, B. Fanget, J.-L. Véron, K. Smith*, J. Armand and M. Grandgeorge

Pasteur Mérieux Sérums et Vaccins, 1541, avenue Marcel Mérieux, 69280 Marcy-l'Étoile, France and
*University of New Mexico, Albuquerque, USA

ABSTRACT

A very high purified FIX concentrate has been produced on a pilot scale (100-200 l plasma) by immunoaffinity chromatography on the metal-ion dependent A7 monoclonal antibody, A7-mAb (Smith & Ono, 1984). The A7-mAb was obtained from biofermentor cultures of hybridoma and was linked to Sepharose^R after purification on four chromatographic steps including a Solvent-Detergent (SD) treatment. The vitamin K dependent clotting factors were isolated by a first anion exchange chromatography and then incubated with a tri (n-butyl) phosphate-Tween 80 mixture (SD treatment). The FIX was subsequently adsorbed on the A7-mAb Sepharose^R column and then eluted by an EDTA containing buffer. Any leached antibody was finally removed by a second anion exchange step. The purified FIX was equilibrated in the final buffer by diafiltration and was lyophilized (without added heparin). The overall FIX yield from the starting cryosupernatant was about 50 per cent. After reconstitution, the final product had a concentration of 50 IU/ml with a specific activity of about 150 IU/mg protein. Neither contaminant FII, FVII, FX, vitronectin nor ATIII was detected. The very high purity of the FIX concentrate was confirmed by crossed-immunoelectrophoresis and Western-blots. Small amounts of degraded FIX (< 20 per cent of the protein on densitometry of SDS-PAGE gels) and high molecular weight material (size exclusion HPLC : < 20 per cent as compared to 65 per cent in heparin affinity purified FIX) were present. There was not detectable thrombin, FXa or FIXa. The product was not thrombogenic when tested at 400 IU/kg in the rabbit stasis-thrombosis model. In non stasis rabbit infusion studies, at 200 IU/kg, no coagulation activation was observed as measured by the following parameters : platelet count, fibrinogen, FV, FVIII, ATIII antigen and fibrin/fibrinogen degradation products. The whole process proved to be effective in eliminating and/or inactivating any possible present virus.

INTRODUCTION

As prothombin complex concentrates (PCC's) are known to induce hypercoagulable state in factor IX (FIX) deficient (hemophilia B) patients, with resulting thromboembolic events and/or disseminated intravascular coagulation, high purity FIX products have been developed in recent years (Clark et al., 1989 ; Burnouf et al., 1989 ; Mannuci et al., 1990 ; Hrinda et al., 1991). Besides FIX, some of the major components of PCC products are other vitamin K dependent factors FII, FVII and FX, native or partly activated as FIX itself, which, together with cell-derived phospholipid contaminants, could disrupt the haemostatic/antithrombotic balance in recipients. Also, the presence of immune globulins in PCC's has been suspected to create immune system impairment (Gomperts et al., 1992).
Heparin-affinity purified FIX and immunoaffinity-purified FIX products have been first developed to reduce thrombogenicity and, more generally to exclude unwanted contaminants. In addition, immunoaffinity chromatography has been shown to have a high potential for removing viral contaminants (Hrinda et al., 1991 ; Addiego et al., 1992). In this study we report about a very high purity FIX concentrate obtained on pilot scale (100-200 l plasma), by immunoaffinity chromatography using A7-mAb, a metal ion-dependent/conformational IgG monoclonal antibody with FIX light chain specificity (Smith & Ono, 1984). The product was treated with Solvent-Detergent (SD) in order to inactivate possibly present enveloped viruses.

MATERIAL AND METHODS

A7-mAb immunoaffinity column

A7-mAb secreting hybridoma cells were cultured in a 150 l biofermentor on defined medium. A7-mAb was purified from culture supernatant by 4 chromatography steps : cation-exchange, anion-exchange, Protein A-affinity after SD treatment and hydroxylapatite.

The anti-FIX activity was 0.98 mg/mg IgG. The IgG monomer level was > 95 per cent in size exclusion HPLC. IgG purity was 100 per cent in SDS-PAGE (reducing conditions, Coomassie blue staining). Contaminants were ≤ 1 ng/mg bovine albumin, ≤ 22 ng/mg bovine IgG, ≤ 10.5 pg/mg DNA, ≤ 3.5 ng/mg Protein A and ≤ 1.2 EU/mg LPS. A7-mAb was coupled to CNBr activated Sepharose^R (Pharmacia) : final concentration, 5.7 mg/ml gel. The FIX capacity was 400 IU FIX/mg gel, i.e. 0.9 mole FIX/mole A7-mAb.

Manufacturing process of Immunopurified FIX

As shown in Fig. 1, FIX was purified from cryosupernatant using a three-step chromatographic procedure. A first anion-exchange chromatography (DEAE-Spherodex^R, Sepracor, France) yielded a PCC which was submitted to a SD treatment. FIX was then isolated by A7-mAb immunoaffinity chromatography using mild elution conditions (EDTA containing buffer). Finally, a second anion-exchange chromatography (DEAE- Sepharose Fast Flow^R, Pharmacia, France) was performed in order to remove traces of leached A7-mAb.

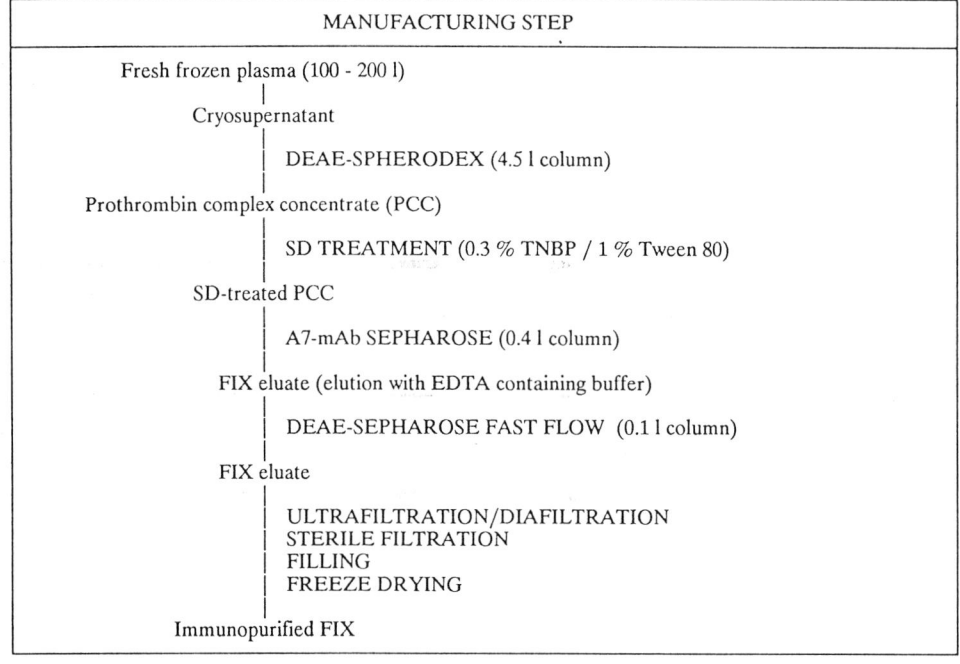

Figure 1. Purification scheme of Immunopurified FIX

Competitor products analysis :
- Heparin-affinity purified FIX (Heparin FIX) from European origin (25 IU FIX/ml),
- Sulfate-dextran affinity purified FIX (S-Dextran FIX) from USA origin (50 IU FIX/ml),
- PCC product from USA origin (30 IU FIX/ml).

Quality control assays

The following tests were performed : FIX activity (FIX : C) by one stage clotting assay ; protein by UV (E 280, 1 per cent = 13.3), (Biuret testing on PCC) ; FIX : Ag by Asserachrom IX : Ag^R ELISA test (Diagnostica Stago, France) ; FII, FVII, FX activities by prothrombin time ; NAPTT according to European Pharmacopeia ; FIXa : Ag by ELISA (Smith, 1988) ; FIIa and FXa activities using S 2238 and S 2222 chromogenic substrates (Chromogenix AB, Mölndal, Sweden) ; heparin by modified Coatest heparin^R test (Chromogenix AB) ; antithrombin III by modified Coamate antithrombin^R test (Chromogenix AB) ; murine IgG by ELISA test ; TNBP by gas chromatography ; Tween 80 by colorimetric assay (cobaltothiocyanate reagent) ; two-dimensional crossed immunoelectrophoresis on 1 per cent agarose plates in veronal buffer against rabbit anti-human serum (Sebia, France) and rabbit anti-human FIX (Diagnostica Stago) ; SDS-PAGE by the method of Laemmli and Western-blot analysis using A7-mAb (anti-FIX

Light Chain-LC), A1-mAb (anti FIX Activation Peptide-AP) and A2-mAb (anti-FIX Heavy Chain-HC) from Smith and Ono (1984) ; size exclusion HPLC analysis on TSK 3000 SWXL column in Na Phosphate 50 mM, NaCl 390 mM, pH 7 buffer.

Preclinical animal studies
Rabbit stasis thrombosis test was performed using a modified Wessler method (Wessler et al., 1960). FIX was injected in central ear artery in ≤ 1.5 min. Contralateral jugular vein segment was ligatured 15 sec. after FIX injection (pre-stasis) and was isolated 15 min. later (stasis) for observation. The scoring was graded from 0 (no clot or fibrin strand) to 4+ (a full clot). Rabbit non stasis study was performed by infusion of FIX and taking blood samples after one hour intervals during a period of 5 hours. The samples were assayed for platelets, fibrinogen, factor V, factor VIII, antithrombin III and fibrin/fibrinogen degradation products.

Viral validation studies
Virus spiking experiments were performed using HBV (DNA, DNA polymerase and HBs Ag), HIV 1 (TCID 50/ml infectivity and p24 antigen), an enveloped model virus (Sindbis virus) and a non enveloped model virus (avian reovirus).

RESULTS

FIX recovery and purification during the chromatography steps.
On 7 consistency batches, FIX specific activity was 2.9 IU/mg protein at the PCC stage and 146 IU/mg in final product. The average yield from starting cryosupernatant was 91 per cent at the PCC stage and 50 per cent for the final product.

Quality control analysis
Some product characteristics obtained on the 7 above mentioned consistency batches are summarized in Table 1. After reconstitution, the final product contained 57.9 IU FIX/ml without detectable FII, FVII, FX, heparin or antithrombin III. The murine IgG level was extremely low i.e. 3 ng/100 IU FIX. NAPTT was satisfactory (Eur. Pharm.) although a somewhat shortened clotting time at the 1 : 10 dilution was observed. No specific activated factors were detected (FIXa : Ag, FIIa and FXa chromogenic).

Table 1 : Product characteristics of Immunopurified FIX

ASSAY	MEAN ± SD (n = 7)
FIX : C (IU/ml)	57.9 ± 6.1
Total protein (mg/ml)	0.396 ± 0.079
Specific activity (IU FIX : C/mg protein)	146
FIX : C after 24 h at room temperature (%)	98 ± 9 %
FIX : Ag (IU/ml)	56.7 ± 8.0
FIX : Ag / FIX : C ratio	0.98
FII : C (IU / ml)	< 0.01
FVII : C (IU / ml)	< 0.05
FX : C (IU / ml)	< 0.01
NAPTT 1 / 10 (sec)	176 ± 12
1 / 100 (sec)	263 ± 22
Control (sec)	297 ± 16
FIXa (ng / 10 μg FIX)	0
FIIa (m U - NIH / ml)	≤ 2
FXa (m IU / ml)	≤ 1
Heparin (IU / ml)	< 0.025
Antithrombin III (IU / ml)	< 0.05
Murine IgG (ng / 100 IU FIX)	3.0 ± 1.4
TNBP (μg / ml)	< 2.0
Tween 80 (μg / ml)	< 20

Two-dimensional crossed immunoelectrophoresis are shown in Fig. 2 and 3. There was no detectable protein against rabbit anti-human serum. However, a symmetric FIX peak was obtained using rabbit anti-human FIX.
Against rabbit anti-human serum, competitor products showed 1 peak for Heparin FIX, 2 peaks for S-Dextran FIX and more than 10 peaks for PCC. Against rabbit anti-human FIX, a single FIX peak was detected for the three products (data not shown).

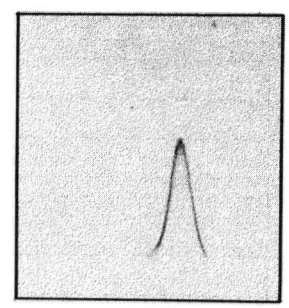

Figure 2 : Immunopurified FIX tested against rabbit anti-human serum

Figure 3. Immunopurified FIX tested against rabbit anti-human FIX

SDS-PAGE and Western-blot analysis are shown in Fig. 4. FIX (71 kDa) corresponds to 85 per cent of the protein on densitometry analysis (either reducing or non-reducing conditions). The five minor bands (15 per cent densitometry) were identified using the 3 specific FIX mAb's and by reference to Lawson & Mann (1991) as : thrombin inactivated FIX (60 kDa), FIX α AP / HC (51 kDa), thrombin inactivated FIX α AP / HC (45 kDa), FIX aβ HC (34 kDa) and FIX aβ (28 kDa). There was no evidence of FIX aβ (activated entire FIX). No significant vitronectin was detected in Western-blot analysis using an anti-vitronectin mAb (Boehring-Mannheim), as opposed to heparin purified FIX (data not shown).

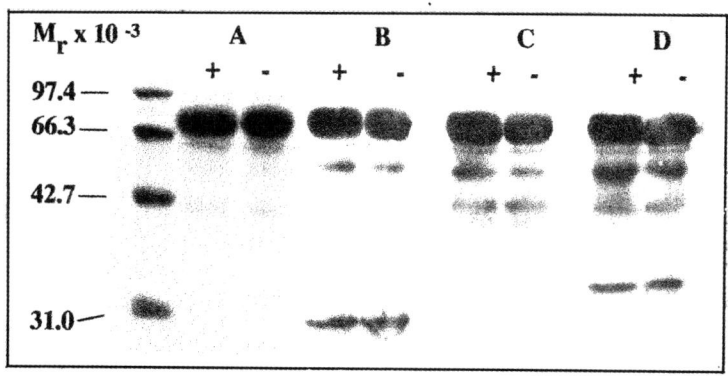

Figure 4 : SDS-PAGE 12 % (reduced +, non-reduced -) of Immunopurified FIX (5 IU FIX) Coomassie blue staining (A), A7-mAb (B), A1-mAb (C), A2-mAb (D).

Size exclusion HPLC analysis is shown in Fig. 5
Not taking into account very low molecular weight peaks, (retention time - RT = 21 - 22 min.) due to stabilizers used, FIX (RT = 15 min.) has a purity of 84 per cent with 16 per cent higher molecular weight components (RT = 10 and 13 min.). With competitor products, purity was 35 per cent for heparin FIX and 69 per cent for S-Dextran FIX (data not shown).

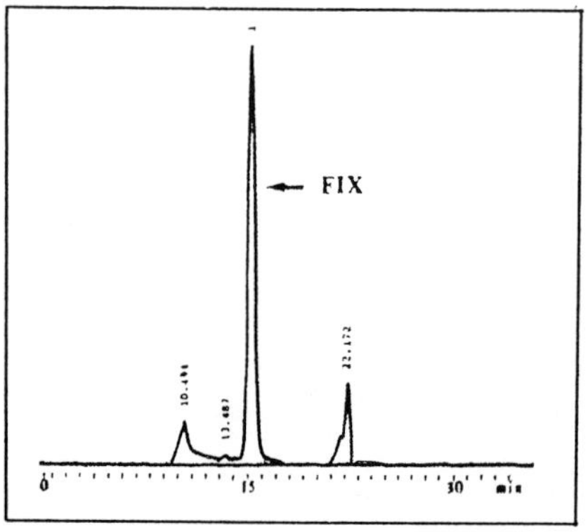

Figure 5 : Size exclusion HPLC analysis of immunopurified FIX. Absorbance at 278 nm is a function of elution time.

Preclinical animal studies

Immunopurified FIX was found not toxic at doses up to 1500 IU/kg, intravenous single injection in mice. No thrombogenicity was demonstrated in the rabbit stasis-thrombosis model at the highest tested dose of 400 IU/kg (3 batches tested with 4 rabbits/batch). No coagulation activation was observed in the rabbit non-stasis model at the dose of 200 IU/kg (2 batches tested with 4 rabbits/batch as compared to 4 rabbits infused with saline-control group). With PCC, at the same dose, clear coagulation activation was observed.

Viral validation of the manufacturing process

As shown in Table 2, beside the SD treatment which is effective on enveloped viruses, the three chromatographic steps, including the immunoaffinity purification, demonstrated a further virus reduction of :

> 4 log 10 for all HBV markers
≥ 8 log 10 HIV 1 infectivity
≥ 5 log 10 avian reovirus infectivity

The SD treatment step was not evaluated in HBV model as it was supposed to have no effect on the markers studied. However, this treatment is well known to inactivate HBV as demonstrated in chimpanzees by the New York Blood Center (Horowitz, 1989). As anticipated, the SD treatment was poorly effective on avian reovirus, a non-enveloped virus.

Table 2 : Virus reduction by key steps of the manufacturing process (log 10 reduction factors)

MANUFACTURING STEPS	ENVELOPED VIRUSES						Non Enveloped Virus
	HBV (plasma from hepatitis B carrier)			HIV 1 (LAV-1-BRU strain)		Sindbis virus (AR 339 - ATCC strain)	Avian Reovirus (Van der Heide strain)
	HBs Ag	DNA polymerase activity	DNA	Infectivity on CEMSS cells	Total p24	Infectivity on MRC 5 cells	Infectivity on Vero cells
First anion-exchange chromatography	> 2.0	> 1.7	0.9	1.5	NT	NT	1.9
Solvent / Detergent treatment	NA	NA	NA	≥ 3.0*	NT	> 3.7**	0.9
Immunoaffinity chromatography	2.0	1.6	2.0	≥ 4.5	2.7	NT	3.4
Second anion-exchange chromatography	0.8	1.3	1.2	≥ 2.1	NT	NT	0
Cumulative loss (log 10)	> 4.8	> 4.6	4.1	≥ 11.1	2.7	> 3.7	6.2

NT : Not Tested
NA : Not Applicable
* : No residual infectivity was found at 30 min.
** : No residual infectivity was found at 1 hour.

DISCUSSION - CONCLUSION

The here described process demonstrated high batch to batch consistency in recovery and FIX quality ; it was found well adaptable to industrial production. The first expected benefit of increased purity of this immunopurified FIX product was reduction of in vivo thrombogenicity in both rabbit tests used. This result could be correlated with the absence of detectable activated factors in the specific assays used for FIXa, FXa and FIIa. Some amydolitic activity towards thrombin-sensitive chromogenic substrate S 2238 was observed with purified human FIXa and FXa : molecular equivalent ratio with respect to FIIa were about 30 : 1 and 180 : 1 for FIXa and FXa, respectively. Therefore, negative testing with S 2238 substrate means absence of these factors, in particular of FIXa which is known as highly thrombogenic (Gitel et al., 1977). The shortened NAPTT test at 1 : 10 dilution was not in accordance with animal thrombogenicity testing ; such result was previously discussed by others (Burnouf et al., 1989 ; Smith, 1992) and renders questionable the use of this test for assaying purified FIX products.

The manufacturing process was shown efficient in inactivating/eliminating HIV 1 and avian reovirus. Apart the SD treatment which was highly efficient on the tested enveloped viruses (HIV 1 and Sindbis virus), the immunopurification step demonstrated a physical elimination capacity for viruses as shown by reduction of avian reovirus infectivity and biochemical markers as HIV1 p24 antigen, HBV DNA and HBsAg.

In conclusion, an immunopurification process was developed for FIX, using the A7-mAb. This monoclonal antibody allows the use of mild elution buffer which helps to produce a high quality FIX, with high yield.

REFERENCES

Addiego, J.E. Gomperts, E. Lin, S.L. Bailey, P. Courter, S.G. Lee, M.L. Neslund, G.G. Kingdom, H.S. & Griffith, M.J. (1992) : Treatment of hemophilia A with a highly purified Factor VIII concentrate prepared by anti-FVIII C immunoaffinity chromatography. *Thromb. Haemost.* 67, 19 - 27.

Burnouf, T. Michalski, C. Goudemand, M. & Huart, J.J. (1989) : Properties of a highly human plasma factor IX : C therapeutic concentrate prepared by conventional chromatography. *Vox Sang.* 57, 225-232.

Clark, D.B. Menaché, D. Gee, D.M. Miekka, S.I. & Drohan, W. (1989) : Coagulation factor IX for replacement therapy in hemophilia B patients. In *Biotechnology of plasma proteins,* ed. Stolz, J.F. & Rivat, C., pp.315-324. Paris : Editions INSERM.

Gitel, S.N. Stephenson, R.C. & Wessler, S. (1977) : *In vitro* and *in vivo* correlation of clotting protease activity : effect of heparin. *Proc. Natl. Acad. Sci. USA* 74, 3028 - 3032.

Gomperts, E.D. De Biasi, R. & De Vreker, R. (1992) : The impact of clotting factors concentrates on the immune system in individuals with hemophilia. *Transf. Med. Rev.* VI, 44-54.

Horowitz, B (1989) : Investigations into the application of tri *(n-butyl)* phosphate / detergent mixtures to blood derivates. *Curr. Stud. Hematol. Blood Transfus.* 56, 83 - 96.

Hrinda, M.E. Huang, C. Tarr, G.C. Wecks, R. Feldmann, F. & Schreiber, A.B. (1991) : Preclinical studies of a monoclonal antibody-purified factor IX, Mononine ^{TM}. *Semin. Hematol.* 28, 6 - 14.

Lawson, J.H. & Mann, K.G. (1991) : Cooperative activation of human factor IX by the human extrinsic pathway of blood coagulation. *J. Biol. Chem.* 266, 11317 - 11327.

Mannuci, P.M., Bauer, K.A. Gringeri, A., Barzegar, S. Bottasso, B. Simoni, L. & Rosenberg, R.D. (1990) : Thrombin generation is not increased in the blood of hemophilia B patients after the infusion of a purified factor IX concentrate. *Blood* 76, 2540 - 2545.

Smith, K.J. & Ono, K. (1984) : Monoclonal antibodies to Factor IX : characterization and use in immunoassays for FIX. *Thromb. Res.* 33, 211 - 224.

Smith, K.J. (1988) : Immunoaffinity purification of factor IX from commercial concentrates and infusion studies in animals. *Blood* 72, 1269 - 1277.

Smith K.J. (1992) : Factor IX concentrates : the new products and their properties. *Transf. Med. Rev.* IV, 124 - 136.

Wessler, S. Reimer, S.M. & Sheps, M.C. (1960) : Biologic assay of a thrombosis-inducing activity in human serum. *J. Appl. Physiol.* 14, 943-946.

Résumé

Un concentré FIX de très haute pureté est produit à partir de 100 à 200 l de plasma par chromatographie d'immunoaffinité sur anticorps monoclonal ion métallique-dépendant A7 (A7-mAb). L'A7-mAb est obtenu à partir de cultures d'hybridomes en biofermenteur et est couplé à du Sepharose^R après purification par 4 étapes chromatographiques incluant un traitement solvant-détergent (SD). Les facteurs vitamine-K dépendants sont isolés du plasma dépourvu de cryoprécipité par une première étape chromatographique d'échange d'anions, puis sont soumis au traitement SD (TNBP/Tween 80). Le FIX est ensuite isolé sur la colonne A7-Sepharose puis élué par un tampon contenant de l'EDTA. Les anticorps relargués par la colonne sont éliminés du FIX par une seconde étape chromatographique d'échange d'anions. Après formulation, le FIX est lyophilisé (en l'absence d'héparine). Le rendement global à ce stade est de 50 per cent. Après reconstitution, la concentration de FIX est de 50 UI/ml avec une activité spécifique voisine de 150 UI/mg. FII, FVII, FX, vitronectine et antithrombine III sont indétectables. La très haute pureté du concentré FIX est confirmée en immunoélectrophorèse bidimensionnelle et en Western-blot. On note cependant une faible quantité de produits de dégradation du FIX (< 20 pour cent en analyse densitométrique - SDS-PAGE) et de composants de haut poids moléculaire (< 20 pour cent en chromatographie HPLC d'exclusion comparés à 65 pour cent pour un FIX purifié par chromatographie d'affinité sur héparine). Aucune trace de thrombine, FIXa ou FXa n'est détectable. Le produit est non thrombogène à 400 UI/kg (test de Wessler modifié) et aucune trace d'activation de la coagulation n'est visible à 200 UI/kg (test de non-stase sur lapin). Le procédé est efficace pour éliminer et/ou inactiver les virus éventuellement présents.

Development and preclinical evaluation of a high-purity factor IX concentrate ('Faktor IX-HPF')

A.H.L. Koenderman, H.G.J. ter Hart, C.T. Hakkennes, E.J. Muller, L. Brands, N. van Duren, H. Hiemstra and J. Over

Department of Product and Process Development, CLB, PO Box 9190, 1006 AD Amsterdam, The Netherlands

SUMMARY:

A single factor IX concentrate ('Faktor IX-HP') was produced using affinity chromatography over Heparin-Sepharose CL6B. Quality control showed the absence of factors II, VII and X and a specific activity of approximately 60 IU factor IX per mg protein. All animal studies (Wessler stasis model, dog and rat model) showed the very low thrombogenic potential of this product as compared to a prothrombin complex concentrate. Preliminary data from the clinical evaluation of this product in hemophilia B patients shows an in vivo recovery and half-life of factor IX similar to those of a prothrombin complex concentrate.

INTRODUCTION:

There are about 300 patients with hemophilia B in the Netherlands. These patients rely for therapy on a prothrombin complex concentrate (PCC) which contains besides coagulation factor IX also the coagulation factors II, VII and X (see Table 1). In the early 70's it became clear that the use of PCC's was associated with very serious side-effects such as DIC (Ménaché et al., 1975). A more recent survey (Lusher, 1991) showed that 72 thrombo-embolic complications were reported in a four year period by 150 physicians treating large numbers of hemophilia B patients.

These unwanted side-effects are probably caused by the presence of activated coagulation factors or by the presence of thrombogenic phospholipids in the product. Furthermore the longer circulation half-life of factors II and X as compared to factor IX could lead to supernormal levels of factors II and X after frequent substitution therapy with PCC. As a consequence surgery in hemophilia B patients is postponed whenever possible due to the thrombo-embolic risk associated with the frequent use of PCC.

The solution for this problem is a single factor IX concentrate, i.e. a product that is characterized by the absence of other (activated) coagulation factors thereby having a very low thrombogenic potential.

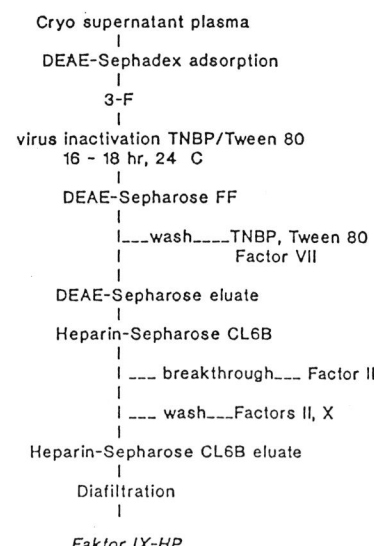

Fig. 1: Schematic production process for 'Faktor IX-HP'

Table 1: Comparison of 'Faktor IX-HP' with 'Protrombinecomplex-SD'

Test	Faktor IX-HP (6 lots 1991) x ± SD	Protrombinecomplex-SD (5 lots 1990) x ± SD
COMPOSITION AND PURITY		
Factor IX (IU/ml)	25.8 ± 5.3	28.5 ± 5.8
Factor VII (IU/1000 IU F IX)	1.3 ± 0.3	365 ± 58
Factor II (IU/1000 IU F IX)	2.3 ± 0.9	931 ±102
Factor X (IU/1000 IU F IX)	0.6 ± 0.6	896 ± 85
Antithrombin III (U/ml)	0.2 ± 0.02	0.13± 0.02
Total protein (g/l)	0.5 ± 0.2	20.3 ± 1.4
Specific activity (IU F IX/mg)	62 ± 26	1.4 ± 0.2
ACTIVATED COAGULATION FACTORS		
NAPTT		
1: 10 dilution (sec)	260 ± 19	220 ± 17
1: 100 dilution (sec)	307 ± 29	254 ± 24
Fibrinogen clotting time		
37 °C	> 6 hr	> 6 hr
room temperature	> 24 hr	> 24 hr

THE CLB SINGLE FACTOR IX CONCENTRATE:

Production process:
For the manufacture of a single factor IX concentrate at the CLB in Amsterdam we have chosen to purify coagulation factor IX by chromatography over Heparin-Sepharose CL6B. The process is based on the work of Burnouf et al. (1989) and was modified on several points to comply with the CLB situation. The manufacturing process is given schematically in Fig 1.

There are four major steps in the manufacturing process. Firstly, factor IX is mass-captured from cryo-depleted plasma by DEAE Sephadex A-50 in a batch-wise fashion. The resulting protein fraction is low in factor VII. Secondly, the factor IX-enriched protein solution is treated with the virucidal chemicals TNBP (0.3%) and Tween 80 (1%) to prevent transmission of viral diseases by the final product. Studies with model viruses showed that the incubation with the virucidal chemicals results in a reduction factor (10 log) of $\geq$ 6.4 for HIV and $\geq$ 7.6 for Pseudorabies virus. Thirdly, the virucidal chemicals are removed by column chromatography over DEAE-Sepharose FF. Trace amounts of factor VII are also removed in this step. Finally, the separation of factor IX from factors II and X is achieved by column chromatography over Heparin-Sepharose CL6B.

Characteristics of 'Faktor IX-HP':
The final product which has been given the provisional name 'Faktor IX-HP' was produced from 250 kg cryo-depleted plasma. Table 1 gives some characteristics of 'Faktor IX-HP' as compared to a classical solvent-detergent-treated PCC ('Protrombinecomplex-SD'). 'Faktor IX-HP' is virtual devoid of coagulation factors II, VII and X (< 5 IU/1000 IU factor IX). The specific activity of the product is about 60 IU factor IX per mg protein based on the Kjeldahl determination. The product contains a small amount of antithrombin III which is added to the final product, but heparin is not added in any stage of the manufacturing process. The results for the global *in vitro* test for activated coagulation factors such as NAPTT and fibrinogen clotting time (FCT) are within the limits specified by the European Pharmacopoeia.

The final product was analysed by means of SDS-polyacrylamide-gel electrophoresis (SDS-PAGE) and immunoblotting using polyclonal and monoclonal antibodies directed against factor IX. SDS-PAGE (under reduced conditions) in combination with immunoblotting did not show the presence of degraded factor IX or activated factor IX in all lots of 'Faktor IX-HP'.

Animal studies to assess the thrombogenic potential of 'Faktor IX-HP':
Figure 2 shows the results of the Wessler (stasis) test in rabbits (Wessler et al., 1959). Injecting PCC into the rabbits results in a measurable thrombogenic response when the dose exceeds 20 - 25 IU factor IX per kg body weight of the rabbit (Wessler score $\geq$ 1). In striking contrast to this, injection of 'Faktor IX-HP' up to 200 - 300 IU factor IX/kg does not induce a thrombogenic response in this animal model.

An alternative for the Wessler test has been developed by MacGregor et al. (1991) which uses a non-stasis model in dogs and measures fibrinopeptide A (fpA) as a very sensitive marker for activation of the coagulation system. Figure 3 shows the response of 'Faktor IX-HP' in this system in comparison with an infusion of a Scottish PCC (low in factor VII) and an albumin infusion. Infusion of albumin results in baseline levels of fpA whereas a PCC infusion results in a rapid rise of fpA during the infusion period. After infusion of 'Faktor IX-HP' (3 lots) in a high dosage there is no significant elevation of the fpA level.

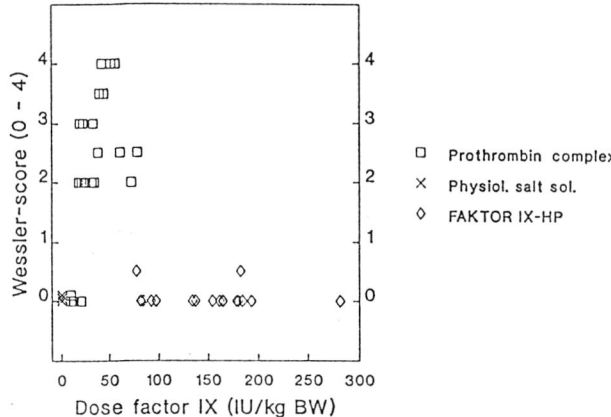

Fig. 2: Thrombogenicity scores of various products as a function of the infused dose (in IU factor IX per kg body weight) in the rabbit stasis model according to Wessler: (x) a physiological salt solution; (□) Prothrombin complex concentrate and (◇) 'Faktor IX-HP'.

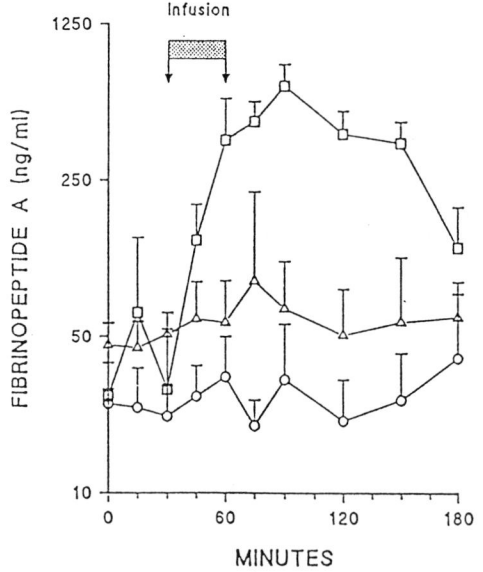

Fig. 3: Plasma fibrinopeptide A after infusion of various plasma products in the dog: (o) albumin solution (250 mg/kg body weight); (□) a Scottish PCC at 120 IU factor IX/kg (low in factor VII) and (△) 'Faktor IX-HP' at 200 IU factor IX/kg; average of 6 transfusions. The shaded box indicates the duration of the infusion.

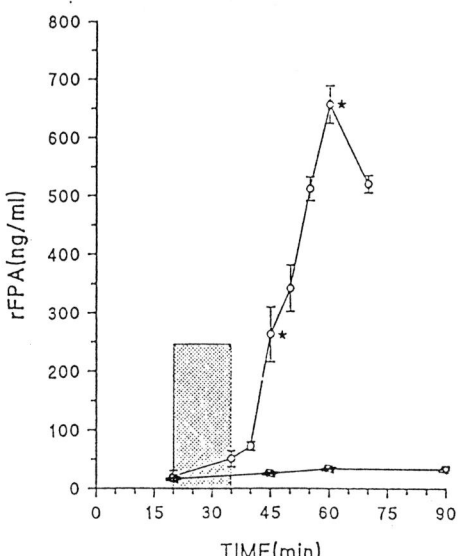

Fig. 4: Plasma rat fibrinopeptide A after infusion of PCC and 'Faktor IX-HP': a Scottish PCC (o, 120 IU/kg) and 'Faktor IX-HP' (▽△, 300 IU/kg). The shaded box indicates the duration of the infusion.

A similar model in rats was developed by McLaughlin et al. (1992). Figure 4 shows that infusion of 'Faktor IX-HP' gives a baseline level of fpA whereas infusion of PCC results in a rise of fpA starting at the end of the infusion period.

Preliminary data of 'Faktor IX-HP' infusions in hemophilia B patients:
The Dutch National Control Authorities gave permission to evaluate 'Faktor IX-HP' in hemophilia B patients. The aim of this study is to assess the clinical tolerance ('well-being', 'allergic' reactions etc.) and pharmacokinetics of factor IX (in vivo recovery, half-life).

In cooperation with the Van Creveld Clinic (Bilthoven, dr. Mauser-Bunschoten) and the Academic Medical Center (Amsterdam, dr. Koopman) six non bleeding hemophilia B patients where infused with 'Faktor IX-HP' using a dosage regime that ranged from 10 to 80 IU factor IX per kg body weight. More patients are still enrolled in this study.

The product was well tolerated by the patients and no adverse effects were observed in the post-transfusion period. The pharmacokinetics of factor IX after infusion of 'Faktor IX-HP' are given in Table 2. The half-life and model-independent pharmacokinetic parameters are similar to those of factor IX from PCC.

CONCLUSIONS:

Conventional chromatography using Heparin-Sepharose CL6B can be used to manufacture a high-purity factor IX concentrate. This single factor IX concentrate is far less thrombogenic than the classical PCC. Pharmacokinetics of factor IX from 'Faktor IX-HP' are similar to those of factor IX derived from 'Protrombinecomplex-SD'

Table 2: Pharmacokinetics of 'Faktor IX-HP' in comparison with 'Protrombinecomplex-SD'

	Faktor IX-HP	Protrombinecomplex-SD
Date of clinical evaluation	ongoing	1988
Number of patients	6	13
In vivo recovery (%) <*>	45 ± 8	38 ± 6
In vivo response (rise [U/ml] per IU/kg BW)	0.011 ± 0.001	0.007 ± 0.002
Half-life factor IX <**>		
Number of patients	3	5
Mono/biphasic decay	0/3	0/5
Distribution half-life (hr)	1.7 ± 1.4	1.7 ± 1.5
Elimination half-life (hr)	19.8 ± 3.6	22.1 ± 2.0
Model-independent pharmacokinetics <**>		
Number of patients	3	5
Mean residence time (hr)	28.3 ± 4.0	31.6 ± 2.7
Clearance (ml/hr/kg)	4.6 ± 0.4	5.2 ± 1.6
Apparent distribution volume (ml/kg)	129 ± 9	171 ± 59

<*> Plasma volume of patient is estimated based on the assumption of a blood volume of 80 ml per kg body weight and on the measured hematocrit.
<**> Calculated using computation method of Messori et al. (1987).

LITERATURE:

Burnouf, T., Michalski, C., Goudemand, M. and Huart, J.J. (1989): Properties of a highly purified human plasma factor IX:C therapeutic concentrate prepared by conventional chromatography Vox Sang. 57: 225 - 232

Lusher, J.M. (1991): Thrombogenicity associated with factor IX complex concentrates. Sem. Hematol. 28 (Suppl. 6): 3 - 5

Ménaché, D., and Roberts, H.R. (1975): Summary report and recommendations of the Task Force members and consultants. Thrombos. Diathes. Haemorrh. 33: 645 - 647

Messori, A., Longo, G., Matucci, M., Morfini, M. and Ferrini, P.L.R. (1987): Clinical pharmacokinetics of factor VIII in patients with classical haemophilia. Clin. Pharmacokin. 13: 365 - 380

MacGregor, I.R., Ferguson, J.M., McLaughlin, L.F., Burnouf, T,. and Prowse, C.V. (1991): Comparison of high purity factor IX concentrates and a prothrombin complex concentrate in a canine model of thrombogenicity. Thromb. Haemost. 66: 609 - 613

McLaughlin, L.F., Drummond, O, and MacGregor, I.R. (1992): A novel rat model of thrombogenicity: its use in evaluation of prothrombin complex concentrates and high purity factor IX concentrates. Thromb. Haemost. 68: 511 - 515

Wessler, S., Reimer, S.M., and Sheps, M.C. (1959): Biologic assay of a thrombosis-inducing activity in human serum. J. Appl. Physiol. 14: 943 - 946

Limitations of *in vitro* thrombogenicity tests applied to high purity factor IX concentrates

I. MacGregor, L. McLaughlin, O. Drummond, J. Ferguson* and C. Prowse

Scottish National Blood Transfusion Service, National Science Laboratory, 2 Forrest Road, Edinburgh, EH1 2QN and *Wellcome Surgical Institute, University of Glasgow, Glasgow, United Kingdom

The non-activated partial thromboplastin time (NAPTT) and the fibrinogen clotting time (FCT) have been used for a number of years as in vitro thrombogenicity assays to determine suitability of batch release for prothrombin complex concentrates (PCC). These assays are now being applied to high purity factor IX concentrates (HP-FIX) but the in vivo studies described here indicate that there are limitations to their usefulness with such products.

We procured a selection of HP-FIX concentrates from 7 manufacturers who used a range of chromatographic methods. These included ion-exchange, affinity, immunoaffinity and metal-chelate chromatography steps. Some of the HP-FIX products passed current EP limits for NAPTT and FCT while some did not as shown for 3 concentrates in Table 1.

TABLE 1

COMPARISON OF HP-FIX PRODUCTS CONTAINING NO HEPARIN OR ATIII:IN VITRO ASSAYS

PRODUCT	NAPTT* at 1/10(s)	FCT 6hr 37°C	FCT 24hr room temp
A	310	PASS	PASS
B	124	PASS	FAIL
C	86	FAIL	FAIL

*NAPTT should be >150s to pass current EP

The concentrates were evaluated in canine and rat non-stasis models of thrombogenicity (MacGregor et al 1991, McLaughlin et al 1992) and some were also tested in a rabbit Wessler stasis model. The results of these in vivo studies were then compared with the known in vitro characteristics of the concentrates in the thrombogenicity assays mentioned above.

The canine model detected significantly increased levels of fibrinopeptide A (FPA), a marker of thrombin activity, after doses of only 50IU/kg of a typical PCC. These elevated levels of FPA reached a peak at 30 minutes after the end of a 30 minute infusion of PCC, indicating that the cause was not traces of thrombin in the product, but generation of thrombin via activation of the coagulation system. In contrast none of the HP-FIX products tested promoted FPA generation after 200IU/kg, see Table 2.

TABLE 2

COMPARISON OF HP-FIX PRODUCTS CONTAINING NO HEPARIN OR ATIII: IN VIVO STUDIES

PRODUCT	NON-STASIS MODELS		STASIS MODEL
	CANINE	RAT	RABBIT WESSLER*
	total FPA generated (ug/ml) after		
	200IU/kg	300IU/kg	Score
A	460	200	0 at 200 IU/kg
B	830	N.D	ED_{50} = 105 IU/kg
C	1420	230	0 at 200 IU/kg
Albumin	710	220	N.D
Typical PCC	17170 (at 150 IU/kg)	3600	2-4 at 50 IU/kg

*Scored as 0 = no thrombus to 4 = full cast thrombus, or as ED_{50} = dose at which thrombi are formed in 50% of the jugular veins observed.

An HP-FIX batch that had very shortened NAPTT and FCT, failing current EP limits, did not elevate FPA in the canine or rat model, nor did it promote thrombus formation in the Wessler model. (Product C, Tables 1 and 2).

In contrast, another batch with shortened NAPTT and FCT did cause thrombus formation in the Wessler stasis model but not in the canine or rat non-stasis models, (Batch 4 Table 3).

TABLE 3

HP-FIX MAY BE THROMBOGENIC IN WESSLER MODEL BUT NOT IN NON-STASIS MODEL.

	NAPTT	FCT		WESSLER STASIS ED_{50} (IU/kg)	CANINE NON-STASIS total FPA generated after 200 IU/kg
		6hr	24hr		
Batches 1 & 2 (Contain heparin)	600	PASS	PASS	>420	750
Batch 3	124	PASS	FAIL	105	830
Batch 4	111	FAIL	FAIL	20	730
Albumin	-	-	-	N.D	710
PCC	177	PASS	PASS	17	17,170

It is likely that low levels of activated clotting factors, which can influence the in vitro assay are less effective in vivo. In the non-stasis models, traces of activated clotting factors may be rapidly inhibited or cleared before causing further activation. Since PCCs with similarly shortened NAPTT/FCT cause marked in vivo activation in the same model, we infer that other components in such products potentiate their thrombogenicity in vivo. We therefore conclude that the current in vitro thrombogenicity assays, or their limits, may be inappropriate for HP-FIX products.

REFERENCES

MacGregor, I.R., Ferguson, J.M., McLaughlin, L.F., Burnouf T, and Prowse C.V. (1991) Comparison of high purity factor IX concentrates and a prothrombin complex concentrate in a canine model of thrombogenicity. Thromb. and Haemostas. 66: 609-613

McLaughlin, L.F., Drummond, O. and MacGregor, I.R. A novel rat model of thrombogenicity: its use in evaluation of prothrombin complex concentrates and high purity factor IX concentrates. Thromb. and Haemostas. (In Press).

Five years of experience in the production and quality control of a highly purified factor IX concentrate

C. Michalski, T. Burnouf and J.J. Huart

Centre Régional de Transfusion Sanguine, 21, rue Camille Guérin, BP 2018, 59012 Lille, France

ABSTRACT

A standardized high-purity factor IX (HP-F IX) concentrate developed for the substitution therapy of hemophilia B was made available for clinical use about five years ago. This concentrate is obtained using a combination of three conventional chromatographic steps based on DEAE chromatography and adsorption on immobilized heparin. Recovery was 30-35 % from 3,000 l of cryo-poor plasma. Enhancement in viral safety, as demonstrated by validation procedures, is achieved through a specific treatment by solvent-detergent as well as through chromatographic purification. Overall clearance factors for these steps were higher than 10 logs for lipid-enveloped model viruses including HIV-1 and 6.3 logs for SV 40, a non-enveloped model virus.
Results obtained on 30 consecutive lots, corresponding to about 27 million units of F IX, are presented.
The product has a specific activity $\geq$ 80 IU F IX/mg, and is essentially free of F VII, F X and F II (less than 0,3 %, relative to F IX). Activated factors were below the detection limits. The product has a significantly lower risk of thromboembolic complications than PCC, as demonstrated "in vivo" by injection of high doses of the product in stasis and non-stasis animal models. The Wessler test as performed at CRTS-Lille is routinely > 500 IU/kg. Infusions in dogs or rats at 200 and 300 IU/kg in the presence of heparin or not, did not induce any rise in FPA. Infusions in human patients at 50 or 100 IU/kg did not reveal any sign of activation of the coagulation cascade as measured by activation peptides. So far, more than 70 million units of this product have been used in hemophilia B substitution therapy, including during major surgery, with good efficacy and safety records.

INTRODUCTION

Hemophilia B patients have long been treated by prothrombin complex concentrates (PCC). However, it soon became apparent that two major risks were associated with PCC therapy (SMITH, 1992 ; LUSHER, 1991 ; BLOOM, 1991) : thrombotic complications possibly due to an overload of factors II and X or presence of activated factors, and the transmission of viral diseases (hepatitis or AIDS) partly explained by the low purification factor from plasma.
In order to avoid these complications, a high-purity factor IX (HP - F IX) concentrate, free of other clotting factors and virus-inactivated by solvent-detergent (SD) treatment, was developed at CRTS-Lille (MICHALSKI et al, 1988 ; BURNOUF et al, 1989). Our experience in the large-scale production and quality control of this product is presented here.

MATERIAL AND METHODS

Preparation of HP - factor IX

The HP - F IX concentrate was purified from 3000 liters of cryo-poor plasma using a three-step chromatographic procedure as described by BURNOUF et al (1989). Briefly, the plasma material was adsorbed on DEAE-sephadex A-50 and a fraction containing the prothrombin complex was eluted.
After treatment with 0.3 % TnBP and 1 % Tween-80 at 25° C for > 6 hours, the mixture was applied on a DEAE-sepharose CL6B FF column to remove TnBP/Tween-80 and clotting F VII by washing the column with the buffer. The resulting F IX eluate was injected on heparin-sepharose CL6B to eliminate the remaining clotting factors II and X and to further purify F IX. After formulation, the F IX concentrate was sterile-filtered, dispensed into 10- or 20- ml vials and lyophilized.

Viral assays

The extent of virus inactivation/elimination during the manufacturing procedure was studied at the Pasteur Institute in Paris following the recommendations from the Biotechnology/Pharmacy working party (CPMP Guidelines, 1991). The viruses studied were human immunodeficiency virus, type 1 (HIV-1) and 4 model viruses : vesicular stomatitis virus (VSV), Sindbis virus, porcine pseudorabies virus and simian virus 40 (SV 40). Infectivity tests were performed following established virological cell culture techniques. The reduction factor in infectivity was expressed in $\log_{10}$. Each step was studied at the laboratory scale under conditions mimicking as closely as possible those used at the production scale.

Coagulation factor assays

Factor IX activity was measured by a one-stage assay using F IX-deficient plasma after predilution of the concentrate in $BaSO_4$-adsorbed cryo-poor plasma. Factor II and X activities were measured using the corresponding deficient plasmas and rabbit thromboplastin. Results were expressed in International Units (IU) given by the first international standard for blood coagulation factor II, IX and X concentrate coded 84/681 (BARROWCLIFFE, 1988). Factor VII activity was measured using F VII-deficient plasma and thromboplastin from bovine (VIIb) or human (VIIc) sources obtained from Stago and Behring, respectively. The F VIIc reference was the first international plasma standard coded 84/665 (BARROWCLIFFE, 1988). NAPTT was determined according to European pharmacopeia (EP).

Activated coagulation factor assays were carried out after complete neutralization of heparin.
Factor IXa, Factor Xa and thrombin were measured on chromogenic substrates S2765 (Biogenic-France), CBS 31:39 and chromo-thrombin (Stago), respectively. F IXa units corresponded to F IX fully activated by F XIa. F Xa units were obtained after activation of normal plasma by Russel viper's venom. Thrombin activity was obtained in nkat/ml. Assuming that whole activity in the samples was due to α-thrombin, results were expressed in NIH units given by the NIH thrombin standard lot J, using the relation 1U NIH = 2000 nkat. F VIIa was evaluated by the ratio of F VIIb to VIIc.
Overall proteolytic activity was measured on the chromogenic substrate S 2288 (Biogenic-France). Results were expressed in variation of absorbance per minute : $\Delta A/mn$.

Protein determination

Protein content was measured as described elsewhere (BURNOUF et al, 1989) using a modified Bradford method and bovine serum albumin as a reference.

Animal models

Rabbit stasis studies were carried out using a modified Wessler method as described elsewhere (MICHALSKI et al, 1988). Results were expressed by the determination of ED 50 : the dose of F IX : c per kg (IU/kg) producing fibrin strands or clots regardless of size in 50 % of the jugular veins tested.
Routinely heparinized F IX concentrates were tested before and after neutralization of heparin.
Dog and rat non-stasis studies were carried out as described in Mac GREGOR et al (1991) and Mc LAUGHLIN et al (1992).

RESULTS

"In vitro" characteristics of the last 30 consecutive lots corresponding to about 27 million units of F IX are given in table 1.

Table 1 : Purity of HP- F IX : comparison to PCC (mean ± SD)

	HP - F IX (n = 30)	PCC (n = 17)
F IX : c IU/ml	50.9 ± 3.4	29.3 ± 8.1
F IX : c specific activity IU/mg	126 ± 32	1.1 ± 0.2
F II : c IU/ml	< 0.10	47.3 ± 10.9
F X : c IU/ml	< 0.15	50.2 ± 8.8
F VII : c IU/ml	< 0.10	17.7 ± 4.7
Added heparin U/ml	5	5
NAPTR 1/10	0.75 ± 0.10	0.78 ± 0.14
1/100	0.96 ± 0.07	1.00 ± 0.05

In contrast to PCC, HP - F IX was essentially free of F II, X and VII. With a mean specific activity of 126 IU F IX/mg, its purity was about 100 - fold that of PCC. NAPTR were similar for both products.

In vitro markers of activation
Potential thrombogenicity of HP - F IX was evaluated in vitro by testing additional activation markers in 10 lots of F IX : see table 2.
Results were compared with those obtained from commercially available conventional and activated PCCs.

Table 2 : "In vitro" markers of activation

ACTIVITY FOR 100 IU F IX	HP - F IX (n = 10)	PCC (n = 3)	FEIBA (n = 2)	AUTOPLEX (n = 2)
F IXa u	< 0.055	0.538 ± 0.106	1.167	15.46
Amidolytic thrombin UNIH	< 0.050	0.290 ± 0.031	0.799	0.894
F Xa u	< 0.04	< 0.04	< 0.04	0.04
S 2288 activity mΔA/mn	< 0.010	0.071 ± 0.043	0.096	0.343
F VIIb/F VIIc	-	10 ± 2.7	13.1	16.0

F IXa, thrombin, F Xa, proteolytic activity and F VIIa were under detection limits in HP-F IX, whereas low amounts of these activities were found in PCC and significantly higher amounts in activated PCC. These results argued strongly in favour of a reduced thrombogenicity of the HP-F IX.

Rabbit stasis thrombogenicity studies
To evaluate the potential thrombogenicity of HP - F IX, further experiments were carried out "in vivo" in the rabbit stasis model. Results from the last 30 consecutive lots are given in table 3.

Table 3 : Rabbit stasis thrombogenicity studies

ED 50 IU F IX/kg	HP - F IX (n = 30)	PCC (n = 3)	FEIBA (n = 2)	AUTOPLEX (n = 2)
Final product	> 500	40-80	15-20	3-6
After heparin neutralization	> 100	5-20	-	-

No clots have ever been observed after infusion of HP - F IX even at the highest dose of 500 IU F IX/kg, showing absence of thrombogenicity in this model. This was not the case for commercially available PCCs containing the same amount of heparin.
Also, after neutralization of heparin, HP - F IX was found to be much less thrombogenic than PCC as indicated by the ED 50 which was routinely greater than 100 IU/kg. This was in accordance with results obtained before addition of heparin.
It must be stressed that, due to the lack of standardization for this model, it is difficult to compare results between laboratories. Only intralaboratory data can be compared.

Dog and rat non-stasis thrombogenicity studies

In order to evaluate any potential delayed thrombogenicity not seen in the Wessler model, HP - F IX was tested in two non-stasis animal models : in dogs (MAC GREGOR et al, 1991) and in rats (Mc LAUGHLIN et al, submitted). Different batches of CRTS HP - F IX were studied, including experimental ones in which no heparin had been added. Results indicated that all were non thrombogenic in both models (table 4).

In the dog non-stasis model, platelet count, fibrinogen levels, activated partial thromboplastin time, fibrinogen degradation products and fibrinopeptide A (FpA) were similar to the albumin control after infusion of 200 IU/kg of HP - F IX, whereas these parameters were significantly changed after infusion of 60 to 180 IU/kg of PCC. Results were the same for samples with and without heparin. Similarly, in the rat non-stasis model, fibrin monomer and FpA were unchanged after 300 IU/kg of HP - F IX, whereas they were significantly increased after 100 to 300 IU/kg of PCC. See table 4 and for FpA levels fig. 1.

Table 4 : Dog and rat non-stasis thrombogenicity studies (Mc GREGOR et al, 1991 ; MC LAUGHLIN et al, submitted)

MODELS	HP - F IX (n = 3)	PCC (n = 3)
Dog non-stasis Platelet count, Fbg, APTT, FDP, FpA	similar to albumin control at 200 IU/kg	＼platelet count, Fbg ／APTT, FDP, FpA at 60 to 180 IU/kg
Rat non-stasis Fibrin monomer FpA	similar to albumin control at 300 IU/kg	／fibrin monomer, FpA at 100 to 300 IU/kg

APTT : activated partial thromboplastin time, FDP : fibrinogen degradation product, FpA : fibrinopeptide A, Fbg : fibrinogen.

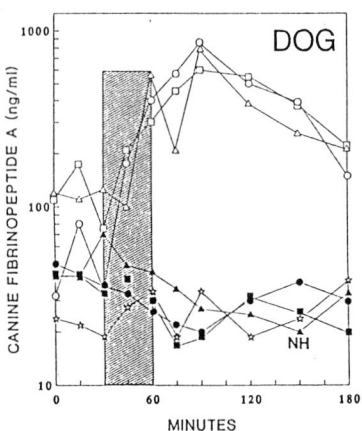
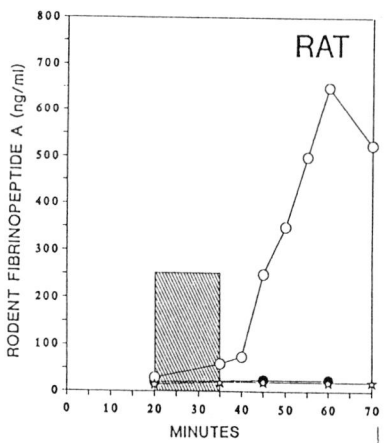

Fig. 1 : Plasma FpA after infusion of HP- F IX or PCC. DOG : ○,□,△ PCC 120 IU/kg ; ●,■,▲ HP-F IX 200 IU/kg ; RAT : ○ PCC 300 IU/kg, ● HP- F IX 300 IU/kg. ✯albumin 250 mg/kg.   NH : non heparinized

Moreover, when tested in the Harbauer model in rabbits, no acute side effects on cardiac function, circulation or respiration were observed at the dose of 100 IU/kg (KOTITSCHKE et al, 1992).

Preclinical study
Reduced thrombogenicity was also observed in a preclinical study in which highly sensitive activation markers were measured (MANNUCCI et al, 1991). These included peptides that are released from zymogens during coagulation : F X activation peptide (F X P), prothrombin fragment 1 + 2 (F1+2), FpA. Also, other haemostasis parameters were measured including platelet count, fibrinogen, antithrombin III and D-dimer.
14 hemophilia B patients were infused with CRTS HP - F IX at a dose of 50 IU/kg or 100 IU/kg. No change in any of these parameters was observed, indicating no activation of the common pathway of the coagulation cascade, even at the highest dose infused.
This was not the case after PCC infusions at 50 IU/kg that induced significant changes in F1 + 2 and in FXP.

Viral safety
The viral safety of HP - F IX was based upon specific virus inactivation treatment with SD as well as upon virus elimination by 3 chromatographic steps conducted under different physico-chemical conditions. Results from validation studies are given in table 5.

Table 5. Clearance factors (log10) of viruses during SD treatment and chromatographic steps.

VIRUSES	SD TREATMENT	DEAE Sephadex A-50	DEAE Sepharose CL6B "FF"	HEPARIN- Sepharose CL6B	TOTAL
HIV 1	> 4.40	2.24	3.10	2	> 11.74
VSV	> 6.16	2.14	1.89	1.92	> 12.11
Pseudorabies	> 3.93	3.37	2.84	5.51	> 15.65
Sindbis	> 4.80	not determined	not determined	not determined	-
SV 40	< 1	1.68	2.21	2.45	6.34

The association of SD treatment with the 3 chromatographic steps gave a total clearance factor higher than 10 logs for lipid-enveloped viruses and 6.3 logs for SV 40, a non-enveloped virus highly resistant to physico-chemical treatments.
An additional filtration step on a 35 nm filter is now being introduced at the industrial scale and has been shown to contribute to the removal of 4 to 6 logs of viruses, including HIV-1 (unpublished), thus further enhancing the viral safety of the product.

Clinical experience
HP - F IX was introduced in France in 1986. Since then, more than 70 million units have been infused in Europe with good efficacy and safety (BARDIN & SULTAN, 1990 ; VERROUST et al, 1992 ; GOUDEMAND et al, 1992).

CONCLUSION

This high-purity factor IX concentrate is a standardized product free of other clotting factors. It carries a much reduced thrombogenic risk compared to PCC and a higher viral safety achieved by the combination of a specific SD treatment and chromatographic eliminations. The lower thrombogenic potential may be explained by the absence of clotting factors II, X and VII as well as the highly reduced content in activated coagulation factors. Five years of clinical experience have confirmed the good tolerance, hemostatic efficacy, and overall safety in hemophilia B substitution therapy.

AKNOWLEDGMENT

The authors thank Dr PROWSE and co-workers at Edinburgh SNBTS for carrying out the dog and rat non-stasis models as well as our colleagues from Lille-CRTS : Dr P. APPOURCHAUX for performing the virus studies, and Mr P. DUVAL for excellent assistance in carrying out the Wessler test. We thank Pr M. GOUDEMAND for his continual interest during the course of this work. Thanks are also due to Mrs G. KACZMAREK for typing the manuscript.

REFERENCES

Bardin, J.M. and Sultan, Y. (1990) : F IX concentrate versus prothrombin complex concentrate for the treatment of hemophilia B during surgery. Transfusion., 30 : 441-443.

Barrowcliffe, T.W. (1988) : Standardization of factors II, VII, IX and X in plasma and concentrates. Report of the ICTH subcommittee on factors VIII and IX, Brussels, July 1987. Thromb. Haemost., 59 : 334.

Bloom, A.L. (1991) : Progress in the clinical management of haemophilia. Thromb. Haemost., 66 : 166-177.

Burnouf, T., Michalski, C., Goudemand, M. and Huart, J.J. (1989) : Properties of a highly purified human plasma factor IX:c therapeutic concentrate prepared by conventional chromatography. Vox sang. 57 : 225-232.

CPMP, Guidelines : Ad hoc working party of biotechnology/pharmacy. Note for guidance "validation of virus removal and inactivation procedures" (III/8115/89-EN), Feb 11-13, 1991.

Goudemand, J., Marey, A., Chiche R., Mizon, P. and Wibaut, B. (1992) : Clinical efficacy of a highly-purified factor IX concentrate (abstract) XX International Congress of the world federation of hemophilia-Athens-Greece-October 12-17, n° 178.

Kotitschke, P., Harbauer, F. and Morfeld, F. (1992) : Purified F IX and F IX complex products : parameters influencing thrombogenic potential. VII kongreβ für Thrombose-und Hämostaseforschung-Heidelberg 9-12 February.

Lusher, J.M. (1991) : Thrombogenicity associated with factor IX complex concentrates. Sem in hemat. 28 : suppl 6, 3-5.

Macgregor, I.R., Ferguson, J.M., Mclaughlin, L.F., Burnouf, T. and Prowse, C.V. (1991) : Comparison of high purity factor IX concentrates and a prothrombin complex concentrate in a canine model of thrombogenicity. Throm. haemost, 66 : 609-613.

Mclaughlin, L.F., Drummond, O. and Macgregor, I.R. (Submitted) : A novel rat model of thrombogenicity its use in evaluation of prothrombin complex concentrates and high purity factor IX concentrates.

Mannucci, P.M., Bauer, K.A., Gringeri, A., Barzegar, S., Santagostino, E., Tradati, F.C. and Rosenberg, R.D (1991) : No activation of the common pathway of the coagulation cascade after a highly purified factor IX concentrate. Br. J. haematol, 79 : 606-611.

Michalski, C., Bal, F., Burnouf, T. and Goudemand, M. (1988) : Large-scale production and properties of a solvent-detergent-treated factor IX concentrate from human plasma. Vox Sang. 55 : 202-210.

Smith, K.J. (1992) : Factor IX concentrates : the new products and their properties. Transf. Med. Rev ; VI : 124-136.

Verroust, F., Ferrer Le Coeur, F., Laurian, Y., Fressinaud, E., Sultan, Y., Gazengel, C. (1992) : Multicentric comparative review of french F IX concentrates in hemophiliacs B during surgery (abstract). XX International Congress of the world federation of hemophilia - Athens - Greece - October 12-17, n° 52.

Résumé

Un concentré de F IX haute pureté (F IX-HP) a été développé il y a environ 5 ans au CRTS de Lille, pour le traitement substitutif de l'hémophilie B. Le facteur IX est purifié à partir de 3000 litres de surnageant de cryoprécipité par l'association de 2 chromatographies d'échanges d'ions et d'une chromatographie sur héparine-sépharose. Le rendement en F IX est de 30 à 35 %. La sécurité virale du produit s'appuie sur un traitement spécifique d'inactivation par solvent-détergent ainsi que sur la capacité du procédé de purification à éliminer les agents pathogènes. Sur plusieurs étapes de production, la diminution totale du niveau d'infectiosité a été supérieure à 10 logs vis à vis de virus enveloppés. Elle a été de 6 logs vis à vis du SV 40, un virus non enveloppé.

Les résultats obtenus sur 30 lots consécutifs, correpondant à environ 27 millions d'unités de F IX sont présentés : l'activité spécifique du F IX y est supérieure à 80 UI/mg. Le concentré contient moins de 0.3 % de F VII, F X ou F II par rapport au F IX. Les taux de facteurs activés sont inférieurs aux limites de détection. Les études de thrombogénicité "in vivo" dans différents modèles animaux avec ou sans stase veineuse, ont montré que le potentiel thrombogénique du F IX HP était fortement réduit par rapport à celui des PPSB. Le test de Wessler tel qu'il est réalisé en routine au CRTS de Lille donne des valeurs de 50 > 500 UI F IX/kg. L'injection de F IX HP chez le chien ou le rat n'augmente pas le taux de FpA plasmatique à des doses de 200 et 300 UI F IX/kg respectivement, en présence ou non d'héparine. La mesure des peptides d'activation après injection chez l'homme à des doses de 50 et 100 UI F IX/kg indique qu'il n'y a pas d'activation du système de coagulation. A ce jour, plus de 70 millions d'unités de ce produit ont été utilisés dans le traitement substitutif de l'hémophilie B, incluant des chirurgies majeures, avec de bons résultats d'efficacité et de sécurité.

Preparation by immunoaffinity chromatography of therapeutic human protein C concentrates

V. Regnault[1], C. Geschier[1,2], M.-E. Briquel[2], C. Rivat[1], P. Alexandre[2] and J.-F. Stoltz[1,2]

[1]INSERM and [2]CRTS, Plateau de Brabois, 54500 Vandœuvre-lès-Nancy, France

ABSTRACT

An immunoaffinity purification method using a monoclonal antibody to human protein C has been optimized for the preparation of therapeutic concentrates. The final degree of purification was 25,000 with a chromatographic recovery of about 80 %. The preparation of highly purified protein C has brought to light the importance of the methodological variables on the evaluation of the molecule. An enzyme immunoassay was developed to quantify protein C antigen and protein C activity was determined by a chromogenic assay. The specific anticoagulant activity of purified protein C was of about 300 U/mg. Sensitive enzyme immunoassays have been developed to measure bovine IgG and protein A levels in antibody preparations and to monitor murine IgG, bovine IgG and protein A leaching from the immunoadsorbent.

INTRODUCTION

Human plasma protein C (PC) which is the precursor of a vitamin K-dependent serine protease, activated protein C (Stenflo, 1976), plays an important role as a naturally occuring anticoagulant protein (Walker et al., 1979; Marlar et al., 1982; Esmon, 1983; Clouse et al., 1986). The physiological relevance of PC in the regulation of blood coagulation derives from the description of recurrent thrombosis associated with hereditary PC deficiency (Griffin et al., 1981; Seligsohn et al., 1984). Thromboembolic complications of PC deficiency may be controlled with PC or activated protein C (APC) replacement therapy. Experiments on the anticoagulating efficacy of purified PC with limited human subjects have shown promising results as one of the most potent therapeutic proteins (Okajima et al., 1990; Dreyfus et al., 1991). The similar physicochemical properties of vitamin K-dependent proteins, the low concentration of PC in normal plasma (about 4 µgml^{-1}), the long time and poor recoveries of a combination of conventional biochemical methods have led to the development of affinity purification procedures (Nakamura et al., 1987; Esmon et al., 1987; Hendl et al., 1991). However, the methods previously reported have used Ca^{2+}-dependent monoclonal antibodies which either crossreact with other plasma proteins or required a barium citrate adsorption as a first step. An immunoaffinity purification method using a monoclonal antibody to human PC (Regnault et al., 1991a) was developed and in an attempt to avoid interference with the recovery of factor VIII or with the classical plasma fractionation, PC was isolated from a prothrombin complex concentrate. The preparation of immunopurified PC has pointed out the problem of PC evaluation in high purity concentrates. Important factors influencing PC antigen and/or activity levels are discussed. With respect to affinity purification techniques, an important safety control concerns the leakage of the ligand. Known contaminants of the antibody solution used for the preparation of the immunoadsorbent as well as the ligand leakage were investigated by means of sensitive enzyme immunoassays.

MATERIALS AND METHODS

Anti-protein C antibody production and purification : A monoclonal mouse antibody (12H8) that reacts with an epitope on the heavy chain of PC (Regnault et al., 1991a) was obtained following widely used procedures. Hybridoma cells were cultured in RPMI 1640 medium (ATGC, France) supplemented with 2 M (v/v) Ultroser HY (Sepracor-IBF, France), 20 mM HEPES buffer, 1 mM sodium pyruvate, 2 g/l glucose, 0.5 % heat-inactivated foetal bovine serum (Institut J. Boy, France) and antibiotics (0.1 g/l streptomycin, 100 000 U/l penicillin). Cell culture supernatants were harvested, the antibodies were concentrated by precipitation with PEG and purified by protein A chromatography. The antibody concentration was measured spectrophotometrically at 280 nm using $A_{1cm}^{1\%} = 14$.

Preparation of the immunoadsorbent : The 12H8 antibody was coupled to Sepharose CL-4B (Pharmacia, Sweden) according to Cuatrecasas et al. (1968). A volume of a 10 % solution of CNBr in distilled water was added to an identical volume of packed Sepharose and the pH was maintained at 11.0 using 10 N NaOH. After extensive washings with distilled water and a 0.1 M sodium bicarbonate, 0.5 M NaCl buffer, pH 8.5, the antibody solution in the same buffer was added to the activated Sepharose and the mixture was left overnight at 4°C under gentle stirring. The immunoadsorbent was then successively washed with the sodium bicarbonate buffer, with 1 M ethanolamine, pH 8.0 for 2 h, with 3 M NaSCN, $NaCH_3COO$, pH 6.0 and finally with 0.05 M Tris-HCl, 0.15 M NaCl, pH 7.4 (buffer A). The immunoadsorbent was stored at 4°C either in buffer A containing 0.02 % NaN_3 or in a 20 % ethanol aqueous solution.

Immunopurification of human plasma protein C : The prothrombin complex concentrate which has undergone viral inactivation using a solvent-detergent solution (Edwards et al., 1987) was applied to the immunoadsorbent equilibrated in buffer A. PC was desorbed with 0.1 M triethanolamine, 1 M NaCl, pH 10.5, concentrated by ultrafiltration using a membrane with a 10,000 MW cut-off and dialysed against 0.15 M NaCl, 0.01 M sodium phosphate buffer, pH 7.2.

Protein C antigen assay : Microtiter plates (Costar) were coated with 100 µl of a 2.5 µg/ml solution of an anti-PC antibody (the C12C5 antibody, Regnault et al., 1991) in 50 mM sodium carbonate, pH 9.6 (coating buffer) at 4°C overnight. All washes were done with 130 mM NaCl, 5 mM Na_2HPO_4 and 1 mM KH_2PO_4, pH 7.2 containing 0.05 % Tween 20 (PBS-Tween). The plates were blocked with 125 µl of 1 % BSA in PBS for 3 h at 37°C. A 100 µl aliquot of sample or standard was added to the wells and incubated for 2 h at 37°C. A purified PC which concentration has been measured by electroimmunoassay (Diagnostica Stago, France) was used as standard. A 100 µl aliquot of a biotinylated anti-PC antibody (12H8) was then added and incubated for 2 h at 37°C. The streptavidin-peroxidase complex was incubated for 15 min at 37°C. After washes with PBS-Tween and 140 mM sodium acetate-citrate, pH 6.0, color was developed with 100 µl of 0.1 mg/ml TMB, 0.01 % H_2O_2 in acetate-citrate. The enzyme reaction was stopped with 25 µl of 2 M H_2SO_4 and the absorbance was measured at 450 nm.

Protein C activity assay : PC activity level was determined by a chromogenic assay (Stachrom Protein C, Diagnostica Stago) using a Chromotimer apparatus (Behring, Germany).

Assays for other coagulation factors : Fibrinogen, factor II, V, VII, IX and X levels were determined by clotting assays. Protein S antigenic level was assayed by electroimmunoassay.

Mouse IgG assay : All buffers and incubation conditions were similar to those described for the PC antigen assay except when indicated. Plates were coated with a 2.7 µg/ml solution of goat anti-mouse IgG antibodies (Tago, USA). The plates were blocked with 125 µl of 0.5 % gelatin (cold water fish skin, Sigma, USA) in PBS for 3 h at 37°C. A pure preparation of a mouse monoclonal antibody which concentration was measured spectrophotometrically was used as standard. Detection was achieved with peroxidase conjugated anti-mouse IgG goat immunoglobulins (Tago) incubated for 1 h at 37°C.

Bovine IgG assay : Coating was performed with anti-bovine IgG rabbit immunoglobulins (prepared in our laboratory) at a concentration of 1 µg/ml. Non-specific binding sites were blocked with gelatin. Bovine IgG purified by ion-exchange chromatography were used as standard. Bovine IgG were detected with biotinylated anti-bovine IgG rabbit immunoglobulins.

Protein A assay : Coating was performed with a human IgG_2 at a concentration of 1 µg/ml. Non-specific binding sites were blocked with gelatin. Commercial protein A (Sigma) was used as standard. Detection was achieved with two antibodies, first, an anti-protein A rabbit serum (Sigma) incubated for 90 min at 37°C and a biotinylated second antibody, anti-rabbit IgG donkey immunoglobulins (Amersham, UK) incubated for 1 h at 37°C.

RESULTS

Optimization of the immunopurification of PC

The high adsorption capacity of the 12H8 antibody and the possibility of total desorption of PC under mild and non toxic conditions has already been reported (Regnault et al., 1991a).

The influence of several parameters on the adsorption capacity of the immunoadsorbent (expressed as the amount of PC desorbed per ml of gel) was studied. Variations in the antibody density on the matrix affect the capacity (Fig. 1) whereas the adsorption is maximum for residence time (calculated as the ratio of the immunoadsorbent volume to the flow-rate) as low as 5 min (Fig. 2). The adsorption yield is dependent on the total amount of PC applied to the immunoadsorbent and optimum results are obtained for amounts of 150 U of PC per ml of gel.

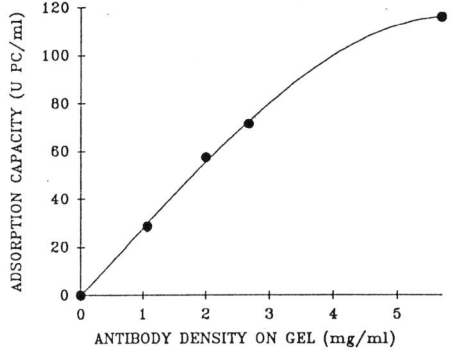
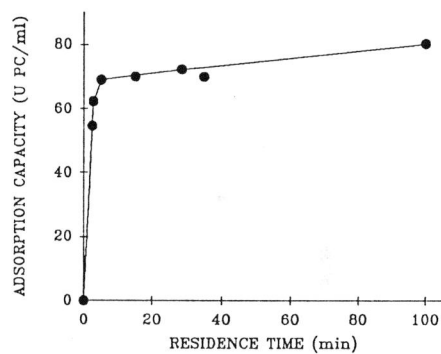

Fig. 1 : *Variation of the adsorption capacity with the antibody density on gel.* Ten column volumes of prothrombin complex concentrate was applied to the immunoadsorbents (1.1 x 3 cm) at a flow-rate of 18 ml/h.

Fig. 2 : *Influence of the residence on the adsorption capacity.* Ten column volumes of prothrombin complex concentrate was applied to the immunoadsorbent (1.1 x 5 cm) at flow-rates ranging from 3 to 125 ml/h.

The immunoaffinity chromatography recovery was about 77 % (Table 1) at a pilot scale (100 ml immunoadsorbent column). Most of the remaining 23 % PC was lost during diafiltration and concentration. About 65 % of the PC in cryoprecipitate-free plasma was recovered in the prothrombin complex concentrate. The overall recovery was then about 50 %.

Table 1 : *Purification of human PC*

	Volume (ml)	Prot.[*] (mg/ml)	PC (U/ml)	Purific. (fold)	Yield (%)
Cryoprecipitate-free plasma	1000	61	0.75	1	100
Prothrombin complex concentrate	16	40	30.5	60	65
Immunopurified PC	9.5	0.13	40.0	25.000	50

[*] Total protein was determined using a bicinchoninic acid commercial kit (Sigma)

Similar values are obtained with immunological and chromogenic PC assays and the specific activity of the purified PC was of about 300 U/mg.

The immunopurification resulted in the isolation of a highly purified PC (Table 2). When analyzed by SDS polyacrylamide gel electrophoresis, the purified PC migrated as a tightly spaced doublet with apparent molecular weights of 62,000 and 59,000 in the absence of reducing agents.

The adsorption capacity of the immunoadsorbent was not altered when it was stored in a 20 % ethanol aqueous solution between uses in order to prevent bacterial contamination. Moreover, the efficiency of the purification remained unchanged over 20 runs.

Table 2 : *Purity of the PC*

	Level
Protein C	9000 % (90 U/ml)
Fibrinogen	< 0.02 g/l
Factor II	< 1 %
Factor V	< 1 %
Factor VII	< 1 %
Factor IX	< 1 %
Factor X	< 1 %
Protein S	0 %

PC antigen and activity evaluation in highly purified concentrates

A comparative study of five functional PC assays from commercial sources has indicated a rather high between-assay variation (Fig. 3). Moreover the discrepancies due to the method this study has brought to light the influence of the prediluent used for purified PC. Dilution of high purity PC concentrates in saline buffer resulted in erroneously low PC values. The activity level of samples tested at multiple dilutions was found to decrease when increasing the dilution in saline buffer. When samples are diluted in a protein milieu, similar results are obtained with immunological and chromogenic assays (Regnault et al., 1991b). A multicenter study was undertaken to evaluate the accuracy of PC assays. High interlaboratory differences are observed and the variations are emphasized for high PC levels (Fig. 4). Careful analysis of the results suggested that the laboratory 1 which used a local pooled normal plasma as standard reported systematically rather high values while the laboratory 4 which diluted samples in saline buffer reported systematically low values.

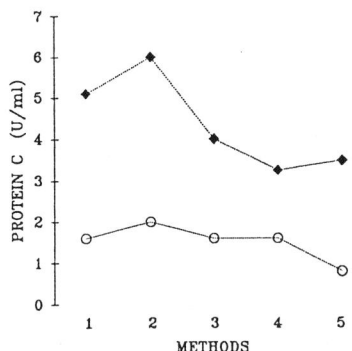 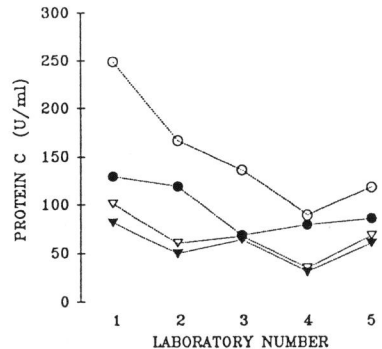

Fig. 3 : *Between-assay variations in PC activity level.* Three clotting assays (methods 1 to 3) and two chromogenic assays (methods 4 and 5) were compared. The purified PC was diluted either in PC deficient plasma (filled diamonds) or in 0.9 % NaCl (open circles).

Fig. 4 : *Interlaboratory variations in PC chromogenic assays.* Lab 2 to 5 used a commercial standard and lab 1 a pooled normal plasma. PC was diluted with PC deficient plasma for lab 1, 3 and 5, with 20 g/l BSA for lab 2 and NaCl for lab 4.

Ligand leakages

The hybridoma cells were cultured in a medium supplemented with foetal calf serum and the antibody was purified by protein A affinity chromatography. The antibody solution used for the preparation of the immunoadsorbent is thus contaminated with bovine IgG purified with murine IgG and with protein A leaching from the affinity sorbent. Murine IgG, bovine IgG and protein A were assayed in the purified monoclonal antibody and in the purified PC.

Table 3 : *Leakages*

	Protein A	Murine IgG	Bovine IgG
Purified antibody	400 ng/ mg of mAb		10 µg/ mg of mAb
Purified PC	< 10 pg/ U of PC	3 to 5 ng/ U of PC	< 0.05 ng/ U of PC

Protein A was present in antibody solutions but was found below the limit of detection in the purified PC (Table 3). Murine and bovine IgG are detected in the purified PC. The bovine IgG level reached values below the limit of detection by adding a polishing step (ion-exchange chromatography) to the purification procedure while the murine IgG level is reduced by half.

DISCUSSION

The potential for the medical application of highly purified PC concentrates for the patients with PC deficiency and with abnormal blood clotting problems should be very promising. Availability of a rapid, specific and high yield method for the purification of PC will allow the preparation of the amounts of PC required for therapeutic uses. With the immunoaffinity chromatography developed purified PC can be obtained in a single step with high recovery and higher purity than that previously reported with other chromatographic procedures or immunopurification methods. Moreover, the possibility of mild elution conditions for the dissociation of the antibody-antigen complex allows the preservation of the biological activity of the purified PC.

Because of the high production cost of immunoadsorbents, the use of this separation technology has been limited to high-valued biologicals. In order for this method to be more economical to use, it will be necessary to maximize the efficiency and the reusability of immunoadsorbents. The optimization of the procedure ensures maximum efficiency and the possibility of multiple uses of the immunoadsorbents has been demonstrated. In order to be in good agreement with correlation between reduced cost and high adsorption capacity an optimum amount of 3-4 mg of antibody would be designed to be immobilized per ml of support. The efficiency of the procedure is unchanged whatever the residence time allowing the use of wide range of flow-rates.

The evaluation of both immunological and functional PC levels in the same manner in highly purified concentrates as well as in intermediate purity samples is essential to monitor the purification and to control the preservation of the biological activity of the molecule. The multicenter study performed on assays for PC has shown significant between-assay and interlaboratory differences. This study has clearly indicated the need for purified PC to be diluted in PC deficient plasma which restaure a total protein level similar to that of normal plasma. In order to improve the accuracy of the results it would advantageous to use well standardized methods and a calibrated purified PC standard concentrate whose molecular integrity has been controlled.

Leakage of the ligand is an unavoidable disavantage of affinity chromatography. Although the murine IgG level in the purified PC concentrate is rather low, 5 µg of antibodies will be present in 1000 units of PC. This amount is greatly lower than the 1 mg amount previously reported as necessary to induce a immune response in patients with therapeutic injections. Nevertheless, the antibody leakage can be decreased by an additional polishing step to the purification procedure without loss of recovery in PC.

With the recognition that infectious viruses may be transmitted from biological products derived from human plasma as well as monoclonal antibodies sources, specific regulatory requirements have been imposed by the legislators. A validation of the master cell bank prepared for the production of the murine monoclonal antibody to human PC has been performed. The possibility of including a validated viral inactivation step in the antibody isolation or in the PC purification procedure to avoid possible contamination with viruses from murine origin without compromising the biological activity of the antibodies should be investigated. Concerning the PC purification, the starting material used offers the advantage to be a validated viral-inactivated concentrate.

One obvious question is whether to administer PC or APC. Substitutive therapy using APC concentrate would allow to immediately halt on going thrombosis. The immunopurification procedure described could be a convenient and efficient method for the purification of APC since the antibody recognize APC as well as PC.

Clinical studies have to be undertaken to evaluate the safety and patient tolerance of PC concentrates.

REFERENCES

Clouse, L.H., Comp, P.C. (1986): The regulation of hemostasis: the protein C system. *N. Engl. J. Med.* 314, 1298-1304.

Cuatrecasas, P., Wilchek, M., Anfinsen, C.B. (1968): Selective enzyme purification by affinity chromatography. *Proc. Natl. Acad. Sci. USA* 61, 636-643.

Dreyfus, M., Magny, J.F., Bridey, F., Schwarz, H.P., Planché, C., Dehan, M., Tchernia, G. (1991): Treatment of homozygous protein C deficiency and neonatal purpura fulminans with a purified protein C concentrate. *N. Engl. J. Med.* 325, 1565-1568.

Edwards, C.A., Piet, M.J.P., Chin, S., Horowitz, B. (1987): Tri(n-butyl) phosphate/detergent treatment of licensed therapeutic and experimental blood derivatives. *Vox Sang.* 52, 53-59.

Esmon, C.T. (1983): Protein C: biochemistry, physiology and clinical implications. *Blood* 62, 1155-1158.

Esmon, C.T., Taylor, F.B., Hinshaw, L.B., Chang, A., Comp, P.C., Ferell, G., Esmon, N.L. (1987): Protein C, isolation and potential use in prevention of thrombosis. *Develop. Biol. Standard* 67, 51-57.

Griffin, J.H., Evatt, B., Zimmerman, T.S., Kleiss, A.J., Wideman, C. (1981): Deficiency of protein C in congenital thrombotic disease. *J. Clin. Invest.* 68, 1370-1373.

Hendl, S., Espana, F., Aznar, J., Estelles, A., Gilabert, J., Griffin, J.H. (1991): Immunoaffinity purification of protein C with a calcium-dependent monoclonal antibody. *Rev. Iberoamer. Tromb. Hemostasia* 4, 25-28.

Marlar, R.A., Kleiss, A.J., Griffin, J.H. (1982): Mechanism of action of human activated protein C a thrombin-dependent anticoagulant enzyme. *Blood* 59, 1067-1072.

Nakamura, S., Sakata, Y. (1987): Immunoaffinity purification of protein C by using conformation-specific monoclonal antibodies to protein C-calcium ion complex. *Biochim. Biophys. Acta* 925, 85-93.

Okajima, K., Koga, S., Inoue, M., Nakagaki, T., Funatsu, A., Okake, H., Takatsuki, K., Aoki, N. (1990): Effect of protein C and activated protein C on coagulation and fibrinolysis on normal human subjects. *Thromb. Haemostasis* 63, 48-53.

Regnault, V., Rivat, C., Pfister, M., Stoltz, J.F. (1991a): Monoclonal antibodies against human plasma protein C and their uses for immunoaffinity chromatography. *Thromb. Res.* 63, 629-640.

Regnault, V., Houbouyan, L., Michalski, C., Vergnes, C., Briquel, M.E., Droulle, C., Delattre, H., Boisseau, M., Alexandre, P., Potron, G., Rivat, C., Stoltz, J.F. (1991b): Etude multicentrique sur les dosages de concentrés de protéine C purifiée et de plasmas à taux définis. *Ann. Biol. Clin.* 49, 345-350.

Seligsohn, U., Berger, A., Abend, M., Rubin, L., Attias, D., Zivelin, A., Rapaport, S.I. (1984): Homozygous protein C deficiency manifested by massive venous thrombosis in the newborn. *N. Engl. J. Med.* 310, 559-562.

Stenflo, J. (1976): A new vitamin K-dependent protein : purification from bovine plasma and preliminary characterization. *J. Biol. Chem.* 251, 355-363.

Walker, F.J., Sexton, P.W., Esmon, C.T. (1979): The inhibition of blood coagulation by activated protein C through the selective inactivation of activated factor V. *Biochim. Biophys. Acta* 571, 333-342.

Résumé

Une méthode d'immunopurification utilisant un anticorps monoclonal anti-protéine C humaine a été optimisée pour la préparation de concentrés thérapeutiques. Le facteur final de purification est de 25 000 et le rendement chromatographique d'environ 80 %. L'obtention de protéine C très pure a mis en évidence l'importance de la méthode utilisée sur l'évaluation de la molécule. Une méthode immunoenzymatique a été mise au point pour le dosage antigénique de la protéine C et l'activité a été déterminée par méthode chromogénique. L'activité spécifique de la protéine C purifiée est d'environ 300 U/mg. Des méthodes immunoenzymatiques ont été développées pour le dosage des IgG bovines et de la protéine A dans les préparations d'anticorps et pour suivre les IgG murines, les IgG bovines et la protéine A rélargués de l'immunoadsorbant.

Biotechnology of Blood Proteins. Eds C. Rivat, J.-F. Stoltz. Colloque INSERM/John Libbey Eurotext Ltd.
© 1993, Vol. 227, pp. 103-108.

Method for manufacturing chemically virus-inactivated, high purity FVIII concentrate with an overall yield of 35%, feasible for small pool production in developing countries

Knut Wallevik, Søren Glavind, Eva Hansen, Jørgen Ingerslev and Jan Jørgensen

Department of Clinical Immunology, University Hospital, Skejby Sygehus, 8200 Aarhus N, Denmark

SUMMARY

Solvent/detergent virusinactivated FVIII concentrate, with a specific activity of 3.7 i.u./mg protein is manufactured in our blood bank at a net yield of 360 i.u. FVIII:C per litre plasma. 1 million i.u. is produced per year. The concentrate (DANATIV S/D) has full clinical activity, no severe adverse reactions have been reported. The method is feasible for FVIII production in developing countries.

INTRODUCTION

Virus safe plasma derivatives produced in the industrialized countries are getting increasingly expensive. The only means by which the developing countries will be able to afford sufficient supplies of virusinactivated FVIII concentrates will be to initiate local production. For economical and educational reasons a production will be based on relatively simple equipment and probably on small plasma pools.
Concurrently with the sophistication of methods for plasma fractionation in the industrialized countries there is a need for design of sturdy, safe fractionation methods, which can function at the premises of the third world.
Our Blood Bank produced from 1986 to 1988 a freeze dried, heat treated, high purity FVIII concentrate (DANATIV) from heparinized plasma, by simple temperature-dependent precipitations in the closed blood pack system (Wallevik et al, 1989). The net yield was 400 i.u. FVIII:C/litre plasma, which was exceptional for a high purity FVIII concentrate.
We have now changed the virusinactivation procedure to the solvent/detergent method using 0.3% TNBP/0.2% cholate. Apart from adding an $Al(OH)_3$ precipitation step, the purification of FVIII is unchanged, but in order to include the more elaborated virusinactivation procedure, it has been necessary to open the system and increase the final batch size.

Method: The manufacturing procedure for Danativ S/D is divid-

ed into two steps which are completely separated in time and can be separated also in location.
- production of "partial batches".
- virusinactivation of pooled "partial batches".

"Partial batch" production: Is visualized in Fig. 1:

FLOW SCHEME FOR PRODUCTION OF PARTIAL BATCH FOR DANATIV

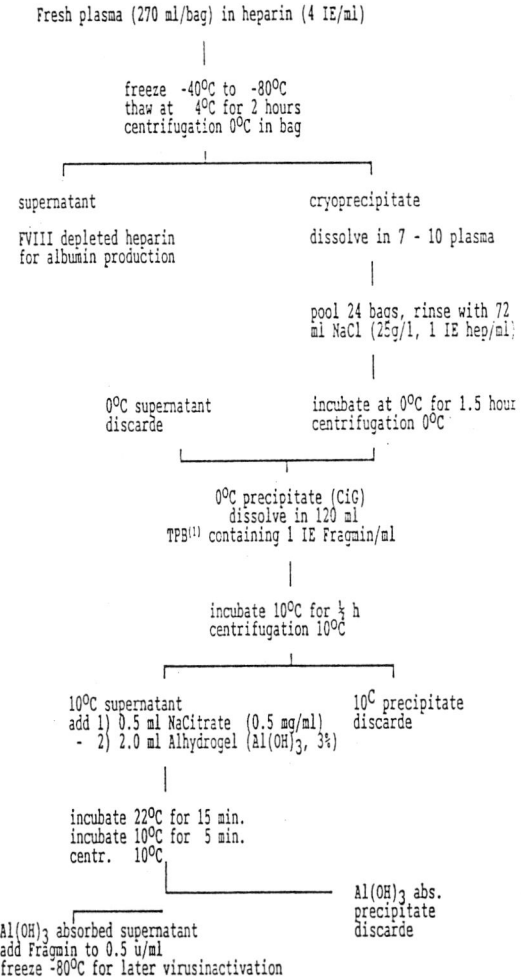

Blood collection in Heparin, pooling of 24 cryoprecipitates in the closed blood bag system, the 0°C and the 10°C precipitations are essential as described by Wallevik et al (1986,-89). However, two changes have been introduced: 1) Heparin has been exchanged with low molecular weight Heparin (Fragmin) in the 10°C Precipitation Buffer (TPB). Fragmin is used also in all solutions from this step onward. The reason is that conventional Heparin was concentrated during the ultrafiltration step following the virusinactivation, resulting in a Heparin concentration in the final FVIII concentrate of 5 u Heparin/ml.

2) Although no thrombin activity can be measured in the partial batches it turned out that it was necessary to add an $Al(OH)_3$ absorption step to avoid activation of FVIII:C during virusinactivation.

$Al(OH)_3$ precipitation step: The supernatant from the "10°C precipitation step" is transferred to a 400 ml dry bag. By means of "Site coupler", 0.5 ml NaCitrate, $3 H_2O$ (0.5 mg/ml) and 2 ml AlhydrogeL 3% (Superfoss, Denmark) is added. The bag is left at room temperature for 15 min and then transferred to the 10°C water bath for 5 min incubation. Centrifuged at 10°C at 3000 g for 15 min.

The resultant 120 ml FVIII concentrate is designated a "Partial Batch" and is frozen and stored at -80°C for later virusinactivation. In our Blood Bank 2-3 partial batches are produced daily as part of the routine blood component preparation.

Virusinactivation: The Solvent/Detergent (S/D), tri-(n-butyl)-phosphate (TNBP)/NaCholate, virusinactivation of pooled "Partial Batches" is performed according to the principles of Horowich et al (1985) licensed by the New York Blood Centre (Fig. 2).

FLOW SCHEME FOR TNBP/CHOLATE VIRUSINACTIVATION OF DANATIV
(according to New York Blood Center)

pool partial batches
↓
filtrate at 35°C
↓
dilute 1/3 with virusinactivation buffer containing 0.6% NaCholate
↓
add TNBP to concentration of 0.3%
↓
virusinactivate at 30°C for 6 h.
↓
2 times oil extraction, room temperature
↓
filtrate at 35°C
↓
Ultrafiltrate (100 KD) with 5 vol of dialysisbuffer
↓
concentrate to 20 u/FVIII:C/ml
↓
sterile filtrate
↓
dispense 25 ml
↓
freeze dry

In our set up, 19 partial batches (2.2 litres) equal to 456 conventional blood donations are included in each final batch and are processed at a 2 week interval. However, the size of the final batch can be adjusted to much larger volumes only restricted by the capacity of the equipment.

RESULTS

In vitro characterization: The protein pattern and the FVIII related parameters of the Danativ S/D FVIII concentrate are depicted in Table I and the general characteristics of 39 consecutive batches in Table II.

Table I: CHARACTERISTICS OF DANATIV S/D FVIII CONCENTRATE (3 batches)

FVIII related parameters (u/ml)	x ± s	Proteins		x ± s
VIIIC	25.4 ± 1.2	Total protein	g/l	7.6 ± 0.9
VIIIAg	27.9 ± 0.9	Fibrinogen	-	1.8 ± 0.1
VIII:Ag/VIIIC	1.13 ± 0.06	Fibronectin	-	2.8 ± 0.2
vwAg	24.0 ± 1.1	Albumin	-	3.2 ± 0.4
		IgG	-	1.1 ± 0.1
		ATIII	-	0.04 ± 0.01
		FII	u/ml	<0.01
		FIX	-	<0.01
		FXIII a.	-	0.11 ± 0.01
		FXIII s.	-	0.12 ± 0.01

Additives, specific activity and yield   (see table 2)

Table II: 39 CONSECUTIVE BATCHES OF DANATIV S/D (~ 45,000 U FVIII:C/BATCH)

	x ± s	Range	
FVIIIC IU/20 ml	507 ± 47	(418 - 584)	
Total protein g/l	6.9 ± 0.9	(4.3 - 9.1)	
Spec. act. u/mg protein	3.7 ± 0.5	(2.9 - 5.3)	
Fibrinogen g/l	1.5 ± 0.3	(1.1 - 2.0)	
Dissolving time min.	2.5 ± 0.5	(1.5 - 3.5)	
TNBP ug/ml (ppM)	1.6 ± 0.7	(<1.0 - 3.7)	
NaCholate ug/ml	14.5 ± 9.3	(<1.0 - 40.0)	
Al^{+++} ug/l	21 ± 7	(9 - 39)	
Heparin (LMW) u/ml:			
until July, 1992	4.8 ± 0.6	(3.9 - 5.7)	Danativ production modified July, 1992 in order to decrease heparin content in final product.
from July, 1992	2.0 ± 0.1	(1.9 - 2.0)	
Net yield FVIIIC u/l plasma	362 ± 36	(312 - 441)	

Compared to the dry heat treated Danativ (Wallevik et al, 1989) the specific activity has increased from 2.2±0.3 i.u. FVIII:C/mg protein (30 consecutive batches) to 3.7±0.5 i.u. FVIII:C/mg protein. This is due to the added fourth precipitation step (the $Al(OH)_3$ absorption) which removes further fibrinogen, fibronectin and IgG, while the Albumin concentration has remained unchanged. Isoagglutinins are low and in most of the batches not detectable. The VIII:Ag/-VIII:C ratio is close to one, indicating mild purification conditions with little denaturation of the FVIII molecule and probably of other contaminating protein molecules as well.

The traces of TNBP, NaCholate and Aluminium are all well below the maximum accepted values set by The Food and Drug Administration (FDA, USA) and the Danish Health Authorities.
The nett yield of FVIII:C has decreased from 400±40 i.u. in the dry heat treated Danativ to 360±40 i.u. per litre Fresh Frozen Plasma. However, this is still a remarkable yield for a chemically virus-inactivated, high purity FVIII concentrate.
During the first 18 months, Danativ S/D was produced with a Heparin/Fragmin content of 200 u anti FXa/1000 i.u. FVIII:C (Table II). As concern has been expressed that this amount of Heparin could result in a bleeding tendency in patients, treated with high doses of Danativ S/D, the production procedure was, as mentioned, slightly modified by substituting conventional Heparin with Low Molecular Weight Heparin (Fragmin). Danativ S/D is today produced with a Fragmin content of 80 u anti FXa/1000 i.u. FVIII:C.
Crude cryoprecipitates and some intermediary purified FVIII concentrates have been demonstrated to inhibit lymphocyttransformation in vitro. Danativ has in clinical FVIII:C concentrations been shown to have no inhibitory or enhancing effect on mitogen- and antigen transformation of lymphocytes isolated form HIV ab. neg. and HIV ab. pos. Haemophilia A patients (Wallevik, 1989).

Clinical characterization: In vivo recovery and turnover of 2500 i.u. Danativ S/D were examined in 4 healthy persons with severe Haemophilia A (Table III).

Table III: IN VIVO RECOVERY AND T/2 OF DANATIV S/D

Patient	FVIIIC u/kg body weight	Recovery % of expected	T/2 hours
1	31.6	93	14
2	28.4	65	9[1]
3	32.5	76	10
4	31.1	76	11[2]

[1] T/2, 1985 Danativ (dry heat treated): 8 hours

[2] T/2, 1985 Nordiocto (dry heat treated): 16 hours

All four were in steady state with plasma FVIII:C below 0.01 i.u./ml. Two had participated in similar turnover studies of dry heat treated concentrates in 1985. In all 4 persons the recovery and the half life of FVIII:C were similar to values found for other commercial FVIII concentrates of good quality. The majority of the 2 million FVIII units produced in our blood bank has been given to one haemophilia patient in "high doses treatment" for a FVIII inhibitor. Danativ S/D was chosen for treatment because the side reactions (nausea, -dizziness) are acceptable for the patient, in contrast to severe reactions in connection to other available FVIII concentrates of similar specific activity. Except for this single patient no adverse reactions to Danativ S/D have been reported.

DISCUSSION

The reported method will be feasible for a small pool production of solvent/detergent virusinactivated FVIII concentrate in a developing country only if a number of prerequisites are fulfilled. A centralized National Blood Transfusion Service must be at function to secure plasma collection. Possibilities for refurbishment to built "clean rooms" must be present. The technical standards of the blood banks must be thoroughly evaluated (water supply, reliable electricity, service for equipment, cold space etc.). The technical and academic staff must be trained to follow GMP guidelines.

In practice it will mean that at least some of the blood banks must have experience in producing liquid cryoprecipitates.

The Danativ method has the advantage that the "partial batches" are produced in a closed blood bag system and only requires ordinary (but good quality) blood bank equipment. Consequently, "partial batches" can be produced in most large blood banks in a Laminar Air Flow bench. When frozen, the "partial batches" can be transported to the "virus inactivation centre" equipped for pharmaceutical production in clean rooms according to GMP principles. Here "partial batches" from different blood banks are pooled and virusinactivated.

"Partial batches" produced from 1 ton plasma have a volumen of 18-19 litre, which means that the virusinactivation procedure will occupy limited space and can be performed using non expensive standard equipment.

REFERENCES

Horowitz, B., Wiebe, M.E., Lippin, A., et al (1985): Inactivation of viruses in labile blood derivatives. I. Disruption of lipid-enveloped viruses by tri(n-butyl) phosphate detergent combinations. Transfusion 25: 516-522.

Wallevik, K., Ingerslev, J., Bernvil, S.S., Kristensen, S.G., Jørgensen, J., and Kissmeyer-Nielsen, F. (1986): Manufacturing in the blood bank of high purity heat-treated factor FVIII concentrate from heparin stabilized blood and its consequence for the red cell and supernate plasma components. In Future Developments in Blood Banking, eds C.Th. Smit Sibinga, P.C. Das and T.J. Greenwalt, pp. 95-101. Martinus Nijhoff Publishing, Boston, Dordrecht, Lancester.

Wallevik, K., Ingerslev, J., Stenbjerg Bernvil, S., Jacobsen, S.E., Harboe, T., and Kissmeyer-Nielsen, F. (1989): Purification of high purity FVIII coagulation protein at a yield of 40% by a three step temperature depdendent precipitation from heparinized plasma. In Biotechnology of plasma proteins, eds J.F. Stoltz, and C. Rivat, pp. 287-294. Collogue INSERM 175.

Wallevik, K. (1989): Influence of factor VIII concentrates of different purity on the in vitro transformation of lymphocytes from haemophiliacs. In Replacement Therapy in Haemophilia. Problems and Solutions, ed P.M. Mannucci, pp. 111-115. University of Milan.

Pilot immunoaffinity purification of Factor VIII/vWF complex (preliminary results)

L. van Wijngaarden[1], H.S. Hoff[1], K. Koops[1], J.J. van Weperen[1], P.C. Das[2] and C.T. Smit Sibinga[2]

[1]Bio-Intermediair B.V., P.O. Box 454, 9700 AL Groningen, The Netherlands and [2]Red Cross Blood Bank Groningen-Drenthe, Groningen, The Netherlands

INTRODUCTION

In 1988 the Red Cross Blood Bank Groningen-Drenthe and Bio-Intermediair, both situated in Groningen (the Netherlands), started the development of an immuno-purification procedure of Factor VIII. This development served as a model study to the purification of plasma proteins by Immuno Affinity Chromatography (IAC) for blood bank application.

The aim is to develop a purification procedure of Factor VIII (FVIII) from small pools of plasma from voluntary, unpaid donors. Strategy is to leave the von Willebrand Factor (vWF) in the end product as a natural stabilizer. Addition of stabilizers, like albumine, would not be necessary. The vWF is adsorbed to, and released from the immuno adsorbent. The FVIII protein stays complexed, and is co-purified with the vWF. The requirements at the starting-point were at least 20 IU/ml FVIII activity and 25 IU/mg total protein specific activity in the endproduct and a yield of > 300 IU/kg plasma.

In the first three years of the work, several stages were passed through (Koops et al., 1990):
- Feasability study; using commercial anti-vWF IgG; setting of a reference method.
- Production of hybridoma cell lines; mice were immunized with purified vWF, and hybridoma cell lines were cloned.
- Selection of monoclonal antibody (MAb); the functionality and suitability of the antibody to IAC.
- Laboratory scale experiments; the immobilization of the antibodies and the purification of the complex.

The results of these stages are summarized in Table 1.

Based to the results of the laboratory scale experiments and experiments to the up- and downstream of the IAC, a standard purification procedure to primary pilot studies was designed.

Table 1. *Results of laboratory scale purification of FVIII/vWF by Immuno Affinity Chromatography. MAb = monoclonal antibody. FVIII:C = FVIII activity (chromogenic substrate assay). Recovery = recovery of FVIII:C compared to plasma.*

MAb-type	: IgG 2a
Resin	: Sephacryl S1000 - CNBr activated
Immobilization	: 5 mg MAb/ml column volume
Capacity	: 80 IU/ml column volume
FVIII:C	: 20 - 30 IU/ml
Specific activity	: > 100 IU/mg total protein
Recovery	: 32%

PILOT PURIFICATION PROCEDURE

The procedure of the pilot scale experiments (Fig. 1) can be distinguished in five steps. The starting material was routine cryoprecipitate of fresh frozen CPDA plasma (I). To remove vitamin K dependent proteins, the cryoprecipitate was treated with 1/10th volume of 3% Al(OH)$_3$-gel (II). The removal of these proteins is of importance to prevent FVIII from being activated, and blocking of the column by clotting. Potentially present viruses are inactivated by treatment with solvent/detergent (III). This was achieved by incubation for 6 hours at 30°C in the presence of 0.3% TnBP and 1% Triton X-100 (Horowitz et al., 1985). Step four is the Immuno Affinity Chromatographic step, which in fact is the most important step of the proces. The last step of the procedure is to desalt the eluate (V). To this, different methods were compared: ultrafiltration, diafiltration, and gelfiltration.

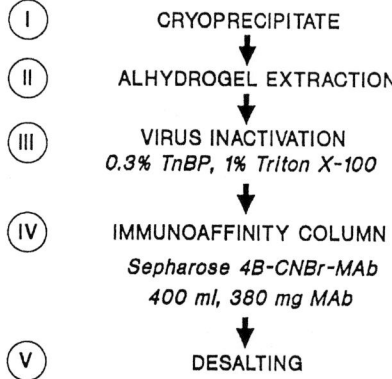

Fig. 1. *Primary pilot scale purification procedure of FVIII/vWF.*

The immuno chromatographic step was performed applying a column of 400 ml Sepharose 4B (CNBr-activated, Pharmacia) containing 380 mg MAb. The FVIII/vWF complex was adsorbed to the column (approximately 2½ hours at 30 cm/hrte). After loading, non-adsorbed proteins and contaminants, like TnBP and Triton X-100, are washed away (2½ hours at 60 cm/hr). The adsorbed complex was released from the column at 30 cm/hr flowrate (40 minutes) using a chaotropic buffer with 1 M KI at pH 6.5 (Hornsey et al., 1987).

Immediately after purifications, FVIII activities were determined using a chromogenic substrate assay (KabiVitrum). Within the purification runs, the column was stored at room temperature.

RESULTS

The results of six pilot purification experiments are presented.

In Table 2, recoveries compared to cryoprecipitate and the yield compared to plasma are shown. The results of desalting are not shown, because in these runs eluates were desalted using ultra- or dia-filtration: most of the FVIII was lost due to adsorption to the membrane of the filter or inactivation. Later experiments using gelfiltration showed good results and prospects.

Table 2. *Recoveries of the first four steps of the pilot procedure. Recovery in percentages compared to cryoprecipitate and in IU/kg plasma.*

Step:	I	II	III	IV	
Run	Cryo (IU)	Al(OH)$_3$ (%)	SD treatment (%)	Breakthr. (%)	Eluate (%)
1	8294	77	78	54	26
2	1971	92	85	28	26
3	3830	115	101	64	29
4	5130	101	95	39	15
5	4835	75	64	43	20
6	4393	121	100	29	17
Perc.:	100%	97% ± 18	87% ± 13	43% ± 13	22% ± 5
IU/kg:	427 ± 56	411 ± 82	369 ± 58	202 ± 49	93 ± 21

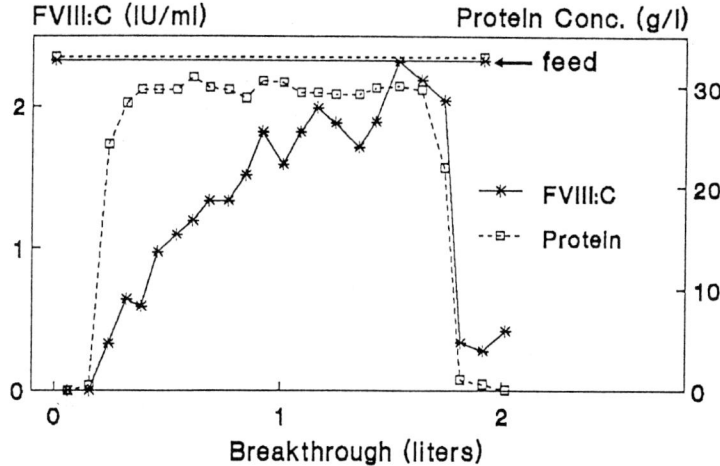

Fig. 2. *Breakthrough curve: FVIII:C and total protein in breakthrough fractions.*

The breakthrough curve of FVIII and total protein (Fig. 2) was determined in breakthrough fractions. During elution, the FVIII:C, total protein and vWF:Ag in elution fractions were determined (fig 3).

The results of the pilot purifications compared to the laboratory scale experiments are presented in Table 3.

Table 3. *Results of pilot scale immunopurification. Recovery = FVIII:C released compared to adsorbed. The amount of TnBP in the eluate was determined in later purification runs.*

Resin	: Sepharose 4B - CNBr activated
Immobilization	: 1 mg MAb/ml column
Adsorption concentration	: 4.7 IU/ml column
Recovery	: 94%
FVIII:C eluate	: 2.2 IU/ml
Specific activity	: 38 IU/mg
FVIII:C/vWF:Ag	: 0.8
Mouse IgG	: < 50 ng/ml
TnBP	: < 4 ppm

N = 6 runs

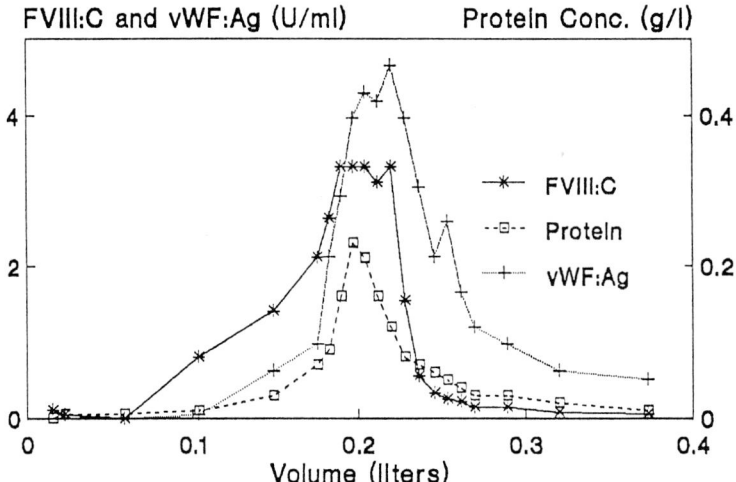

Fig. 3. *Elution pattern: FVIII:C, total protein and vWF:Ag determined in elution fractions.*

DISCUSSION.

During these primary pilot scale experiments, information was obtained for further development of the procedure.

There are good prospects to the improvement of the yield of FVIII. The yield was largely determined by the amount of FVIII collected in the breakthrough fraction: 43% (Table 2). Improving the breakthrough curve, and loading the column with no excess of FVIII, the yield can be enhanced to approximately 40%. Experiments are needed to confirm this. The most crucial factor to the yield remains the cryoprecipitation step: 427 IU/kg plasma (Table 2). However, the cryoprecipitate used in this experiments, was originally not intend to FVIII production. In four runs, 93% of the adsorbed FVIII:C was released from the column (Table 3). In two runs, run 4 and 6, the recovery was significantly lower.

To enhance the loading efficiency (minimal FVIII in the breakthrough fraction at maximum adsorption) the breakthrough curve has to be improved (Fig. 2). Ideal would be a zero FVIII potency in the breakthrough fraction until the column is saturated, followed by a sharp increase. Parameters like the choice of column material and adsorption concentration, FVIII:C and protein concentration at the feed, the flowrate and the column dimensions are of influence.

The adsorption concentration of the column was 4.7 IU/ml column, and the FVIII:C in the eluate was 2.2 IU/ml (Table 3). Compared to the column used at laboratory scale, these results are very poor. Using a CNBr-activated Sephacryl S1000 column, containing 5 mg MAb/ml column, the adsorption concentration was 80 IU/ml column (capacity of 16 IU/mg MAb). The FVIII:C in the endproduct was 20 - 30 IU/ml. Optimal concentration of the immobilized MAb and the choice of the column material and coupling chemistry of the MAb are of influence on the adsorption concentration. Although the elution peak (Fig. 3) will be higher, the volume of elution will be larger due to peak broadening.

To the eluate and the end product, several assays to quality control and validation are performed. The specific activity of the end product was 38 IU/mg (Table 3) which is more than the requirement at the starting-point. The ratio FVIII:C/vWF:Ag was 0.8. The concentration of mouse IgG in the eluate leaked from the column was < 50 ng/ml. IgG will be removed by an additional chromatographic step. Laboratory experiments to this are continuing. The amount of TnBP in the eluate was detected at < 4 ppm, which is acceptable. However this value will be decreased after gelfiltration and an IgG removal step. The set up of additional assays to the quality control, for example Triton X-100 determination, vWF ristocetin cofactor activity and characterization of the FVIII and vWF proteins, has already been started.

FUTURE DIRECTIONS

New pilot purification experiments are planned with modifications to the procedure (Fig. 4). To lower the total protein concentration and improve filtration of the cryoprecipitate, a fibrinogen and fibronectin precipitation step by zinc and heparin (Foster et al., 1983) will be included. Before virus inactivation the cryoprecipitate will be sterile filtered using a 0.45 μm filter. The eluate will be desalted using a Sephadex G-25 column. Finally, the end product will be freeze dried. To this experiments, an immunosorbent is available now of 100 ml of Sephacryl S500, CNBr activated, containing 500 mg MAb. The adsorption capacity of this column is approximately 80 IU/ml column.

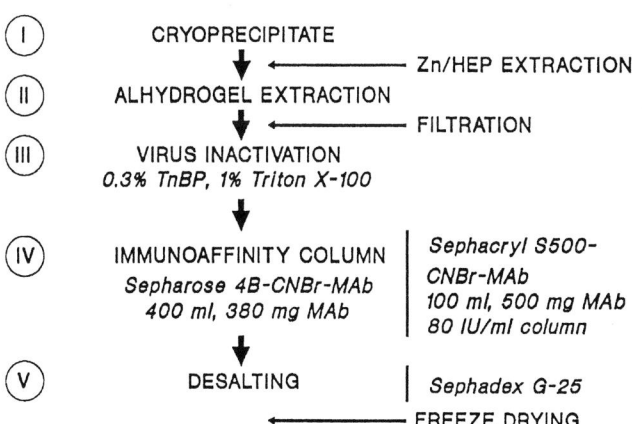

Fig. 4. Set up of the modified pilot scale purification procedure. On the left the original procedure as shown in Fig. 1 and on the right the modifications.

The requirements stated at the starting-point of the project are still attainable. Using a Sephacryl S500 column (80 IU/ml column), the FVIII:C in the end product will be 20-30 IU/ml, as was shown at laboratory scale experiments. A yield of 300 IU/kg plasma is attainable by improving the cryoprecipitation step and adsorption kinetics of the complex to the column (breakthrough curve).

The developments to the immunoadsorbent and the Up- and Downstream are proceeding. Good Manufacturing Practices continuosly is a point of attention and preliminary work to registration is started. During the project assays to the quality control are developing and validated.

The end product will be a highly purified, virus safe, Factor VIII preparation stabilized by the natural von Willebrand Factor, without addition of albumine.

Acknowledgment

We would like to thank Dr. D.S. Pepper, Dr. R.V. McIntosh and Dr B.D. Griffin (Scottish National Blood Transfusion Service, Edinburgh, Scotland) for their support and help to the development of the immunoadsorbent and the up- and downstream of the pilot procedure.

REFERENCES

Foster, P.R., Dickson, I.H., MacLeod, A.J., and Bier, M. (1983): Zinc fractionation of cryoprecipitate. *Thromb. Haemostas.* 50,117.

Hornsey, V.S., Griffin, B.D., Pepper, D.S. ,Micklem, L.R., and Prowse, C.V. (1987): Immunoaffinity purification of Factor FVIII complex. *Thromb. Haemostas.* 57,102-105.

Horowitz, B., Wiebe, M.E., Lippin, A., and Stryker, M.H. (1985): Inactivation of viruses in labile blood derivatives. *Transfusion* 25,516-522.

Koops, K., Hoff, H.S., Weperen, J.J. van, Das, P.C., and Smit Sibinga, C.Th. (1991): Immunoaffinity purification of Factor VIII/von Willebrand Factor complex. In *Coagulation and blood transfusion: Developments in hematology and immunology. Vol. 26*, ed Smit Sibinga, C.Th., Das, P.C., Mannuci, P.M., pp. 103-117. Dordrecht: Kluwer Academic Publishers.

Purification and depyrogenation of antihemophilic FVIII:C from human plasma

M. Ezzedine[1], F. Lawny[2] and M.A. Vijayalakshmi[1]

[1]*Laboratoire d'Interactions Moléculaires et de Technologie des Séparations, Université de Technologie de Compiègne, B.P. 649, 60206 Compiègne Cedex, France and* [2]*Centre National de Transfusion Sanguine (CNTS), Les Ulis, France*

SUMMARY

The human serum anti hemophilic factor A (FVIII:C) was specifically retained on histidine coupled agarose gels at pH 6.0 and at low ionic strength and eluted by Glycine 0.1 M, Lysine 0.3 M $CaCl_2$ 0.3 M, pH 7.0. The purified preparation contained almost 100% of the injected FVIII:C and ≈ 60% of VWf injected. Only fibronectine and fibrinogene were found as trace umpurities. The histidine ligand recognises specific sites both on the FVIII:C and on the Von Willebrand factor. Hence, the purified factor VIII contains the Von Willebrand factor intact. The light chain of the FVIII:C was found to contain the immobilised histidine recognition site. Moreover, the purified FVIII can be depyrogenated by using the same column, as the desorption conditions for FVIII:C + VWf were different than those for desorbing the pyrogens.

INTRODUCTION

The antihemophilic factor A (FVIII:C) is a glycoprotein of ≈ 330000 dalton and is found in a normal plasma at a low concentration (100 to 200 µg/l). The molecule is bound to Von Willbrand factor (VWf) by noncovalent forces. This FVIII-Von Willebrand factor complex dissociates at 20 mM calcium or at high ionic strength.

Due to its very low concentration in plasma and due to the difficulties encountered in the stability of the molecule, chromatographic methods are better choice than the different precipitation methods. The pseudobiospecific adsorbents are known to be better alternatives to the more selective immunoadsorbents (Vijayalakshmi, 1989). These adsorbents are based on ligands having potential sites for multiple interactions with proteins. Further it has been shown that the combined hydrophobic and ionic sorbents such as aminohexyl Sepharose could be used for the purification of FVIII:C from either plasma or from cryoprecipitate (Austen et al., 1982; Ruttyn et al., 1989).

Recently histidine coupled matrices are reported to be retaining several proteins with high selectivity as a function of adsorption conditions, based on a combined hydrophobic and ion pairing complementarity (Vijayalakshmi 1992). With the added advantage of being a ligand of biological origin histidine represents a potential ligand for the purification of several plasma proteins.

MATERIALS AND METHODS

The different starting materials, plasma, solvent-detergent treated, dialysed cryoprecipitate and an ion exchange prepurified FVIII preparation (THP) having specific activities of 0.014 ; 1.59 and 150 respectively were from CNTS, France. Sepharose 4B and Sephacryl S1000 were from Pharmacia, Uppsala, Sweden and fractogel TSK HW-65 was purchased from Merck, (Darmstadt, FRG). All other chemicals were of analar grade, either from Merck or from Sigma

Preparation of adsorbents

The epoxy activation using either epichlorhydrin or 1.4 butanediol diglycidyl ether as described by Sundberg and Porath (1974) was used as may be the case. Then L-histidine was coupled as described by Kanoun et al., 1986 . The coupled ligand concentration was determined based on the nitrogen assay described by Kjeldahl.

Chromatography

For the initial optimisation of the adsorption and desorption conditions, all the chromatographic experiments were run at ambient temperature using a (2.5 x 30 cm) column filled with about 30ml of the adsorbent, with a linear flow of 36 $cm.h^{-1}$. The adsorption buffer was 20 mM Tris-acetate at pH 6.0. After the optimisation studies, the scaled up chromatography was run using a (2.5 x 110 cm) H-B-Seph-4B column and ion exchange prepurified FVIII preparation as the starting material. Typically 20 U FVIII/ml adsorbent were injected except in experiments for the determination of maximum adsorption capacity.

Determination of Factor VIII:C activity and other plasma proteins

The Factor VIII:C content of the starting materials as well as that of the individual purified fractions were determined using a chromogenic assay developed by the hemostasis laboratory of CNTS. This assay is based on the chromogenic substrate CBS 4803 for the Factor VIII:C kit of Diagnostica Stago, Franconville, France.
The antigenic activities of FVIII and of VWf were determined by a sandwich ELISA technique developped by the hemostatic laboratory of CNTS using the kit from Diagnostica Stago, Franconville, France. Fibrinogen and fibronectin were equally determined by an ELISA method using the reagent kit from Diagnostica Stago, Franconville, France.
The total protein concentration was determined by the BCA protein assay as described by the manual from Pierce Chemical Company, Illinois, USA. The standard curve was determined using a 70mg/ml monotol solution.
Albumin and immunoglobulins were determined by the laser nephelometric method using Behring reagents (Behring, FRG).

Electrophoresis

SDS-PAGE with a linear gradient for 6 to 12% polyacrylamide gel was used both for testing the homogeneity of the purified fractions as well as for the determination of the light and heavy chains of FVIII:C before and after dissociation with EDTA and binding to H-B-Seph-4B adsorbent. Both comassie blue or silver nitrate staining were used.

Pyrogen estimation

The "Limulus Amebocyte Lysat (LAL)" in vitro test, based on the amidasique activity on a chromogenic substrate with C terminal arg. linked to p.nitroaniline (PNA) was used as described by Baggerman et al., 1984 and Bussey and Tsuji 1984. The samples to be tested were incubated with LAL at 37°C. The PNA released due to the enzyme attack at the C terminal arg. gives a yellow colour with λ_{max} at 405 nm. This PNA release is proportional to the endotoxin

present in the mixture. The test is sensitive to 0.01 to 0.30 ng endotoxin/ml. Further the presence of fungus or yeast or other gram positive bacteria upto 105/ml does not interfere with the test (Pearson et al., 1984).
However, the presence of Ca^{2+}, Zn^{2+} or EDTA inhibits the enzyme. Hence, all the eluted fractions were dialysed free of traces of calcium ions before applying the test.
In order to confirm the data from this test, a rabbit in vivo assay was performed on the pooled fractions. Strictly selected rabbits taking into account their age, body weight, diets administered etc. were used. The pooled fractions to be tested were injected to these rabbits and the raise in their body temperature was followed. It is known that the endotoxins when injected provoque a biphasic fever in rabbits (Milner 1973) ; whence the name "pyrogens". It is to be noted that only the "rabbit test" is validated by the french pharmacopia (French Pharmacopia x edition 1983).

RESULTS AND DISCUSSION

The FVIII from an alumina adsorbed solvent-detergent treated and dialysed cryoprecipitate was retained on a histidyl Sepharose 4B (H.Seph.4B) column at pH 6.0 and was eluted almost quantitatively using the same buffer added with 0.1 M Gly + 0.03 M Lys + 0.3 M $CaCl_2$. A 2100 fold purified FVIII with ≈ 18% yield as compared to the initial plasma and 99% yield as compared to the material injected onto the column were obtained (Fig 1, Table I). However, the capacity and through put of the Sepharose coupled with histidine using simple epichlorhydrin activation was not very high. Hence, we studied different support matrices with a longer spacer arm using bisoxirane coupling method.

Table I.: PURIFICATION OF DIALYSED CRYOPRECIPITATE ON A H-SEPHAROSE 4B COLUMN. (See text for details).

Fractions	FVIII:C (U/ml)	Volume (ml)	Total Units	Yield %	AS	Purification factor
Plasma	1	4000	4000	100	0.014	1
Dialysed Cryo-precipitate	4	100	400	/	1.59	113
Non retained on H-Sepharose 4B	<0.05	118	0	/	/	/
Eluted from H-Sepharose 4B	16.8	23.5	394.8	18 (99)*	29.5	2100

* Note : 18% yield with reference to plasma ; but 99% with reference to material injected onto the column (dialysed cryoprecipitate).

As shown in Table II, His-Biosoxirane Sepharose-4B (H-B-Seph. 4B.) gives a good compromise with a 18.5 fold purified preparation and a high capacity of 60U FVIII:C/ml adsorbent, in spite of the fact that the coupled ligand concentration is not as high as in the sephacryl matrix. Apparently the acrylamide groupes in the sephacryl matrix are quenching the interaction between the ligand and the FVIII. Nevertheless the specificity to FVIII was unimpaired in all the cases.

Gel using	Concentration of histidine coupled μmole/ml gel	Capacity of FVIII (U/ml)	Purification factor	Specific activity (U/mg)
Histidyl-bisoxirane sepharose 4B	150	60	18.5	29.5
Histidyl-bisoxirane sephacryl S1000	350	75	6.7	10.7
Histidyl-bisoxirane fractogel TSK HW-65	24	8	7.5	12
Histidyl-epoxy-sepharose-4B	40	30	35.7	56.9

Table II. : COMPARATIVE EFFICIENCIES AND CAPACITIES OF THREE DIFFERENTS GELS USED FOR FVIII:C PURIFICATION

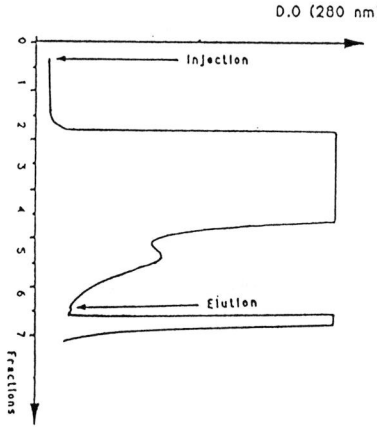

Fig. 1. : CHROMATOGRAPHY OF DIALYSED CRYOPRECIPITATE ON H-SEPHAROSE 4B COLUMN.

Influence of the quality of injected material

Histidine coupled matrices are in general weak affinity sorbents with dissociation constants in the range of 10^{-4} to 10^{-6} M (3.6×10^{-5} M for FVIII, Ezzedine 1990). Moreover the versatile capacity of the sorbent to recognize other plasma proteins depending upon the adsorption conditions may reflect in differences in the level of other contaminant proteins in the purified fraction, as a function of the composition/purity of the material injected to the column.

So in order to ascertain the place of H-B-Seph.4B. in a general purification scheme for FVIII:C we studied the chromatography of two preparations having 4U/ml (dialysed cryo precipitate) and 30U/ml (cryo precipitate prepurified on an ion-exchanger) FVIII:C respectively.

The respective composition of the two starting materials and that of the fraction purified on H-B-Seph.4B are shown in Table III While in both the cases 100% of FVIII:C and 60 to 70% of VWf were recovered the ion exchange prepurified preparation gave a very high specific activity 850 U with only fibronectine and fibrinogen as trace contaminants. No immunoglobulines or albumin could be detected in the final product. From these data we can note that fibronectin and fibrinogen are the two major components competing with the FVIII for binding to histidine ligands under the adsorption and desorption conditions used.

	Dialysed cryoprecipitate			THP (ion exchange purified		
	Before	After	%	Before	After	%
Total Protein mg/ml	2.51	0.57	22	0.2	0.04	20
F VIII:C (U/ml)	4.00	4.00	100	30	30	100
F VIII:C Ag. (U/ml)	5.20	5.00	100	65	35	54
VWf : AG. (U/ml)	9.00	6.48	72	17	10	59
Fibrinogen (mg/ml)	0.12	0.02	15	0.05	0.015	30
Fibronectin (mg.ml)	0.17	0.30	>100	0.027	0.01	37
IgG (mg/ml)	0.40	0.02	5	0.12	BT	BT
IgA (mg/ml)	0.10	0.02	20	<0.025	BT	BT
IgM (mg/ml)	0.03	0.05	>100	BT	BT	BT
Alb (mg/ml)	0.90	BT	BT	BT	BT	BT

Table III : INFLUENCE OF THE DEGREE OF PURITY OF THE FVIII PREPARATIONS INJECTED ON H-SEPH-4B ON THE FINAL PURITY OF THE ELUTED PRODUCT.
(BT:Below Threshold)

Stability of the purified FVIII

A major inconvenience with many of the previously reported purified FVIII preparation was their stability and activation. On the other hand it is known that the FVIII is stabilised by complexing with Von Willebrand factor. We have seen from Table III that our purified preparations have ≈ 60 to 70% VWf. This should ensure good stability of the FVIII. In fact the fractions purified on the H-B-Seph.4B. were subjected to stability tests with and without added albumin to ensure stability as described by Ruttyn et al., 1989. We observed that the preparation were stable for more than 24 hours at 25°C even without the addition of protein stabiliser (e.g.albumin.).

Binding site

The factor FVIII-VWf complex is known to dissociate in the presence of calcium (Tuddenham et al., 1979) The purification scheme worked out here uses 0.3 M $CaCl_2$ in the eluting buffer. Hence, a priori we are eluting the FVIII separated from VWf.

The FVIII:C protein is composed of a heavy chain of Mr 210 kDa. and a light chain of Mr 80kDa. linked by a calcium. It was important first to know whether the binding of FVIII-VWf complex occurs at FVIII:C or at the VWF part of the protein complex. Hence we injected separately, immunopurified preparations of FVIII:C and that of VWf (Bihoreau et al., 1989) on a H-B-Seph-4B column. We found that both FVIII and VWf can bind independently to this sorbent with a somewhat tighter binding of VWf. Furthermore, we tried to identify the recognition site on the FVIII:C by adsorbing onto H-B-Seph.4B, the light and heavy chains of FVIII:C separated by immunoadsorption using the antilightchain epitope-Ac463-A8- as ligand followed by dissociation with EDTA. As shown in Fig 2 only the light chain was seen to bind to H-B-Seph-4B. So, at least in the case of FVIII:C binding to the adsorbent, we can the binding site is located in the light chain. The light chain corresponding to 80 Kd has many potentiel sites for recognising the immobilized histidine due to ion-pairing and hydrophobic interactions. Hence, at this present stage of investigation, it is difficult to attribute the binding to any specific peptide sequence in the light chain. However, it is clearly demonstrated that the FVIII:C binds to H-B-Seph-4B at the light chain.

Depyrogenation

One of the important qualities of injectable purified plasma protein preparations is their pyrogen free nature. Pyrogens are endotoxins secreted by gram negative bacteria (e.g. *E.Coli*) which can be the contaminants during the different steps of the purification process. Hence, it was very important to include a final depyrogenation step in the obtention of purified FVIII preparation.

It is known that immobilized histidine and histamine are good adsorbents for endotoxins (Minobe et al., 1982). So, it was all the more important to study the adsorption and desorption conditions for the endotoxins on the H-B-Seph-4B used for preparing high purity FVIII:C. The Table IV shows the influence of different buffer composition at pHs ranging from 5.5 to 7.0, on the retention of endotoxins on the column. A 10 ml solution having 200 EU/ml was injected in each case. We find that ≈ 95% of the injected endotoxins were retained on the column at pH 6.0 using Tris-HCl buffer. But we have to note that, this pH with the same Tris-HCl buffer is also the adsorption pH for the FVIII:C. However, the elution buffer containing 0.1 M Glycine + 0.03 M Lysine and 0.3 M $CaCl_2$ at pH 7.0 was able to elute only FVIII and not the endotoxins as shown in Table V. Only 7 EU of the 250 EU of endotoxins from the injected preparation were found with eluted fractions decreasing the endotoxin/FVIII ration from 5 to 0.23. It is to be noted that the endotoxins assay in the eluted fraction was realised after eliminating the calcium ions by dialysis, as the latter interfere in the assay method. To ensure the validity of this data, a rabbit test was performed as described in Materials Methods section. The rabbits did not show any increase in their body temperature. We have also, analysed the material bound to the column, after stripping it with 0.5 M NaOH, and accounted for the rest of the endotoxins.

The observed strong affinity of endotoxins from different strain of *E.Coli* and *Salmonella* can be attributed to the hydrophobic complimentarity between the endotoxins and the immobilized histidine.

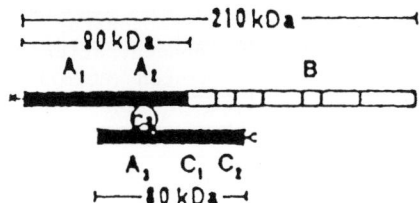

Heavy chain : A1, A2 Domain
Light chain : A3, C1, C2 Domain

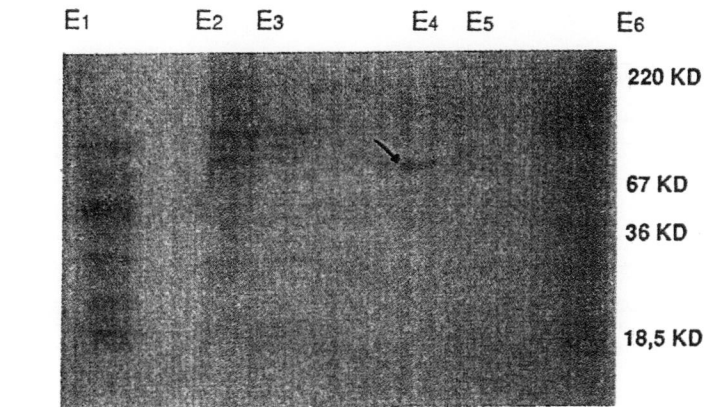

80 Kd band corresponding to light chain

E1, E6 : Molecular weight markers
E2 : 150µl - immunoadsorbent with FVIII:C (both light and heavy chains)
E3 : 150µl - immunoadsorbent + FVIII:C (heavy chain removed by EDTA after adsorption)
E4 : 150µl - H-B-Seph.4B gel after incubation with FVIII:C light chain.
E5 : 150µl - H-B-Seph.4B gel after incubation with FVIII:C heavy chain.

pH	Buffer	Endotoxines retention %	Endotoxines concentration eluted (EU/ml)
5.5	Tris-HCl	50	40
6	Phosphate	92	10
7	Phosphate	50	27
6	Tris-HCl	95	7
7	Tris-HCl	10	80

Table IV. : INFLUENCE OF pH AND BUFFER COMPOSITION ON THE RETENTION OF ENDOTOXINS ON H-B-SEPH-4B. (10 ml ≈ 200EU/ml endotoxins injected in each case)

Fractions	FVIII:c (U/ml)	Volume (ml)	Endotoxines (EU/ml)	% FVIII:c	% Endotoxines	Endotoxine/ FVIII
Initial extract	50	10	250	100	100	5
Non absorbed	<0.05	30	0.19	<0.1	0.1	0
Eluted	30	20	7	99	7	0.23

Table V. : PURIFICATION OF FVIIIC AND ENDOTOXIN REMOVAL USING H-B-SEPH-4B (See text for details)

In conclusion we can say that the H-B-Seph-4B is an excellent alternative chromatographic sorbent for the efficient purification of pyrogen free FVIII from plasma. Moreover, the purified preparation contains about 60% of the VWf, thus ensuring good stability of the preparation.

References

Austen, D.E.G., and Smith, J.K. (1982): Thromb. Haemost. Stuggart. 48, 46.

Baggerman, C., and Kannegieter, L.M. (1984) : Appl. Environ. Micorbiol. 48, 662-664.

Bihoreau, N., Sauger, A., Yon, M.J., and Van de Pol, H. (1989) : Eur. J. Biochem. 185, 111-118.

Bussey, D.M. and Tsuji, K. (1989) : J. Parenter. Sci. Techn. 38, 228-233.

Ezzedine, M. (1990): Thèse de docteur 3ème cycle, Université de Technologie de Compiègne.

Milner, K.C. (1973) : J. Infect. Dis. Suppl. 128, S237-S245.

Minobe, S., Sato, T., Tosa, T., and Chibata, I. (1982) : J. Chrom. 248, 401-408.

Pearson, F.C., Dubczak, J., Nakashima, C., and Carpenter D.F. (1984) : J. Parenter. Sci. Techn. 38, 196-198.

Ruttyn, Y., Brandin, M.P. and Vijayalakshmi M.A. (1989): J. Chrom. 491, 299-308.

Sundberg, L., and Porath, J. (1974) : J. Chrom. 90, 87-98.

Tuddenham, E.G.D., Trabold, N.C., Collins, J.A. and Hoyer, L.W. (1979) : J. Lab.Clin.Med. 93, 40-53.

Vijayalakshmi, M.A. (1989): Tibetch. 7 (3), 71-76.

Vijayalakshmi, M.A. (1992) : in"Practical Protein Chromatography" ed. Kenney, A. and Fowell, S. Methods in Molecular Biology vol. 11, 33-44.

Résumé

Le facteur anti-hémophilique A du plasma humain a été retenu de façon spécifique à pH 6.0 à faible force ionique sur des gels d'agarose couplés avec de l'histidine. Une élution avec un tampon contenant Gly 0.1 M, Lys 0.3 M et CaCl2 0.3 M, pH 7.0 a été efficace pour récupérer la quasi totalité du FVIII:C injecté avec ≈ 60% de VWf. Seuls fibronectine et fibrinogène sont des contaminants présents en très faibles quantités. Le ligand histidine immobilisé, semble reconnaitre le FVIII:C et le VWf indépendamment à des sites spécifiques. De plus, le site d'association entre le ligand immobilisé et le FVIII:C se situe sur la chaine légère de FVIII:C.
Le complexe FVIII:C + VWf ainsi purifié a pu être dépyrogénéisé en utilisant la même colonne, car les conditions de désorption de FVIII:C - VWf et celles de pyrogènes sont différentes.

The effect of monosaccharides glucose and fructose during 80°C heat treatment of a factor VIII concentrate

A. Knevelman and H.J.C. de Wit

Red Cross Bloodbank Friesland, Leeuwarden, The Netherlands

INTRODUCTION

Since july 1991 a factor VIII concentrate, heat treated at 80°C during 72 hours in dry state, is manufactured in 3 Dutch bloodbanks. In these centres intermediate products of 4 additional bloodbanks are manufactured into the finished product. The fractionation of ca. 15 liter plasma results in a batch of 10 bottles containing 200-400 IU of factor VIII each. The total production of ca. 5 miljon IU each year is distributed to hospitals and haemophiliacs for home treatment.

Method * Cryoprecipitation
* Precipitation of contaminating proteins with glycine
* Precipitation of factor VIII with sodium chloride
* Diafiltration against freeze drying buffer
* Freeze drying
* Heat treatment, 72 h, 80°

The 80°C dry heat treatment has a good safety record with regard to the transmission of the Hepatitis C virus (NANBHV) and HIV by coagulation factor concentrates (Pasi et al., 1990; Watson et al., 1992). The effect of this virucidal method on the labile factor VIII protein is a resultant of several factors :

Product formulation after freezing * proteins (cryoprecipitation and purification)
* additives (freezedrying buffer)
* crystal size (freezing method)
Freezedrying process

Sucrose is added to the freeze drying buffer of severely heated factor VIII concentrates in order to act as a stabilizer of factor VIII (Winkelman et al., 1989;

McIntosh et al., 1987, 1990). In this article, it will be demonstrated that a partial hydrolysis of sucrose into glucose and fructose can cause a very detrimental effect during the heat tretament of the producton the factor VIII yield and resolution behaviour. Finally, the effect of glucose during the validation of the virus reduc-tion will be discussed.

THE EFFECT OF GLUCOSE AND FRUCTOSE DURING PRODUCT DEVELOPMENT & PRODUCTION

During the development of the severely heated factor VIII concentrate a freeze-drying buffer was used composed of 2% (w/v) sucrose, 2.5mM calciumchloride, 15mM tris and 20mM tri sodium citrate. The conversion from unsterilized to autoclaved freezedrying buffer caused a substantial decrease in yield during the heattreatment of the product (table 1, A and B). The impaired yields could partly be reversed by lowering the shelf temperarature from 0°C to -20°C during primary drying (table 1, C). Best results were obtained using unsterilized freeze-drying buffer and a low shelf temperature during primary drying (table 1, D).

Table 1.

Batches	A (n=4)	B (n=3)	C (n=2)	D (n=2)
Autoclaved buffer	no	yes	yes	no
Shelf temp.primary dr.	0	0	-20	-20
Shrinking/collaps	yes	yes	no	no
Resolution time	2 min.	4-6 min.	3-4 min.	1-2 min.
Solution	clear	d.yellow	yellow	clear
Yield FVIII over FD/HT	80-90%	35-45%	60-63%	88%

Based on kinetic considerations, a buffer was prepared containing 1% sucrose and a modified heat treatment of 100°C during 1 hour was applied. The products prepared with this buffer showed a high yield of factor VIII (88%) over freeze-drying and heattreatment. This buffer is currently used in routine production in combination with the low shelf temperature of -20°C during the primary drying of the product.

The analysis of non-heated and heated buffers showed a partial, temperature dependent hydrolysis of sucrose in the heated buffers (Table 2.)

Table 2.

	Buffer 1 (batches A,D)	Buffer 2 (batches B,C)	Buffer 3 (production)
Thermal treatment	not heated	120°C, 20 min	100°C, 1 h
Sucrose % (w/v)	2%	2%	1%
Sucrose (g/l)	20.34	19.88	10.02
Glucose (g/l)	-	0.110	0.019
Fructose (g/l)	-	0.096	0.014

The detrimental effect of concentrations of fructose and glucose as low as 0.1-0.2 g/l was confirmed by freezedrying and heattreating products spiked with increasing levels of these monosaccharides (table 3).

Table 3.

	Vial X Control	Vial Y Spiked 50µl	Vial Z Spiked 100µl
Sucrose (g/l)	10.00	10.00	10.00
Glucose (g/l)	0.02	0.12	0.22
Fructose (g/l)	0.02	0.12	0.22
Colour, cake	white	cream	light brown
Dissolutiontime	2.30'	7.00'	unsoluble
Colour, solution	clear	yellow	brown
Debris	no	some	thick clot
FVIII yield, FD/HT	56%	22%	7%

THE EFFECT OF GLUCOSE DURING THE VALIDATION OF VIRUS REDUCTION

Glucose can also interfere with the dry heattreatment during the in-vitro validation of the virusreduction. It is present as a substrate in the medium for the host-cells during the cultivation of the virus, and the non-metabolized residual is added to the product with the virus.

Validation of virus reduction
- * Production of a high titer virus inoculum from a host cell culture
- * Spiking of the product
- * Simulation of freeze drying and heat treatment processes
- * Reconstitution of product and determination of residual virus levels (TCID$_{50}$)

The results of the validation study loose much their value if the virus inoculum should alter product characteristics. In order to investigate the effect, vials of a routine production batch were spiked after fill with two solutions.

Solution 1 : fresh RPMI 1640 medium
Solution 2 : supernatant of a culture of host cells for HIV-1 in RPMI 1640 after a cultivation cycle that is known to produce a high titer HIV-1 inoculum (PFC, Edinburgh)

In products spiked with fresh medium a correlation was found between the volume added and the decrease in yield, the loss of solubility and the degree of discolouration of the plug and the solution after reconstitution. In products spiked with supernatant medium used to grow HIV-host cells for 4 days there was no effect on yield, a slight increase in dissolution time at high spiking level and only a slight discolouration of the solution after reconstitution (table 4).

Table 4.

	Control	Fresh 1/20	Fresh 1/10	Spent 1/20	Spent 1/10
Colour of plug	white	cream	cream	white	white
Resolution time	1.40'	-	-	1.45'	3.00
Colour of solution	clear	dark yellow	yellow brown	slight yellow	yellow
Debris	no	small clots	brown clot	no	no
FVIII yield over FD/HT	69%	48%	<20%	68%	67%

Before the actual validation of the reduction of HIV-1 and Sindbis as a model virus for HCV, the laboratory that was contracted to perform the study simulated the cultivation procedure that was used for the production of the high titer HIV-1 and Sindbis inocula with uninfected host cells.

The host cells for cultivating Sindbis were grown in EMEM medium, containing originally 1 g/l D-glucose. In the supernatant medium however no residual level of glucose could be detected, and therefore during the validation of the inactivation of this virus during 80°C heattreatment no special precautions were taken.

The HIV-1 host cells were cultivated in RPMI 1640, containing originally 2 g/l D-glucose. In this case, in the supernatant of the cell culture a substantial level of glucose was determined (1.65 g/l). At the intended spiking volume of 10%, it can be expected from table 3 that this level would give rise to altered product characteristics. In this case it therefore was necessary to implement a procedure to remove glucose and other low M.W. substances from the virus inoculum.

ACKNOWLEDGEMENTS

The authers would like to thank B. Griffin, H. Hart and R.V. McIntosh (Protein Fractionation Centre, Edinburgh); J.M. de Bruijn (C.S.M. Suiker BV, Central laboratory); D. Vacante and M. Meseck (Microbiological Associates, Rockville, USA)

REFERENCES

Pasi K.J., Evans J.A., Skidmore S.J. and Hill F.G.H. (1990): Prevention of hepatitis C virus infection in haemophiliacs. In Lancet 335: 1473-1474.

McIntosh R.V., Docherty N., Fleming D. and Foster P.R. (1987): A high yield factor VIII concentrate suitable for advanced heat treatment. In Thromb. Haemostas 58:306.

McIntosh R.V. and Foster P.R. (1990): The effect of solution formulation on the stability and surface interactions of factor VIII during plasma fractionatin. In Transfusion Science 11: 55-66.

Watson, H.G., Ludlam C.A., Rebus S. et al. (1992): Use of several serological assays to determine the true prevalence of hepatitis C virus infection in haemophiliacs treated with non-virus inactivated factor VIII and IX concentrates. In Br. J. Haematology 80/4: 514-518.

Winkelman L., Owen N.E., Evans D.R., Haddon M.E., Smith J.K., Prince P.J., Williams J.D. and Lane R.S.: Severely heated therapeutic factor VIII concentrate of high specific activity. In Vox Sang 57: 97-103.

Three year experience with plasma derived factor VIIa concentrate

F. Verroust[1], Y. Laurian[3], J. Chabbat[3] and M.-J. Larrieu[2]

[1]Bio-Transfusion, Zac Paris Nord II, 117, avenue des Nations, BP 60079, 95973 Roissy CDG Cedex; [2]Hôpital de Bicêtre, 78, avenue du Général Leclerc, 94275 Le Kremlin-Bicêtre Cedex and [3]CNTS, avenue des Tropiques, BP 100, 94943 Les Ulis, France

SUMMARY :

Eighteen severe hemophiliacs (15 A, 3B) with high responder inhibitors participated in a 3 year study of a plasma derived FVIIa concentrate, solvent detergent treated. The kinetic study measured half life about 2 hours. Prothrombin time was significantly shortened (2-4 seconds from initial value). The efficacy was evaluated on 220 hemarthroses and hematomas, partly on home treatment. The following guidelines are suggested : each treatment should include 2 infusions at 4-6 hour interval; the dose should be 200 U/kg/infusion in moderate bleeds (large volume, target joint, trauma or late treatment >6h) and 150 U/kg/infusion in mild bleeds. With these conditions, 82% of good results were observed. Ten severe bleedings received higher doses, mainly with excellent results. No DIC nor thromboses occured. Anamnestic response was only observed in 1 hemophiliac B at 10 BU. Provided the suggested guidelines were followed, efficacy was good in minor, moderate and most severe bleeds with an excellent tolerance and viral safety (HIV=0/7). Further study is needed to determine dosage during severe bleeds and surgery.

In hemophilic patients, the development of an inhibitor remains a major complication of substitution therapy. Several first generation products (for instance Feiba and Autoplex) have been available for 10 years. Nevertheless their use is not always satisfactory;

We describe a 3 year study of a plasma derived activated factor VII concentrate (Acset). Factor VIIa concentrate is obtained from the supernatant of cryoprecipitate after a chromatographic step described by J. Chabbat[1]. It is virally inactivated by a solvent detergent procedure. Eighteen hemophilic patients with anti factor VIII or anti factor IX inhibitor were included in this study. All were high responders. The protocol was submitted for ethical committee approval and patients and children's parents gave an informed consent. The protocol involved two different steps :

- *Phase I* : Nine participated in a pharmacokinetic study. When not bleeding, they received one Acset infusion of 78 to 168 U/kg. Clinical and biological tolerance was excellent. Significant shortening of the prothrombin times was observed (2-4 secondes of initial values).

- The *Phase II* study was itself subdivided into several parts :

a) A _prospective protocol_ was followed <u>for minor bleeds</u> : A Case Report Form detailed site of the bleed, severity, delay since first symptoms, and asked if the bleed was spontaneous or post-traumatic and if it occured in a target joint. Results were evaluated on objective and subjective criteria : pain, mobility and enlargement of the joint or the muscle.

Thirteen patients participated in this trial while 220 bleeding episodes (hemarthroses and muscle hematomas) were recorded in 18 months. Doses of 68 to 300 U/kg/injection were infused once or twice, at 4 to 6 hour-intervals. Satisfactory results (excellent or good) were observed in 71 percent of total cases. Site of hemarthrosis had no effect on efficacy.

In the first part of the trial, episodes were treated with a **single infusion** of VIIa. The incidence of "excellent" and "good" results increased as dosages rose from 70 U/kg to 200 U/kg. Other episodes were treated with **2 infusions**. The incidence of good and excellent results increased with two infusions administered at a short interval (below 6 hours). Best results were obtained when an **early treatment** was followed by a repeat dose performed 4 hours later. Especially with hemarthroses, *early treatment* is the key to the best results. In hematomas results were similar whatever the severity of the bleeding. In contrast, efficacy of Acset on the hemarthroses treatment was far better in mild and moderate bleeds compared to severe bleeds

b) Once the efficacy of Acset had been confirmed in phase IIa, *home treatment* was practiced by 2 outpatients. Within one year, more than 30 bleeding episodes were recorded. Excellent clinical tolerance and "excellent" or "good" results were recorded in most episodes.

c) During the 18 months of study, some *limb-threatening bleeding episodes* occurred and Acset was infused with good results in most of them : four ilio-psoas hematoma (2 with femoral palsy), a severe calf hematoma, two episodes of bleeding in a pelvic pseudo-tumour, wound of the wrist needing a suture, a femoral fracture.without developing a thigh hematoma. No bleed occured when intra-femoral pins were removed.

CONCLUSION

This plasma derived VIIa concentrate (Acset) was convenient to use with 10 to 30 ml per infusion and therapeutic dose was administered within 5-10 minutes. Clinical tolerance was always "excellent". No biological signs of in vivo thrombogenicity were observed in all the tests performed. Most of the bleeds recorded in this study on efficacy of Acset were mild or moderate. Efficacy was evaluated at 24 hours: 71 percent had "excellent" and "good" results. Increasing efficacy was observed with :

- Short delay between first symptoms and treatment, mainly for hemarthroses.
- Dose above $\geq$ 150 U/kg per infusion and a systematic second injection performed at 4-6 hours.

Anamnesis was only observed in 1 out of the 3 hemophilia B patients and none in hemophilia A patients. None of the 7 HIV negative patients seroconverted. Efficacy was good in minor, moderate and in most (9/10) limb-threatening bleeds treated. Nevertheless further study is needed to determine dosage and frequency of injections for severe hemarthroses and emergency surgery.

REFERENCES :

1 - Chabbat J., Hampikian-Lenin S. et al. 1989
   A human factor VIIa concentrate and its effects in the hemophilic A dog.
   Thromb. Research, *54,* 603-612.

2 - Laurian Y., Verroust F. et al 1990
   Human plasma derived factor VIIa (Acset) for treatment of hemophilia A or B patients with inhibitors
   World Federation of Hemophilia. Washington. (abstract n°46).

3 - Laurian Y., Verroust F. et al 1992
   3 Year experience with plasma derived activated factor VII (Acset)
   World Federation of Hemophilia. Athens (abstract n° 353).

Résumé

Dix-huit hémophiles sévères avec inhibiteur fort répondeur ont participé à l'étude d'un concentré plasmatique de facteur VIIa traité par solvant détergent. La demi-vie est environ 2 heures. Un raccourcissement notable du temps de quick est observé (2-4 secondes de la valeur initiale). L'efficacité a été appréciée sur 220 hémarthroses et hématomes. Pour un traitement efficace, les consignes suivantes sont proposées : chaque traitement doit comporter 2 injections administrées à 4-6 heures d'intervalle à la dose de 200 U/kg/injection pour les accidents modérés (volumineux, traumatiques ou traités tardivement > 6h, articulation cible) et 150 U/kg/injection suffit pour les accidents mineurs. Dans ces conditions, 82% de bons résultats sont enregistrés. Dix accidents sévères ont reçu des doses plus fortes. Aucune CIVD ni thrombose n'est survenue, une seule réponse anamnestique a été observée chez un hémophile B à 10 UB. Dans les conditions précitées, l'efficacité a été bonne dans les accidents mineurs, modérés et la plupart des accidents graves avec une tolérance excellente et une innocuité virale (VIH : 0/7). Reste à définir les doses efficaces lors d'accidents graves et lors de la chirurgie.

III. Purification of IgG
and albumin

III. *Purification des IgG
et de l'albumine*

Application of chromatography system in plasma protein fractionation on pilot scale

Zhao Shuliang, Zhong lu, Zhou Quing, Luo liang, Li Shujin and Chen Chunsheng

Research Department of Plasma Derivatives, Chengdu Institute of Biological Products, Chengdu, China

Abstracts

The Clinical demand increasingly of both variety developing and quality improving for plasma derivatives has urged us to seek new technique for plasma protein fractionation.

In recent years, based on the chromatography procedure by Curling etc. we have finished laboratory research and steped in pilot scale chromatography with part of import devices fitted with most domestic equipments and utilities to form a complete set. After getting success of trial run author tried to do some comparative research for process procedures and parameters related so as to make this system more efficiency and consumate, then were ready for the successive running by combining the main chromatogr phy technique of ionexchange and gelfiltration with membrane filtration technique.

The batch size was enlarged from 16 L to 64 L of plasma. By means of quality control, biochemical and immunological analysis of albumin and IgG from above system, the results indicated that the quality accorded with the requirment of Chinese Regulation for Biological Products and WHO Stipulation related. The recoveries of albumin and IgG after sterilfiltration are 2.47gm and 0.65gm / per 100ml plasma respectively. The stability observation of albumin under 4–8 ℃, 25℃ and 37℃ for one to five month showed its good stability without polymer except small ammount of dimer (<3%) at 37℃ for one month. Only anti–HCV, HBsAg and anti–HIV negative plasma pooling was used for manufacture; the resource plasma contained high titer of anti–HBsAg as well. Heat treatment (60℃, 10 hours) for final albumin products and unfinished IgG is another effective step for virus inactivation. In addition we have explored inactivation or elimination effect of distributing and diluting as well as heating. Above trial the Sindbis, VSV, Polio, CMV, Mumps viruses etc. were taken as virus markers of which the titer in plasma was 10^7 TID 50 / ml. Preliminary result has expressed there is difinite efficiency for the safey of the products in our process procedure.

1 Method

1.1 Process Procedures

We take Pharmacia Chromatography system for plasma protein fractionation.

1.1.1 Pretreatment of human plasma

The plasma was desalted and followed by euglobulin removing. For liquid–solid separtion, the filtration was used instead of centrifugation. The pH adjustment was finished with adding the buffer.

1.1.2 DEAE–Sepharose chromatography

The plasma pretreated as above was applied on this column and eluted the albumin fraction with pH 4.5 acetate buffer.

1.1.3 CM–Sepharose chromatography

The DEAE–albumin was applied directly on CM–column, After eluting the albumin fraction the CM–albumin was concentrated through an ultrafiltration unit.

1.1.4 The adsorption of CM–albumin at low pH

The CM–albumin was adjusted pH to 4–4.5 by adding dilution of HCl followed mixing the filter aids to 2% (W / V). After stirring about 20 minutes, the mixture was pumped through a filter.

1.1.5 Gelfiltration

The CM–albumin filtrate was furtherly purified on the Sephacryl S–200 column with several application.

The monomer of albumin was collected and adjusted pH to 6.8–7.0.

1.1.6 Ultrafiltration and formulation of albumin solution

1.1.7 The post treatment of albumin solution

The concentrated albumin would be followed by sterilfiltration, filling, Pasterizing and quanantining.

1.2 Study for some process procedures of albumin   separation with chromatography system.

1.2.1 The series experiment for desalting effect of different application amount of plasma.

The condition of experiment was as follow: column dimension (2.6× 60cm), flow rate: (20ml / min). The proportion of plasma sample / column (v / v) was 6–18% . The plasma fraction from column was detected for protein concentration and conductivity.

1.2.2 Optimization of pH for euglobulin precipitation. Salt poor plasma was taken every 50ml in series at pH 5.0, 5.1, 5.2, 5.3, 5.4, 5.5, then analyized for supernatant and precipitate.

1.2.3. Study of some parameters related to the acidic adsorption of CM–albumin

In order to improve the appearance of final albumin products and choice optimal condition, three group experiments of acidic adsorption had been finished. It included pH series (pH 3.0, 3.5, 4.0, 4.5, 5.0); concentration series of adsorbents (1%, 2%, 3%, 4%, 5%, adsorbent / volume of CM–albumin = g / 100ml); different kinds of adsorbent series. Then analysis and quality control would followed for above samples.

1.2.4. Optimization of application frequency of CM–albumin in Sephacryl S–200 chromatography

Usually for 64L / batch, the gelfiltration would lasts 32–36 hours through BP 252 column series packed with Sephacryl S–200. In order to shorten this period and get good resolution We tryed to compare different application points of sample in several cycles.

1.3 Quality control of biochemical and immunological analysis for chromatograpy albumin

Above detection and analysis were finished according to the " Regulation of Chinese Biological Products" (1990, vol ist edition) and routine methods in the laboratories.

1.4 Immunogenity analysis of chromatography albumin

The albumin products from Cohn and chromatography methods were immunolized in rabbits. Then we made several analysis as the methods in 1.3 with the albumins and rabbit antiserum against corresponding albumins individually.

1.5 Study for the biological half life of albumin in vivo (rabbit)

The albumin products from Cohn and chromatography methods marked with ^{125}I were injected introvenously in rabbits, blood samples drawed out at different interval time (1.3.6 hours and 1.3.5.4.5.7.9 days) respectively were furtherly analyized for the radio activity and the "half life" was calculated as well.

1.6 The preliminary evaluation of virus safty for chromatography albumin

The proportion of starting materia vs viruses were 9/ 1 (v / v). This mixture contained virus titer to 10^7TCID 50 / ml. The first group had made for the effection of the distribution and viruses depletion during the process. The second experiment was only for the elimination of viruses in Sephacryl S–200, and the heat treatment was finished for viruses inactivation with Polio. VSV, Mumps viruses etc. Samples were taken every step.

The detection of above viruses had made complying with general tissue (cell) culture methods. The procedures of both the cell culture with BHK cell–line and EIA were used for Sindbis and VSV. Hep–2 cell–line human 2BS cell and vero cell–line were used for the titer detection of Polio–I Sabinal strain, CMV–AD 169 Strain and Mumps–WM 84 Strain respectively.

2 Result

2.1 Purification result of albumin for each step in different scale of chromatography

The efficiency of every chromatography procedure are expressed as the purities (%) by acetate cellulose electrophoresis (ACE) as Table 1 and Fig · 1.

Table 1   The purity results of every chromatography procedure by ACE

No. of batch	Purity	Process steps of chromatography				
		Pretreatment	DEAE–	CM–	acidic adsorption of CM–albumin	gelfitration
92–4	%	69.44	93.14	96.56	92.03	99.14
92–5	%	70.50	90.20	96.80	97.45	99.80
92–6	%	66.88	92.55	96.64	97.30	99.33
average	%	68.94	91.96	96.67	97.26	99.42

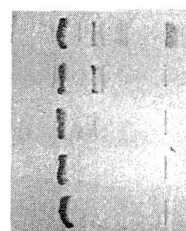

Saltdepletion plasma

DEAE-alb

CM-alb

CM-alb adsorpted at low pH

Final product of alb

Fig · 1 The pattern of every chromatography step by ACE

The chromatogram of albumin separation in various scale of plasma per batch showed that all above chromatogram of corresponding step were identical, if the hight of column, linear flow rate, ratio of sample vs the bed volume of matrix and buffer system etc. are same.

2.2 Some results of the parameters optimization for process procedures of albumin
2.2.1 The effect of different oppication amount of sample in desalting step. (Table 2)

Table 2 The compareson of desalting effect for different application ratio of plasma

ratio of application* (V/V)	6%	8%	10%	12%	14%	16%	18%
Volume of application (ml)	21.6	28.8	36.0	43.2	50.4	57.6	64.8
recovery of protein %	98%	98.3%	97.6%	97.2%	96.1%	95.2%	94.3%
pH	7.89 ± 0.06	7.89 ± 0.04	7.90 ± 0.03	7.96 ± 0.04	7.96 ± 0.03	8.00 ± 0.01	8.00 ± 0.04
Conductivity (ms)	0.42 ± 0.07	0.48 ± 0.01	0.64 ± 0.02	0.68 ± 0.03	0.89 ± 0.02	1.13 ± 0.02	1.35 ± 0.05

* each proportion was tested for five times

Above result showed the desire proportion of smaple / column is about 10–12% at which both the volume of sample application and recovery are rather high and the conductivity of plasma fraction meet the range needed next step for removing impurity.

2.2.2 The optimal pH for preciptating of residual proteins (Table 3)

Table 3 The results of ACE for the fractionsand weighting of precipitate after precipitating salt-deplection plasma

pH (± 0.05)	Wt. of pricitate (g)	Supernant		
		$\gamma(\%)$	$\alpha+\beta(\%)$	A(%)
5.00	1.92 ± 0.10	25.9 ± 1.7	15.7 ± 1.1	58.0 ± 0.6
5.20	1.54 ± 0.06	28.8 ± 1.0	12.7 ± 0.7	58.3 ± 1.0
5.40	1.40 ± 0.04	27.2 ± 0.7	16.2 ± 1.9	56.5 ± 0.8
5.6	1.32 ± 0.05	23.2 ± 0.8	18.8 ± 09.	58.0 ± 0.6
5.80	1.25 ± 0.06	23.0 ± 08	19.2 ± 0.8	57.8 ± 0.5
6.00	1.20 ± 0.04	20.4 ± 0.6	21.4 ± 0.6	58.2 ± 0.6

The optimal pH for impurity depletion is 5.20 ± 0.5 at which the impurities ($\alpha + \beta$) were largely removed, and the losing of albumin and γ-globulin was at lowest degree.

2.2.3 The result of removing lipids by acidification and adsorption (Table 4, 5, 6 and Fig. 2, 3)

Table 4 The result of acidification for CM-albumin at different pH*.

result	pH for acidification	3.0	3.5	4.0	4.5	5.0
losing of CM-Alb after adsorption (%)		4.82	4.40	3.57	3.05	2.45
appearance of final albumin	without treating	++	++	++	++	++
	after treating	–	–	–	–	–
	quarantine	–	–	–	–	±
	shaking 14 days	±	±	–	–	+

* the absorbent is 2.5% filter aids. "–": clear; "+":cloudy and particles; "++": more particles

Table 5 The result of different concentration of adsorbent for CM-albumin*

resnlts	Concentration of absorbent	0.5%	1%	2%	3%	4%
losing of CM-alb after adsorption (%)		1.73	2.14	2.83	3.64	4.86
appearance of final albumin	without treating	++	++	++	++	++
	after treating	–	–	–	–	–
	quarantine	+	±	–	–	–
	shaking 14 days	±	+	–	–	–

* the pH after acidification was 4.5 with the filter aids as adsorbent

139

Table 6 The adsorption results of different adsorbents *

results	adsorbent	2% filter aids	2% charcoal	2%** filter aids +charcoal
losing of CM−ale after adsorption (%)		2.62	2.84	2.75
appearance of final albumin	without treating	++	++	++
	after treating	−	−	−
	quarantine	−	−	−
	shaking 14 days	−	±	−

* the pH of acidification was 4.5   ** 1% for each

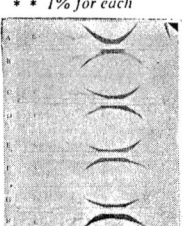

A, B, C: the altumin products of 92~4, 92~5, 92~6 without adsorption; D, E, F: the same batches as above which were acidified and asorpted; G: chromatography albumin made in other country; H: Cohn's albumin.

Fig·2 The pattern of immunoelectrophoresis for albumin

From Fig. 2, some faint precipitate lines were visible at α, β position, and mainly disappeared for the albumin from the CM-alb acidified and adsorpted.

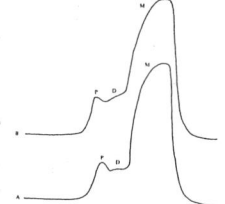

A: CM−alb without treatment;   B: CM−alb adsorped at low PH;   P: polymer;   D: dimer;   M: monomer

Fig. 3 The chromatogram of Sephacryl S-200 for different condition of CM-albumin

As Fig·2 more dimers of CM-albumin appeared after adsorption at low pH than that of CM−alb without adsorption.

According to above results, We choiced optimal parameters of acidification and adsorption as follow: the optimal pH = 4.0−4.5, adsorbent: filter aids or the mixture of filter aids and charcoal, concentration of adsorbent: 2%. After adsorption about 20 minutes at low pH, the albumin molecule extends and releases out the residual lipids which were eveloped in original molecule. Then it was absorbed on the filter aids and removed by filtration. So that the apprearance of final albumin was improved remarkablly.

2.2.4 Chromatography results of different application points for CM−albumin on Sephacryl S−200 column

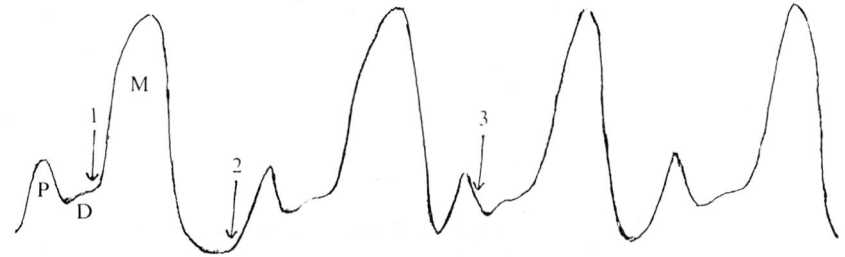

Fig·4 Chromatogram of different application position on Sephacryl S−200 column;
P: polymer;   D: Dimer; M: Monomer;   1, 2, 3: The points for application of sample;

From the chromatogram as above, the optimal application position of smaple for S-200 column is at the back part of polymer peak (3) where we obtained both the desire separation effect and the shortest running time (18-20 hours less than before).

2.2.5 The result of pyrogen monitoring for distill water (DW) and protein fractions by Limulus polyphemus test and rabbit test.

Having monitored successively more than fifteen batches for pyrogen of DW and protein fractions in pilot scale, we have never found the pyrogen contamination problem.

2.2.6 The result indicated that the main parameter HETP of all the columns still conformed to the requirement for nice resolution.

2.3 The result of quality control for albumin products of 17 batches from chromatography process all meet the "Regulation of P.R. China" (1990, Vol. I)

2.4 Various biochemical and immunological analysis illustrated that the quality of our chromatography albumin was perfectly consilent with the albumin from other procedures. The identity of above albumins had been confirmed as well. (Fig. 5, 6, 7, 8)

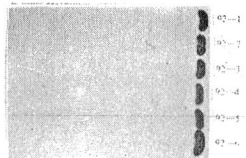

Fig · 5 The PAGE pattern of chromatography albumin

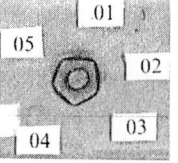

Fig · 6 The pattern of double-dimersion immunodiffusion
01: chro-alb 92-4; 02: chr-alb 92-5; 03: chr-alb 92-6; 04: chr-alb (made in other country); 05: Cohn-alb; centrol hole: rabbit antisera against Cohn-albumin

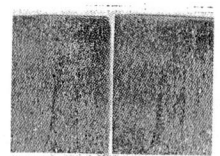

A: chr-alb 92-5; rabbit antisera. against chr-albumin in the agarose
B: chr-alb 92-5; rabbit antisera against Cohn-albumin in the agarose

Fig · 7 The pattern of Cross-immunoelectrophoresis for chromatography albumin

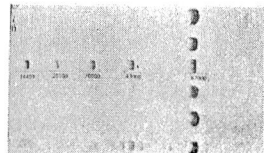

Cohn-alb
chr-alb (made in other country)
standard proteins
chr-alb 92-2
chro-alb 92-1
plasma

Fig · 8 The pattern of SDS PAGE for albumins

The estimation of chr=alb (92-1, 92-2) according to Fig.8 is about 6.7KD showed no difference from Cohn-alb and chr-alb made in other country.

2.5 The result of Circular dichroism analysis for albumin (Fig · 9, 10)

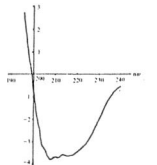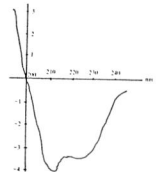

Fig · 9-10 The pattern of circular dichroism

distance of optical path: 0.02 cm; concentration: 0.2 mg / ml; sensitivity: 2×10^{-3}. (Fig.3: Chromatography albumin (chro-alb) Fig.4: (ohn's-albumn (cohn-alb)

.From Fig·9 and Fig·10 the secondary conformation of our chromatography albumin is almost consistant as that of Chon's albumin in our institute. For chro-alb the α-helix, β-plate sheet as well as unregular roll are 50.11%, 22.51%, 27.38% respectively, the corresponding parameters for Cohn's-alb are 50.26%, 21.47%, 28.27%, which are fairly similar as that in reference.

2.6 The result of biological half-life for albumin in vivo of rabbit (Fig·10)

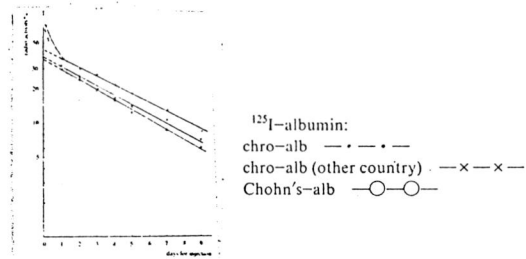

Fig·11 The attenuation curve of ^{125}I-albumin in vivo (rabbit)

Comparing albumin produced by our pilot scale with Cohn's albumin and other chromatography albumin, the results are 96.11 ± 0.01hrs, 95.95 ± 9.62 hrs, 90.00 ± 1.69hrs respectively, which accounts for the similar quality and stability. However, our albumin overpasses the other two control albumins a little in attenuation and stability.

2.7 The basically establishment for the virus inactivation and elimination in chromatography procedures.

The viruses titer of both Sindbis and Polio were removed $10^7 TCID50$/ ml from starting plasma to CM-albumin and only Sephacryl S-200 step respectively.

For the 60°C 10hrs treatment; Polio-I, Sindbis, Mumps and VSV would be eliminated $10^5-10^7 TCID$ 50 / ml after one hour. Howerver, all above viruses included CMV were inacted after more than 3hrs at 60°C.

2.8 The result of stability for chromatography albumin

Three batches of albumin (92-1, 92-2, 92-3) were kept at 4°C, 25°C, 37°C for five month and one month respectively, Some vials of albumin were shaken for 14 days at room temperature. (4hrs per day). Then analysis and observation were followed. There is a litter dimer of albumin (<3%) in the products without polymer. The appearance of albmin meet the regulation (light-yellow-transparent without precipitate). So the stability of our chromatography albumin is satisfied.

(The researchers who had attributed for this subject are as follows: Lu Xiandeng, Chen Maogong, Cai Jun, Huang Yaping, Chen Shuo, Chu Yibo, Liang Quan. And the authors are sincerely grateful to Mrs Li Nanling and Wang Chengshu for their help on biochemical and biological analysis in this subject.)

Development of a process for the preparation of human serum albumin using chromatographic methods

H.B. Yap, I.F. Young, V. Micucci, R.W. Herrington, P.J. Turner and J.R. Davies

Blood Products Development Group, CSL Limited, 45 Poplar Road, Parkville, Victoria 3052, Australia

INTRODUCTION AND SUMMARY

CSL Limited, an Australian bio-pharmaceutical company, is presently constructing a plasma fractionation facility. In this plant, albumin will be purified by chromatographic techniques based on the method developed by Curling et al., (1977). This plant has been designed to process at least 250 tonnes of plasma per annum, with the capability of increasing to 500 tonnes per annum. The chromatographic approach was selected over Cohn fractionation because it is readily automated and results in a product with higher purity, yield and monomer content. Additionally the process can be further developed for the isolation of other plasma proteins. A pilot plant has been established at CSL to evaluate the process, manufacture material for clinical trials and establish design criteria for the new fractionation plant. Evaluation of intermediate fractions and final product showed the process to be extremely reliable. The product was routinely $\geq$ 98% albumin and showed excellent stability with respect to monomer content, pH, aluminium levels, and appearance. Prekallikrein activator (PKA) showed a tendency to increase during storage and the method of manufacture was subsequently modified to overcome this problem. Data from the pilot plant indicate yields will be 25 to 28 grams of albumin per litre of plasma processed.

MATERIALS AND METHODS

Processing methods. Ultrafiltration was conducted using a 50 square foot Millipore Hellicon PHSAT SS50 cartridge (nominal MW cutoff: 30,000). All chromatographic steps were conducted using columns and chromatographic media from Pharmacia, Uppsala, Sweden. Ion-exchange chromatography was conducted on 16 litre Pharmacia KS370 columns (37 cm diameter x 15 cm) using DEAE Sepharose Fast Flow and CM Sepharose Fast Flow (FF) media at a flow rate of 60 litres per hour. Size-exclusion chromatography was performed on a 96 litre (6 x KS370 columns) of Sephacryl S200-HR resin at a flow rate of 24 litres per hour.
Final product was dispensed in neutral type I glass bottles purchased from St. Gobain Desjonqueres, France.

Plasma was processed by Cohn fractionation to remove Fraction I and Fraction II + III. The II+III filtrate was concentrated and diafiltered against 5 mM sodium acetate pH 6.8 to remove ethanol, salts and low molecular weight proteins. This solution was adjusted to pH 5.2 at 4°C, the resulting precipitate removed by filtration and the filtrate applied to the DEAE Sepharose FF column equilibrated in 0.02 M sodium acetate pH 5.2. Following loading (640 grams of protein per cycle) the column was washed with 1.8 column volumes of equilibration buffer. Albumin was eluted directly onto CM Sepharose FF using 0.025 M sodium acetate pH 4.5 and the CM Sepharose FF column washed with 1.8 column volumes of the same buffer. Albumin was then eluted with 0.11 M sodium acetate pH 5.5. For all regeneration steps on the ion exchange columns the direction of flow was reversed. The DEAE Sepharose FF column was regenerated by washing with 1.5 column volumes of 0.15 M sodium acetate pH 4.0. The CM Sepharose FF column was regenerated by washing with 1.5 column volumes of 0.4 M sodium acetate pH 8.0. Every third cycle both the CM and DEAE columns were washed with a column volume of 1 M sodium hydroxide followed by 0.15 M sodium acetate pH 4.0. The ion exchange eluate was then concentrated to approximately 14% w/v protein solution and applied to Sephacryl S200-HR column equilibrated with 0.05 M sodium acetate pH 6.8 at a load of 4 litres per cycle. Eluted albumin monomer was collected using either Method 1 or Method 2 (indicated in Fig. 5). Albumin monomer was diafiltered against water, formulated as 5% w/v or 20% w/v albumin solutions then sterile dispensed and pasteurised.

Analytical methods. Immunoelectrophoresis was conducted according to the method of Laurell (1966) using antisera purchased from Dakopatts, Denmark and plasma standards purchased from Behring, Germany. PKA was determined using the chromogenic substrate S2302 (Kabi Vitrum, Sweden) and a procedure based on that of Hojima et al., (1980). PKA-C1 esterase inhibitor complex was determined by radioimmunoassay based on the method of Bakker et al. (1990). Levels of this complex were expressed as PKA potential which represents the PKA level reached if all complex dissociated and released active PKA. Aluminium levels were determined by Graphite Furnace Analysis. Protein content was determined by Biuret. Albumin content was determined by immunoelectrophoresis except for the results presented in Table 1 which were determined by cellulose acetate membrane electrophoresis (CAME) as specified in Appendix IIIf of the British Pharmacopoeia. Albumin monomer and polymer content was determined by high performance size exclusion chromatography. PKA was prepared from Fraction II+III filtrate using a procedure based on that of Tankersley et al., (1980).

RESULTS

Albumin yield and purity. Protein yield and albumin purity achieved during the purification are presented in Fig. 1. The data illustrate most albumin purification occurs on removal of Fraction II+III and processing on the ion exchange columns. Pilot plant data to date indicate that the process will routinely yield 25 gram of albumin per litre of plasma processed.

Protein composition Intermediate fractions were also analysed for the presence of plasma proteins which are relatively abundant and have isoelectric points similar to albumin. The results are presented in Fig. 2 and show most α_2 macroglobulin is removed with Fraction II+III. Apolipoprotein A was almost entirely removed during the isoelectric precipitation step and further reduced by ion-exchange chromatography. Haptoglobin, transferrin, α_1 acid glycoprotein, and most α_1 proteinase inhibitor were removed by ion-exchange chromatography. Size-exclusion chromatography removed remaining traces of α_2 macroglobulin.

Comparison of 5% albumin produced by chromatographic methods and cold ethanol precipitation (Cohn) methods.

The properties of albumin solutions prepared by either the chromatographic method described or by cold ethanol (Cohn) fractionation are compared in Table 1. Chromatographic albumin exhibited a higher purity and monomer content and a lower aluminium content. PKA and PKA potential (PKA-C1 esterase inhibitor complex) levels were slightly higher in the chromatographic product. Transferrin, haptoglobin and α_1 acid glycoprotein were detected in albumin produced by Cohn fractionation but not in the chromatographic product. Both products contained α_1 proteinase inhibitor with the chromatographic product containing higher concentrations of this protein. Apolipoprotein A was detected at very low levels in the chromatographic product.

Table 1: Comparison of albumin solutions

For each product data were derived from approximately 10 batches with the exception of data on the analysis of specific proteins indicated by an asterix (*). The latter were derived from the analysis of 4 chromatographic batches and one batch produced by Cohn fractionation.

COMPONENT	COHN PROCESS	CHROMATOGRAPHIC PROCESS
Albumin (% w/w)	96.8 ± 1.14	97.6 ± 1.6
Monomer content (% distribution)*	95.4 ± 0.5	98.4 ± 1.2
PKA (IU/mL)	1.1 ± 0.3	2.4 ± 0.9
PKA Potential (IU/mL)	3.9 ± 4.7	7.6 ± 3.3
Endotoxin (EU/mL)	0.11 ± 0.12	0.51 ± 0.39
Pyrogens (°C)	0.38 ± 0.23	0.43 ± 0.33
Aluminium (μg/L)	33 ± 19	10.9 ± 6.2
Transferrin (g/L)*	0.23	<0.014
Haptoglobin (g/L)*	0.16	<0.018
α_1 proteinase inhibitor (g/L)*	0.008	0.035 ± 0.006
α_1 acid glycoprotein (g/L)*	0.13	<0.014
α_2 macroglobulin (g/L)*	<0.033	<0.033
Apolipoprotein A (g/L)*	<0.007	0.027 ± 0.024
Inter-α-trypsin inhibitor (g/L)*	<0.012	<0.012

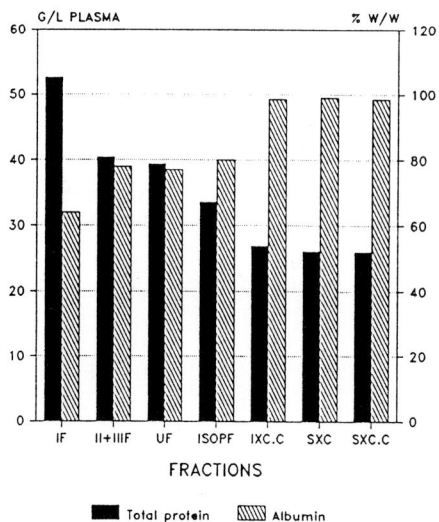

Fig. 1: Characterisation of intermediate fractions: Albumin yield and purity.
Intermediate samples from 2 batches were assayed to determine protein yield (g/L of plasma processed) and albumin purity (%w/w).
Fractions: Fraction I filtrate (IF); Fraction II + III filtrate (II+IIIF); Ultrafiltrate (UF); isoelectric precipitate filtrate (ISOPF); ion-exchange chromatography eluate concentrate (IXC.C); size-exclusion chromatography eluate (SXC); size-exclusion chromatography eluate concentrate (SXC.C).

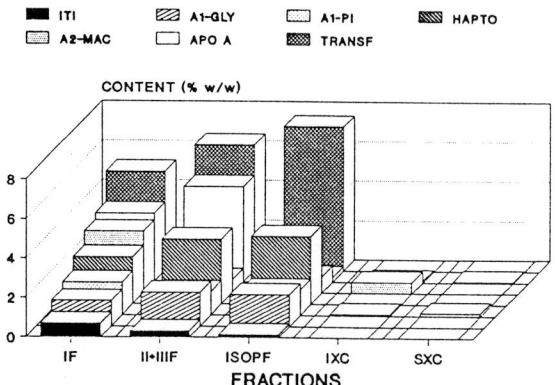

Fig. 2: Characterisation of intermediate fractions: Protein composition.
Intermediate samples from 4 batches were analysed by Laurell immunoelectrophoresis for the presence of inter-alpha-trypsin inhibitor (ITI); Alpha-1-glycoprotein (A1-GLY); Alpha-1-proteinase inhibitor (A1-PI); Haptoglobin (HAPTO); Alpha-2 Macroglobulin (A2-MAC); Apolipoprotein A (APO A); Transferrin (TRANSF).
Fractions: Fraction I filtrate (IF); Fraction II + III filtrate (II+IIIF); isoelectric precipitate filtrate (ISOPF); Ion-exchange chromatography eluate (IXC); size-exclusion chromatography eluate (SXC).

Stability of chromatographic albumin. The final product was shown to be stable with respect to pH, aggregate and monomer content, and appearance when stored at 8°C, 27°C or 37°C over 60 weeks. Aluminium levels showed some increase during storage with increases more rapid at higher temperatures (Fig. 3). Analysis of product stored upright (i.e. not in contact with the stopper) confirmed aluminium was leaching from the glass and not the stoppers used. PKA levels increased in a temperature dependent fashion in some batches of 5% chromatographic albumin solution but remained below the limit of 35 IU/mL (Fig. 4). At 37°C the PKA level increased and then decreased. Our data to date indicate that the maximum level of PKA is reached after 20 to 26 weeks at 27°C and 50 to 60 weeks at 8°C.

PKA and PKA potential in albumin solution: Separation of PKA complexes from monomeric albumin by size-exclusion chromatography. Evaluation of our ultrafiltration processes have shown that free PKA is removed by these steps indicating that PKA (MW 28000) is permeable to the membrane we are using (30,000 MW cut off). Hence the presence of PKA in our final products is likely to be derived from PKA complexes. PKA is known to form complexes with other plasma proteins such as C1 esterase inhibitor (Bakker et al. 1990) and albumin itself (Simonianova and Hrkal 1990). Furthermore it is possible for such complexes to dissociate during storage releasing active PKA (Bakker et al. 1990). To avoid this possibility it is desirable that such complexes be removed from albumin preparations.
 The gel filtration process was evaluated as a method for removing PKA complexes. The results (Fig. 5) show that PKA activity elutes with the high molecular weight protein, albumin dimer and in the later half of the albumin monomer peak. The interpretation of this data is that PKA eluting with the high molecular weight protein was derived from PKA associated with α_2 macroglobulin and/or albumin aggregates. Alpha-2 macroglobulin, which has a molecular weight of 725,000 (Travis and Salvesen 1983), is present after cation exchange chromatography (ca 0.3% of total protein) and is removed by processing on Sephacryl S200-HR. PKA in the dimer region was likely to be derived from PKA associated with C1 esterase inhibitor (MW 110,000) and/or albumin. The final PKA peak, eluting at the tail end of the albumin peak, was free PKA.

Figure 5 suggests stability in relation to PKA levels should be improved by changing the point at which the collection of the monomeric peak is begun to reduce levels of PKA complex in this fraction. When the mode of collection in the pilot plant used was Method 1, (see Fig. 5), the PKA potential averaged 23.4 ± 12 IU/mL (n=7) compared with 7.6 ± 3.3 IU/mL using Method 2. Yields using the Method 2 were approximately 25 gram/Litre of plasma processed. By delaying the collection of the monomeric peak past the point indicated in Method 2 further reduction in PKA potential is expected. This approach will impact on yield and necessitate rework (by size exclusion chromatography) of the ascending side of the monomeric peak.

Performance of chromatographic media. The gel life of DEAE Sepharose FF, CM Sepharose FF and Sephacryl S200-HR is currently being evaluated by monitoring the performance of the chromatographic albumin process as conducted in the pilot plant. No changes attributable to the deterioration of column gels have been detected after

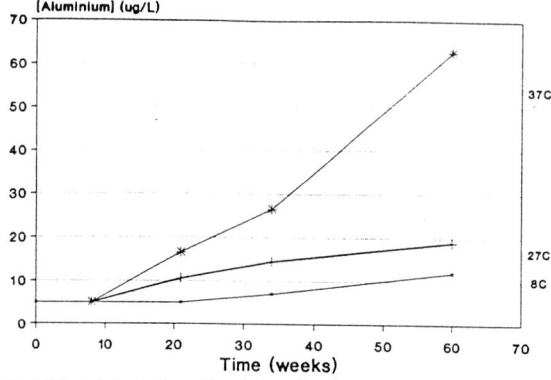

Fig. 3: **Stability trial studies: Aluminium levels.**
Aluminium levels were measured in 4 batches of 5% chromatographic albumin solutions that have been stored at 8 °C, 27 °C, and 37 °C over a period of 60 weeks.

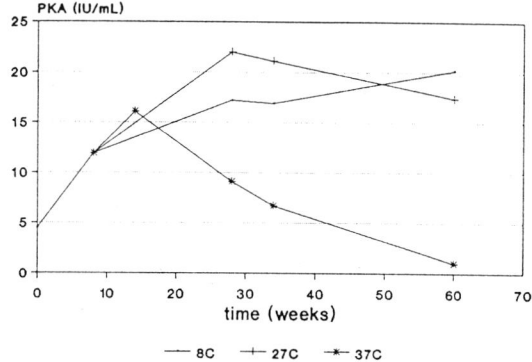

Fig. 4: **Stability trial studies: PKA levels.**
PKA levels were measured in a single batche of 5% chromatographic albumin solutions that have been stored at 8 °C, 27 °C, and 37 °C over a period of 60 weeks.

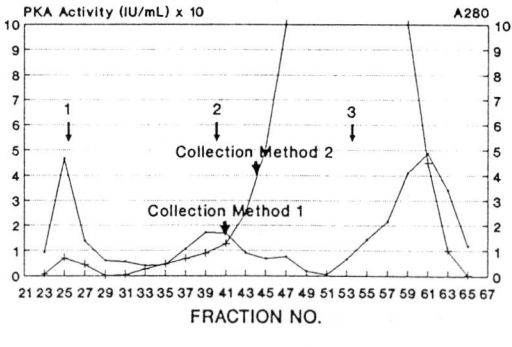

Fig. 5: **Separation of PKA-complexes and albumin monomer by chromatography on Sephacryl S200-HR**
Chromatogram of albumin on S200-HR (3 cm diameter x 53 cm). Albumin eluted from the cation exchange step (980 mg in 7 mL) was spiked with PKA prepared as described in Materials and Methods. This preparation containing 67 IU/mL PKA and 15 IU/mL PKA potential (PKA-C1 esterase inhibitor) was chromatographed at a flow rate of 2 mL/minute. The elution positions of aggregated albumin (1), albumin dimer (2) and albumin monomer (3) are shown in the chromatogram. Also shown are the elution positions of PKA activity. Collection of albumin monomer was performed by either Method 1 or Method 2 as indicated above.

conducting in excess of 240 cycles on the ion-exchange resins or 180 cycles on the Sephacryl S200-HR resin as assessed by chromatogram overlays, column yield data and the final product testing.

CONCLUSIONS

The chromatographically derived albumin solutions were consistently of higher yield, purity and monomer content than product produced by the Cohn fractionation process. Chromatographic albumin solutions stored at 8°C, 27°C and 37°C exhibited excellent stability over a 60 week period. Aluminium levels increased slowly on storage due to leaching from type I glass but remained well below 200 µg/Litre (the British Pharmacopoeial limit for use in dialysis patients and neonates). PKA levels increased in some batches during storage and this was probably due to the presence of PKA complexes. Optimisation of the gel filtration step should remove PKA complexes from the albumin monomer and thus improve the stability of the product with respect to this parameter. The gel life has important ramifications with respect to the economics of the process described above. No changes attributable to deterioration of column gels have been detected after conducting in excess of 240 cycles on the ion-exchange resins or 180 cycles on the Sephacryl S200-HR resin.

REFERENCES.

Bakker J. Stekkinger P, Nuijens J, Radema H, Duivis-Vorst C, Bluken WK Hack CE (1990) Detection of prekallikrein activator bound C1-esterase inhibitor
in albumin solutions. International Symposium on Blood Transfusion, Los Angeles.

Curling JM, Berglof J, Linquist LO, Eriksson S (1977). A chromatographic procedure for the purification of human plasma albumin. Vox Sang. 33: 97-107.

Hojima Y, Tankersley DL, Miller-Anderson M, Pierce JV, Pisano JJ (1980). Enzymatic properties of Human Hageman Fragment with Plasma Prekallikrein and Synthetic Substates. Thrombosis Res. 18: 417-430.

Laurell CB (1965) Antigen-antibody crossed electrophoresis. Anal. Biochem. 10: 358
Simonianova E, Hrkal Z (1990) Separation of the Hageman Factor fragment from human serum albumin by chromatography on Blue Sepharose CL-6B. Biomedical Chromatography (1990) 4: 152-153.

Tankersley DL, Fournel MA, Schroeder DD (1980). Kinetics of activation of Prekallikrein by Prekallikrein Activiator. Biochem. 19: 3121-3127.

Travis J, Salvesen GS (1983) Human plasma proteinase inhibitors. Ann. Rev. Biochem. (1983) 52: 655-709.

Our initial experience with large scale chromatography for plasma fractionation

Vijaylaxmi Ray and M.V. Kamath

National Plasma Fractionation Centre, K.E.M. Hospital Complex, Parel, Bombay 400 012, India

The National Plasma Fractionation Centre in Bombay was established in March 1990. The chief aim of this centre is to make available & provide Quality Assured Virus Safe Plasma Fractions. Presently blood fractions are being imported in India. The Fractionation process is totally based on Chromatography. This method is very convenient in our situation since there is a chronic shortage of voluntary blood donors. The batch size varies from 50-150 lts/wk. The product produced are Albumin, Gammaglobulin and F IX complex.

Collection of Plasma:
The blood is collected from voluntary donors & is screened for HBsAg, anti-HIV & VDRL. Whole blood is seperated into different components as shown in Fig.1.

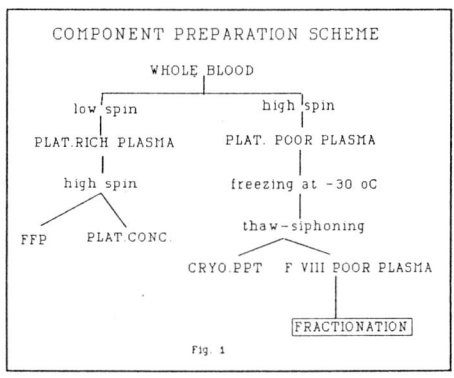

Fig. 1

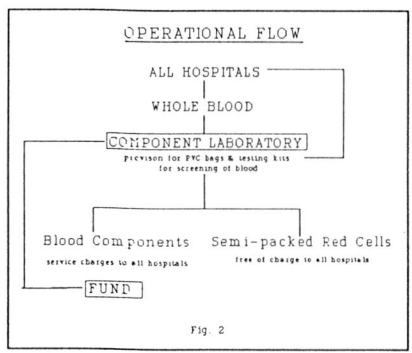

Fig. 2

The left over plasma after cryoprecipitate separation is send to NPFC for fractionation.

The policy for input of blood from different blood banks to component laboratory is shown in Operational Flow, Fig 2.

Fractionation Process

The chromatography process is imported from Pharmacia AB, Sweden. The process involves mainly gelfiltration & ion exchange chromatography. The process is computer controlled. The chromatography system comprises of three basic units ie. Control unit, Liquid handling module & Chromatography column.

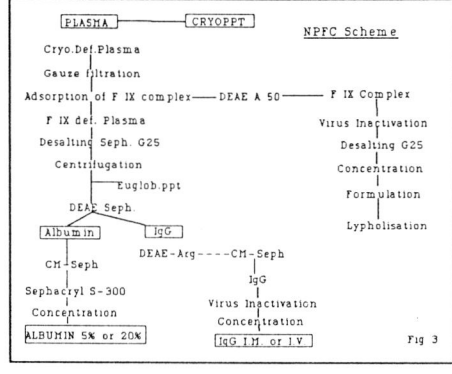

Fig 3

The fractionation of batch takes a week to complete. The process is carried out in a clean environment of class 100,000. The final product filling preparations and filling is done in class 10,000 & class 1000 rooms respectively. The actual filling is done under laminar air flow bench of class 100. The fractionation scheme followed at NPFC is shown in Fig 3. The virus inactivation is carried out in a dedicated room with separate set of equipments so as to prevent any cross contamination.

Viral Safety

The viral safety precaution begins with raw material ie donor screening and in-process screening by ELISA. The final product are made virus safe by heat pasteurization for Albumin at 60°C for 10 hrs. The Gammaglobulin and F IX complex is made virus safe by solvent-detergent technique of NYBC.

Product Quality Control

The in-process and final products are tested in in-house quality control laboratory. Besides Pharmacopeial requirements the patterns of FPLC & PAGE is used to confirm the purity of final products. The Albumin founds to be > 99% monomeric. The IgG contains < 2% of dimers and aggregates. F IX complex shows three peaks pattern on FPLC & PAGE analysis

Product Recovery

Table 1. shows the recovery of Albumin, IgG & F IX complex.

TABLE 1.
Batch size: 46-47 lts
Total Protein: 65-70 gms/lt

	ALBUMIN		IgG		F IX complex	
% YIELD	1990 60.2%	1992 65.6%	1990 52.0%	1992 52.2%	1990 N.A.	1992 48.5%
No of bottles/batch	200 bottles 5% 100 ml & 100 bottles 20% 50 ml		I.M. 1000 vials 10%, 2 ml. I.V. 400 vials 5%, 10 ml.		20 bottles 200 I.U./Bottle	

The product like 5% & 15% Albumin, Gammaglobulin I.M. grade and F IX complex is available and already in use. The clinical trial on intravenous grade Gammaglobulin is under process.

Initial Problems Faced with Fractionation

While standardizing the chromatographic process the problems faced were:

1. Pyrogens in buffer because of static water in pipelines & deadends which was subsequently rectified.
2. Particles leaching from rubber bung into filled product for which intense washing procedures were adopted.
3. The stability of 20% Albumin: precipitation after heat pasteurization or on keeping for few months. An extra step has been devised to solve this problem.
4. Sterile filtration of IgG which is still a problem though minimized by serial filtration.

Cost of Process

The production cost of a 50 lts batch is approx. $ 2,900/- (1 $ = 30 Indian Rupees)

We can conclude from our initial experience that the cost effectiveness of such fractionation unit will depend on the number of product rather than on the amount of plasma being fractionated.
We hope to make use of the total potential of chromatography in near future.

Design of a large scale chromatographic plant for the purification of human albumin

V. Micucci, I.F. Young, H.B. Yap, J.R. Davies, R.W. Herrington, B.R. White, G. Naylor and P.J. Turner

CSL Limited, 45 Poplar Road, Parkville, Victoria 3042, Australia

CSL Limited an Australian bio-pharmaceutical company is presently constructing a new plasma fractionation facility at Broadmeadows in Melbourne. Construction commenced in 1989 and it is estimated to be completed by early 1993. The plant is expected to be fully operational by December 1993.

The task of designing the new facility was given to a CSL led project team. The team, composed of a number of design consultants, CSL engineering and process staff as well as a number of contract staff numbered 150 people at the peak of the design phase.

The facility has been designed to process up to 250,000 litres of plasma per annum with the potential to scale up to 500,000 litres per annum. When complete this facility will meet all Australian blood products requirements as well as those of neighbouring countries like New Zealand.

The products to be manufactured in the Broadmeadows facility include:

    Prothrombin Complex Concentrate
    High purity Factor IX
    Factor VIII
    Immunoglobulin products
    Human serum albumin
    Antithrombin III
    α_1-proteinase inhibitor

The manufacture of human serum albumin will be by a chromatographic process based on the method developed by Curling et al (1977). The process will be substantially automated, providing for a high degree of reliability and traceability in a clean paperless environment.

Purification of Human Serum Albumin

Work at CSL on the chromatographic process for the purification of human serum albumin has been ongoing since 1981, first at bench scale and from late 1982 at the pilot scale using 16 litre column segments. Figure 1 outlines the process as developed by CSL.

The purification process is a combination of Cohn cold ethanol precipitation, with ion exchange and gel filtration chromatography. The II + III precipitate is removed by filtration and the filtrate concentrated and diafiltered to reduce ethanol and salt levels. The pH of the filtrate is then adjusted to 5.2 which results in a precipitate.

The precipitate is removed by filtration and the filtrate loaded in approximately 200 litre aliquots onto two 200 litre DEAE - Sepharose FF columns. Each column is 1200mm in diameter and 175mm in height. These columns are run independently and in parallel to each other. The albumin is bound onto the DEAE - and is later eluted directly onto two CM-Sepharose FF columns. The CM-columns are also 200 litre each, and are connected in series with the corresponding DEAE-column (See Fig 2). In line heat exchangers ensure that the entire process is carried out at 15°C.

The CM - eluate is concentrated and loaded onto 3 x 233 litre Sephacyrl - S200 HR columns (acting as a single column).

For the processing of 5000 litres of plasma equivalent 24 x DEAE/CM runs and 30 x S200 runs are required. This takes a total of approximately 4 days to process.

The monomeric Albumin from the S200 columns is collected, further concentrated and then diafiltered against cold pyrogen free water. The protein solution is then dispensed and pasteurized.

Buffer Preparation

The chromatographic albumin plant is serviced by a dedicated buffer supply system which comprises two preparation (1500 litre and 3500 litres respectively) and eleven storage vessels. The chromatographic process requires 150,000 litres of various sodium acetate, sodium hydroxide and sodium chloride solutions to process a 5000 litre batch of plasma to pure albumin (See Figure 3). Each sodium acetate buffer is prepared by accurately mixing together predetermined ratios of 1M sodium hydroxide and 1M acetic acid, then diluting with cold pyrogen free water.

All buffers are filtered through a 0.2u membrane during transfer to the storage vessels. Each of the storage vessels is dedicated to a single buffer and is continuously topped up as the buffer is required. Each of the buffers is pumped to the chromatography columns as required.

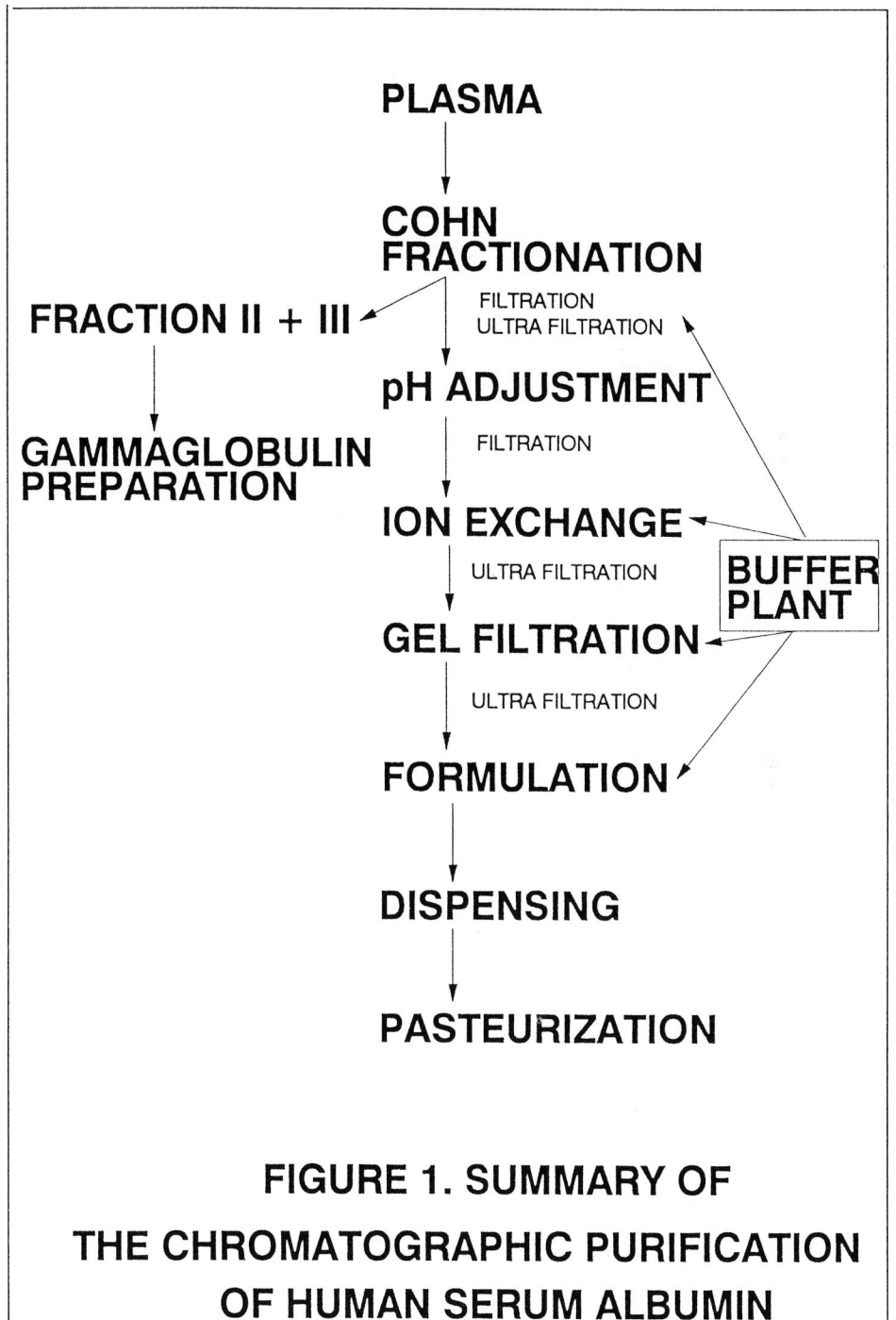

FIGURE 1. SUMMARY OF THE CHROMATOGRAPHIC PURIFICATION OF HUMAN SERUM ALBUMIN

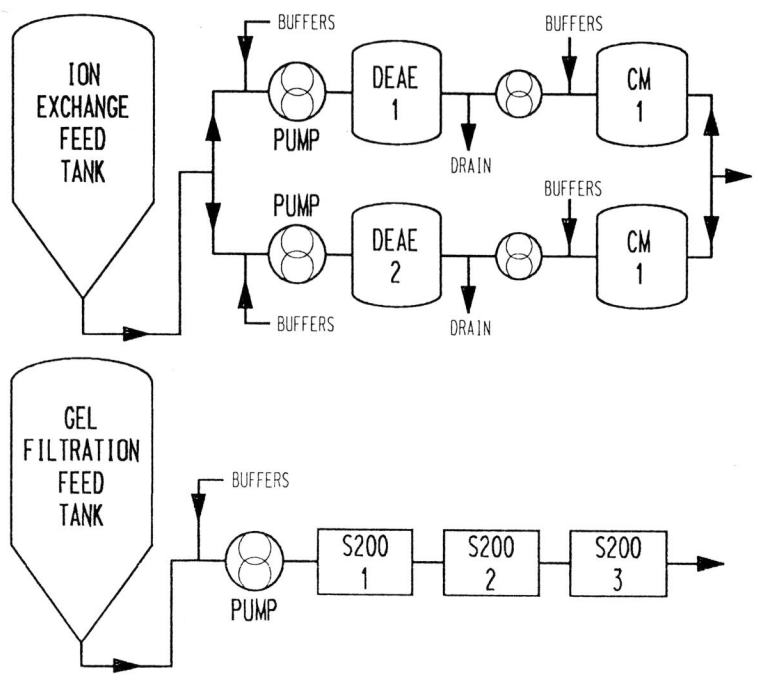

FIGURE 2. ARRANGEMENT OF THE ION EXCHANGE AND GEL FILTRATION COLUMNS

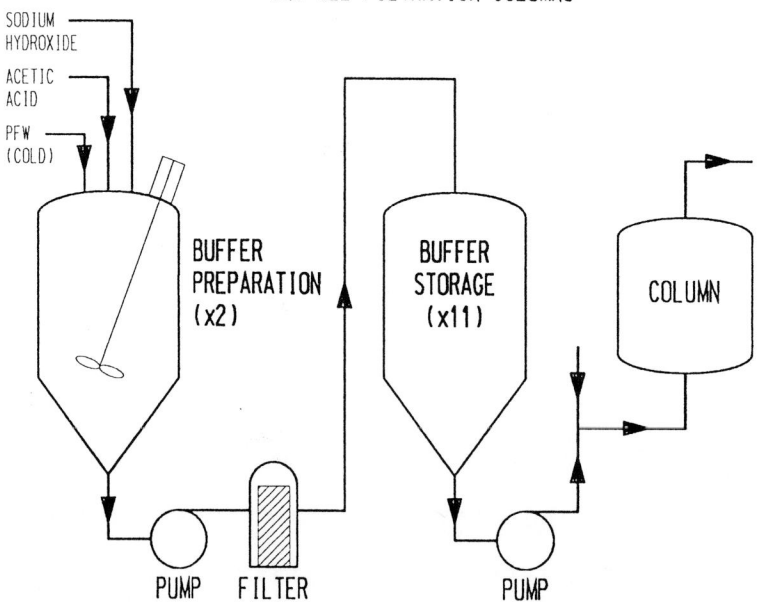

FIGURE 3. BUFFER PREPARATION, STORAGE AND DELIVERY

Reticulated Services.

Reagents required by the albumin plant (including the Buffer System) are supplied to the point of use via reticulated systems. The reagents include sodium hydroxide, acetic acid, hydrochloric acid, cold (15°C) and hot (85°C) pyrogen free water (PFW).

The PFW plant produces 765,000 litres (290,000 litres hot and 475,000 litres cold) of water per week distributed to 131 consumer outlets throughout the facility. 5MW of cooling is required to keep the PFW at 15°C. Ozone is used to sanitize the cool PFW, and UV is used to destroy the ozone prior to the point of use. The PFW plant has 60,000 litres of storage capacity.

Other services such as -8°C glycol, steam, nitrogen and compressed air are also supplied to the point of use.

Process Hygiene

To meet with CSL's stringent quality standards, the chromatographic plant has been designed as a closed system, hard piped, able to be fully cleaned in place (CIP).

In line filtration systems (some of which are steamed-in-place (SIP)), ensure product integrity during processing.

Furthermore the plant incorporates a number of other design features such as:

- metal surfaces in contact with product are electro-polished 316L stainless steel.
- in-line and tank instrumentation have tri-clamped fittings.
- all pipework is free draining
- extensive use of zero dead leg valves to eliminate pockets in pipework
- valves in contact with product are of the sanitary diaphragm type.
- process areas are supplied with Hepa filtered (0.22u) air resulting in Class 3,5000 (AS-1386), equivalent to Class 100,000 (US).
- regular sanitization of the chromatography gels with sodium hydroxide.

Automation

The automation system used in the CSL facility is based upon a proprietary Distributed Control System with some functionality being provided by a mini computer. This system controls all process, CIP and service plants. Additionally there are approximately 100 standalone control sub-systems, primarily associated with equipment such as freeze driers and autoclaves. The system is extensive having a total input/output count of 15,000.

The chromatographic albumin process is suitable for automation as it is largely a 'straight through' process with buffer preparation and column runs being highly repetitive.

Software specification and development for the albumin process is expected to take in excess of 6 labour years. The albumin plant (with buffer preparation) contains 30% of all instrumentation in the facility and requires 25% of the control hardware.

Monitoring of the process is achieved via numerous screens. Some of these are located in a central control room whilst others are mobile units out on the process floor.

CSL's objectives for using an automated plant were:

- to improve productivity through the provision of reliable unattended services allowing increased production capacity with existing staff and equipment.

- to enforce processing within validated limits and where this is not possible provide the documentation to give a basis for an informed product sign off decision.

- to improve the sanitation of the process by reducing, human involvement by "closed manufacturing techniques" and eliminating paper and other particle shedding materials from process areas.

- to aid personnel and batch safety via condition monitoring, and alarm broadcast systems.

- to improve process traceability in manufacturing in compliance with GMP regulations.

Quality Standard

CSL has adopted the International Standards for Quality Systems, the ISO-9000 series (AS-3900) as the most appropriate standard for the project. CSL applied ISO-9001 to the CSL lead project team throughout the preparation of a project quality manual and project procedures.

In key project areas, such as process software, commissioning and validation, specific quality manuals and procedures were also prepared.

The specifications for contract packages required each contractor to identify the quality system under which they would operate and CSL would specify the quality level. Where possible each contractor was audited before commencement of work and any differences rectifed.

Prior to any work commencing CSL required each contractor to submit for approval an inspection and test plan and their company's Quality Manual. During the progress of the work CSL enforced compliance with the approved standards, manuals and procedures by a programme of planned and random audits, document reviews and progress meetings.

The Quality System for the operational facility will build on what we have learnt from the project and although CSL intends to rigidly comply with the requirements of ISO-9000, cGMP and TQM, the methods used will be flexible enough to allow for new initiatives and continuous improvement.

Summary

CSL Limited is building a new fractionation plant. Human serum albumin will be manufactured by a chromatographic procedure which incorporates the latest process and control technologies, and embraces stringent quality standards and phylosophies.

Design and development of the chromatography plant and indeed of the whole facility, has been a major undertaking with significant cost implications. However, CSL firmly believes that this will be outweighed by the substantial benefits gained.

References

Curling, J.M, Berglof, J.H, Lindquist, L.-O, Eriksson, S. (1977)
A chromatographic procedure for the purification of human plasma albumin. Vox Sang 33, 97 - 107.

Chromatographic purification of plasmatic human albumin

Ilias Stefas, Marcel Rucheton and Hubert Graafland*

*Laboratoire Rétrovirus-Parasites, ORSTOM, 911, avenue Agropolis, BP 5045, 34032 Montpellier Cedex 1 and *Institut d'Hématologie, Centre Régional de Transfusion Sanguine, 240, avenue Emile Jeanbrau, 34000 Montpellier, France*

Abstract. Human Albumin was purified by single perfusion through a chromatographic support, after appropriate treatment of either Cohn's Supernatant IV or Precipitate V. Under the circumstances utilized, most of the impurities remain fixed on the gels. The Albumin is directly recovered in the effluent, in a single-step process. Both the chromatographic yield and the final Albumin purity approximate 100%. The Albumin product is exempt of polymers, and stable even after the heating at 60°C for 10 hours. Material responsible for the thermal instability of the Albumin is thus mostly removed. This procedure is simple, quick and then spares work, time and material.

INTRODUCTION.

Since the Cohn cold-ethanol method, various ion-exchange chromatography (Curling, 1980; Tayot et al, 1980; Saint-Blanchard et al, 1981) procedures have been used to purify the plasmatic human Albumin. In these, Albumin is retained on a support. In the one-step procedure described below, contaminants are fixed on the support and purified Albumin is recovered in the effluent of the columns.

Principle.
Human Albumin was purified by a single-step perfusion through a chromatographic support after appropriate treatment of either Cohn's Supernatant IV or Precipitate V.
This Procedure is described by a PATENT registered in FRANCE by care of Cabinet Peuscet in Paris.

RESULTS.

Starting Material: Cohn's Albumin. Human plasma was fractionnated according to the method of Kistler and Nitschman (1962) to obtain the Cohn fractions, either Supernatant IV or Precipitate V.

SCHEME I: THE PURIFICATION STEPS OF THE ALBUMIN.

--Starting material:
  Supernatant IV or Precipitate V of Cohn

--Preliminary steps:
  Adaptation from Cohn's fractions
  to 20% w/w Albumin, pH 7,0, Na+ 0.15M,
  ionic strength, osmolarity .
  Ultrafiltrated Albumin

--ONE-STEP PERFUSION :
  through the chromatographic material
  Recovery of effluent Albumin

--Final steps
  Concentration to 20% or dilution to 4%
  Addition of sodium caprylate.
  Heating at 60°C for 10 hours.

  THERAPEUTIC ALBUMIN

Process: The different steps of the Albumin purification are illustrated in scheme I. The Albumin from either Supernatant IV or from Precipitate V was dialysed, then concentrated to 20% by ultrafiltration, adjusted for physical parameters and Na+ concentration. The ultrafiltrated Albumin was then perfused in a one-step procedure through chromatographic material. Under the described circumstances, the Albumin does not fix on the support, but reappears in the effluent and is adapted for different uses.

* **Characteristics of Chromatographied Albumin.**
a) <u>Purity:</u> By cellulose acetate electrophoresis, as in fig.1, the purity of the final product approximates 100%, whereas the purity of the Albumin from Supernatant IV or ultrafiltrated Precipitate V is by average of 97%.
b) <u>Denatured protein and Albumin polymers:</u> Ultrafiltrated and processed Albumin were submitted to gel filtration on Sephacryl S 400 HR. Fig. 2. shows the elimination of impurities by the process. There are no polymers after the heating of the processed Albumin (60°C, 10 hours), such as is not the case of the ultrafiltrated Albumin.
c) <u>Heat stability of Albumin:</u> The treated effluent Albumin, after perfusion through chromatography, shows, in fig. 3, a much lower turbidity than the ultrafiltrated Albumin in course of time at 60°C.
* **Yield:** The yield from the whole process approximates 100%. On a laboratory scale, the production range was of 23-24g Albumin per initial liter of plasma when the process was applied to Paste V common Albumin samples, towards 26-28g for Supernatant IV samples. More than 20 experiments have been performed in each case.
* **Haem:** In the case of the Albumin treated by chromatography, there is no absorbance peak at 403 nm. In fact, the pigments and the haem recurring in a classic ultrafiltrated Albumin are retained on the support.
* **Colour:** The pale yellow colour of the 20% Albumin obtained by this chromatographic method is much less intense, even after 10 hours of heating at 60°C, than that of a classic Albumin.

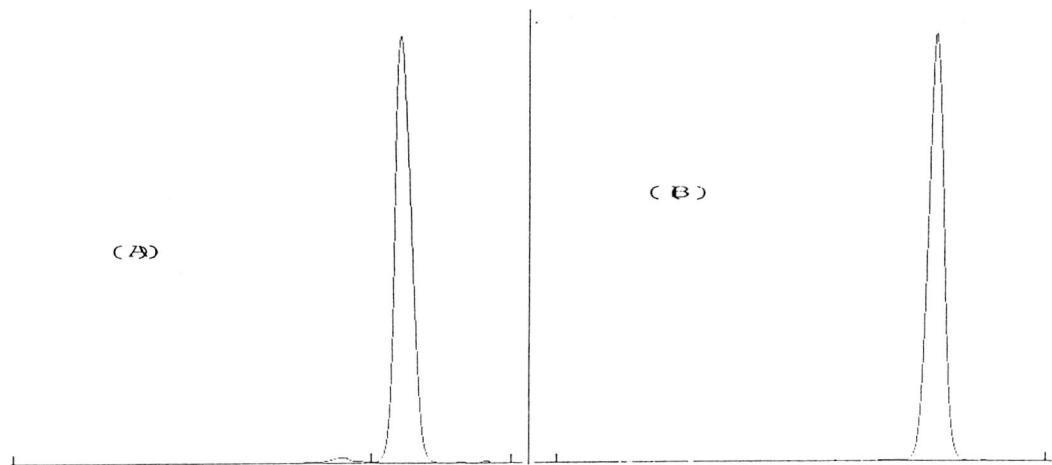

Fig. 1 : Cellulose acetate electrophoresis of 20% Albumin solutions : ultrafiltrated (A); then chromatographied (B).

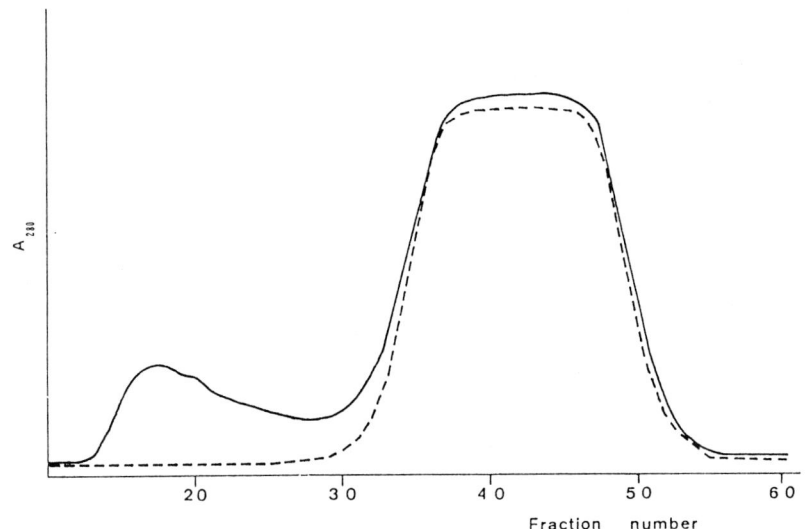

Fig. 2 : Gel filtration on Sephacryl S400 HR of plasma 20% Albumin solution after final heating (60°C, 10 hours): ultrafiltrated (-), then chromatographied (- - -);

* **Neoantigens:** In immunoelectrophoresis after Grabar's method, there is a precipitation line around the deposit resevoir in the case of ultrafiltrated Albumin after pasteurization. This phenomenon originates in new antigenes appearing in course of heating of the Albumin, the so-called "neoantigens" (Cohen and Roelands, 1976; Ring et al, 1979). The chromatographied Albumin does not show any neoantigen.
* **Dilution effect:** The ultrafiltrated Albumin is diluted 1.15 times by the chromatographic process.

* **Recycling of Column Material:** more than 50 passages have been performed with the same material without any observable change in the quality of the Albumin.

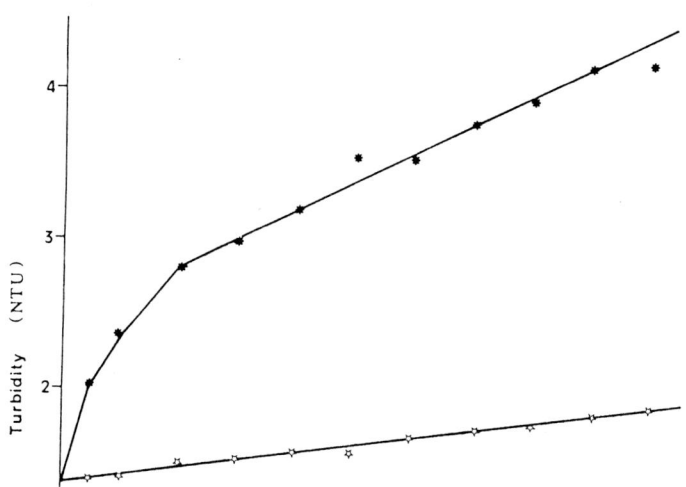

Fig. 3 : Time course of turbidity of a caprylate added, 60°C heated 20% Albumin : ultrafiltrated (*---*), then chromatographied (+---+).

DISCUSSION.

The method presented here for a chromatographic treatment without retention of Albumin from Supernatant IV or Paste V gives yield and purity of Albumin near to 100%, as neither losses nor impurities could be detected at a significant level by current technics.
This chromatographied Albumin is more stable during prolonged heating than ultrafiltrated Albumin. Polymers are mostly removed. Material responsible for the thermal instability of the Albumin is thus mostly removed. The method insures elimination of the pigments and the haem, and gives a clear yellow final product. This chromatographic process also increases the homogeneity of the final product.

Preparations of plasmatic Albumin contain a certain amount of polymers, depending notably on the nature of the plasma and on the procedure adopted, appearing during the plasma fractionnation, pasteurization and storage (Friedli and Kistler, 1970; Finlayson, 1965). The addition of stabilizers (Edsall, 1984) is used to prevent their appearance. Alternatively, other methods have been proposed,such as thermocoagulation or chromatographies (Curling, 1980; Tayot et al, 1980; Schneider et al, 1975; Harvey, 1980). The thermocoagulated Albumin shows a strong decrease in the free cysteine group per Albumin molecule (Peters, 1975; Morgenthaler and Nydegger, 1985), indicating a certain alteration of the Albumin

SCHEME II   TWO WAYS OF USING THE PERFUSION PROCESS

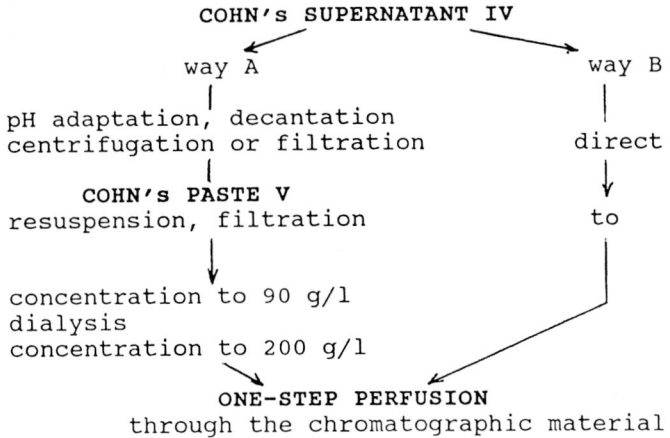

Final production
Albumin weight per initial liter of plasma

way A	way B
23-24g	26-28g

molecule. The purification of Albumin by retention chromatographies are heavy and consume huge amounts of buffers and top quality water.

The procedure described above is applicable to both Cohn's Supernatant IV and Paste V, as illustrated in sheme II, and combines security with practical advantages. The empiric security of the Cohn's fractionation (Stolz et al, 1987) is effectively increased here by the addition of the chromatography and the elimination of neoantigens. The described process, where Albumin does not fix on the gels, offers multiple other advantages: -a volume of gel corresponding to 0.13 volume of initial plasma, thus 4 to 10 times weaker compared to current chromatographic retention procedures; -no change of buffers or pH; - thus minimal amount of chemicals and expensive distilled water (calculated 20 to 50 times smaller) and a reduced number of solutions for chromatography and recycling. Furthermore, the Albumin treated by this chromatography, even at 20%, presents a very good filterability through $0.2\mu m$ filters. Rejected Albumin samples due to troubles or precipitation have been succesfully treated by this procedure.

Finally, starting this procedure from Supernatant IV instead of from Paste V gave an identically pure Albumin but a substantial improvement in the Albumin yield and would at the industrial scale spare installations, work, time and materials.

REFERENCES.
Cohen, P.; and Roelands, J. F.: Detection of an antigen in Albumin subjected to repeated heating. Vox Sang. 31: 332-336 (1976).
Curling, J.M.: Albumin purification by ion exchange chromatography. In "Methods of Plasma Protein Fractionation" Ed. J. Curling, Acad. Press, 77-91 (1980).

Edsall, J. T.: Stabilization of serum Albumin to heat, and inactivation of the Hepatitis Virus. <u>Vox Sang. 46</u>: 338-340 (1984).

Finlayson, J. S.: Effects of long-term storage on human serum Albumin. II. Follow-up of chromatographically and ultracentrifugally detectable changes. <u>J. Clin. Invest. 44</u>: 1561-1568 (1965).

Friedli, H.; and Kistler, P.: Polymers in preparations of human serum albumin. <u>Vox Sang. 18</u>: 542-546 (1970).

Harvey, M. J.: The application of affinity chromatography and hydrophobic chromatography to the purification of serum Albumin. In <u>"Methods of Plasma Protein Fractionation"</u> Ed. J. Curling, Acad. Press, 189-200 (1980).

Kistler, P.; and Nitschman, H.S.: Large scale production of human plasma fractions. Vox Sang. 7: 414-424 (1962).

Morgenthaler, J. J.; Nydegger, U. E.: Preservation of structure and function during isolation of human plasma proteins. In <u>"Plasma fractionation and Blood Transfusion"</u> Ed. C. Th. Smit Sibinga, P. C. Das and S. Seidl, in Martinus Nijhoff Publishers. 127-138 (1985).

Peters, T. Jr.: Serum Albumin. In <u>"The Plasma Proteins"</u> vol. I Ed F. W. Putnam, Acad. Press, 133-181 (1975).

Ring, J.; Stephan, W.; Brendel W.: Anaphylactoid reactions to infusions of plasma protein and human serum Albumin. <u>Clin. Allergy 9</u>: 89-97 (1979).

Saint-Blanchard, J.; Fourcart, J.; Limonne, F.; Girot, P.; and Boschetti, E.: Nouveaux échangeurs d'ions Trisacryl: intérêt et application au fractionnement des proteines du plasma humain. <u>Ann. Pharm. Fr. 39</u>: 403-409 (1981).

Schneider, W.; Lefevre, H.; and Mccarty, L.J.: An alternative method of large scale plasma fractionnation for the isolation of the serum Albumin. <u>Blut 30</u>: 121- 134 (1975).

Stoltz, J.F.; Rivat, C.; Geschler, C.; Colosetti, P.; Sertillanges, P.; Tondon, J; et Regnault, V.: Purification chromatographique de l'albumine plasmatique humaine à l'échelle pilote. <u>Bio-Sciences. Vol.6-N°4</u>:103-106 (1987).

Tayot, J.L.; Tardy, M.; Gattel, P.: Ion exchange and affinity chromatography on silica derivatives. In <u>Methods of Plasma Protein Fractionnation</u> Ed. J. Curling, Acad. Press, 149-160 (1980).

Résumé

L'albumine obtenue par ultrafiltration du surnageant IV ou du precipité V de Cohn a été purifiée par simple perfusion a travers un support chromatographique. Dans les conditions utilisées seules sont retenues des impuretés responsables de l'instabilité thermique de l'albumine. Le rendement et la pureté de l'Albumine, obtenue directement dans l'effuent, approchent 100%. L' Albumine 20% produite est exempte de polymères et bien plus stable lors de la pasteurisation. Ce procédé simple et rapide et permet d'economiser temps, travail et produits.

Large scale albumin fractionation by chromatography

Stephen B. Marrs

The South African Blood Transfusion Service, P.O. Box 9326, Johannesburg 2000, Republic of South Africa

The South African Blood Transfusion Service (SABTS), in May 1980, commissioned the first column chromatography plasma protein fractionation unit for the large scale recovery of Human Serum Albumin for intravenous use.

The method was developed by Curling *et al*, Pharmaćia, Sweden, who constructed and supplied the original equipment and methodology.

PLASMA FRACTIONATION METHOD

The SABTS salvages plasma for protein fractionation by the aspiration of plasma from outdated voluntary donated whole blood, unused blood returned from hospitals and from cryoprecipitate poor plasma recovered in the production of Factor VIII. The plasma received may be pyrogenic, non-sterile and slightly haemolysed.

Plasma for processing is kept frozen at minus 20°C until required. It is thawed between 4 to 10°C.

The plasma is crudely filtered, to remove lumps of fibrin, by passing the material through a stainless steel sieve. The plasma is then applied to a continuous flow centrifuge where it is clarified before being filtered through a 3 micron filter.

GEL PERMEATION CHROMATOGRAPHY SEPHADEX G25C

The plasma is applied to a 75l Sephadex G25C column where desalting takes place. Our experience with this media has shown that it is a rugged gel and can withstand the processing of large volumes of raw plasma. The media in this column was replaced after six years (after processing approximately 70,000l of material). The reason for changing the media was due to an increase in column pressure, decrease in flow rate and poor separation even after repeated cleaning procedures.

The desalted plasma is adjusted to pH 5.2 and Polyethylene Glycol 4000 added to a concentration of 5 per cent. The material is mixed for 1 hour and placed in a cold room at 4°C overnight. The following day the supernatant plasma is applied to the continuous flow centrifuge and the precipitate discarded.

In our experience PEG treatment reduces the level of Hepatitis B surface antigen and removes large molecular weight proteins, adding considerably to the life-span of the gel.

The plasma is filtered after centrifugation through a 3 micron pre-filter and finally through a nominal 0.2 micron filter. The material is then applied to the Ion Exchange Chromatography Systems.

ION EXCHANGE CHROMATOGRAPHY

Treated plasma is applied to an anion column, DEAE Sepharose FF media at pH 5.2 to 5.4. The first fractions, consisting mainly of gammaglobulins and transferrin, are discarded. The second fraction contains albumin and haemoglobin and is eluted off the column at pH 4.45. The column is regenerated at pH 3.8 and ceruloplasmin is washed off.

The DEAE Sepharose column is a very important stage of the process as it is primarily here where endotoxins in the product are removed and extreme care must be taken in the subsequent stages not to contaminate the product.

The second fraction is applied directly onto the cation CM Sepharose Fast Flow Media at pH 4.7 to 4.8. Albumin is eluted off at pH 5.5 and haemoglobin at pH 8.

ULTRAFILTRATION

The albumin is filtered through a 0.5 micron filter before being applied to the ultrafiltration system at pH 6.5.

Membranes with a 10,000 dalton cut-off are used to concentrate the albumin to a concentration of 5 per cent before it is applied to a Sephacryl column in the Gel Filtration Stage.

GEL PERMEATION CHROMATOGRAPHY

Approximately $5l$ of 5 per cent albumin is applied to a $200l$ Sephacryl S200 column in order to reduce polymer levels. One cycle takes two hours to complete.

The albumin is then adjusted to pH 6.7 to 7.3 and concentrated on the ultrafiltration system to above 20 per cent (m/v).

Throughout production we strive to achieve acceptable levels of Good Manufacturing Practice.

After samples have been evaluated by the quality assurance department, and found to meet the required specifications, the product is transferred to a Class 1000 clean room.

The pH, protein concentration and pyrogen levels are checked. Sodium caprylate is added (to 0.04M) as a stabilizer to the product.

The albumin is then sterile filtered into prepared sterile bottles in a laminar flow work station using aseptic technique.

The albumin is pasteurized in a water bath at 60°C for 10 hours and held in quarantine at 32°C for 14 days.

Initially 100 litres of plasma was processed per week using DEAE and CM Sepharose CL6B media, however, production volumes increased with increased therapeutic demand for the product.

Sepharose Fast Flow media was introduced and it was found that the size of the tubing and valves needed to be increased from ¼ to ½ inch. New pumps had to be installed to increase flow rates up to $5l$ per minute.

Problems were encountered with the KS370 columns as after repeated packing under pressure (using nitrogen) several columns distorted and cracked. These have been replaced with large Amicon stainless steel columns. These are easy to pack and allow flexibility in packing media volumes from 20 to 100 litres.

At present the DEAE FF column is loaded with 100 litres of diluted plasma containing approximately 800 grams of albumin. Sixty litres of media packed in the column is used to separate protein at flow rates of 5 litres per minute at 60kpa column pressure. A cycle is performed in 3 hours. Life expectancy of the anion exchange media is 14 to 16 weeks with continuous operation, producing between 6000 and 8000 units of albumin with yields of up to 80 per cent from citrated plasma containing 30g/l albumin.

The upgrading of the ultrafiltration stages became a necessity as the small Pellicon system was taking too long to process material. Delays in the processing of material can lead to contamination. The Millipore Prostak System was introduced to speed up the ultrafiltration stages. Fifteen Prostak modules with a total of 150ft^2 of 10,000 dalton cut-off membrane surface area have been installed and 800 litres of post CM albumin can now, for example, be processed in under 1 hour, thus enabling the material to move more quickly to the next processing stage.

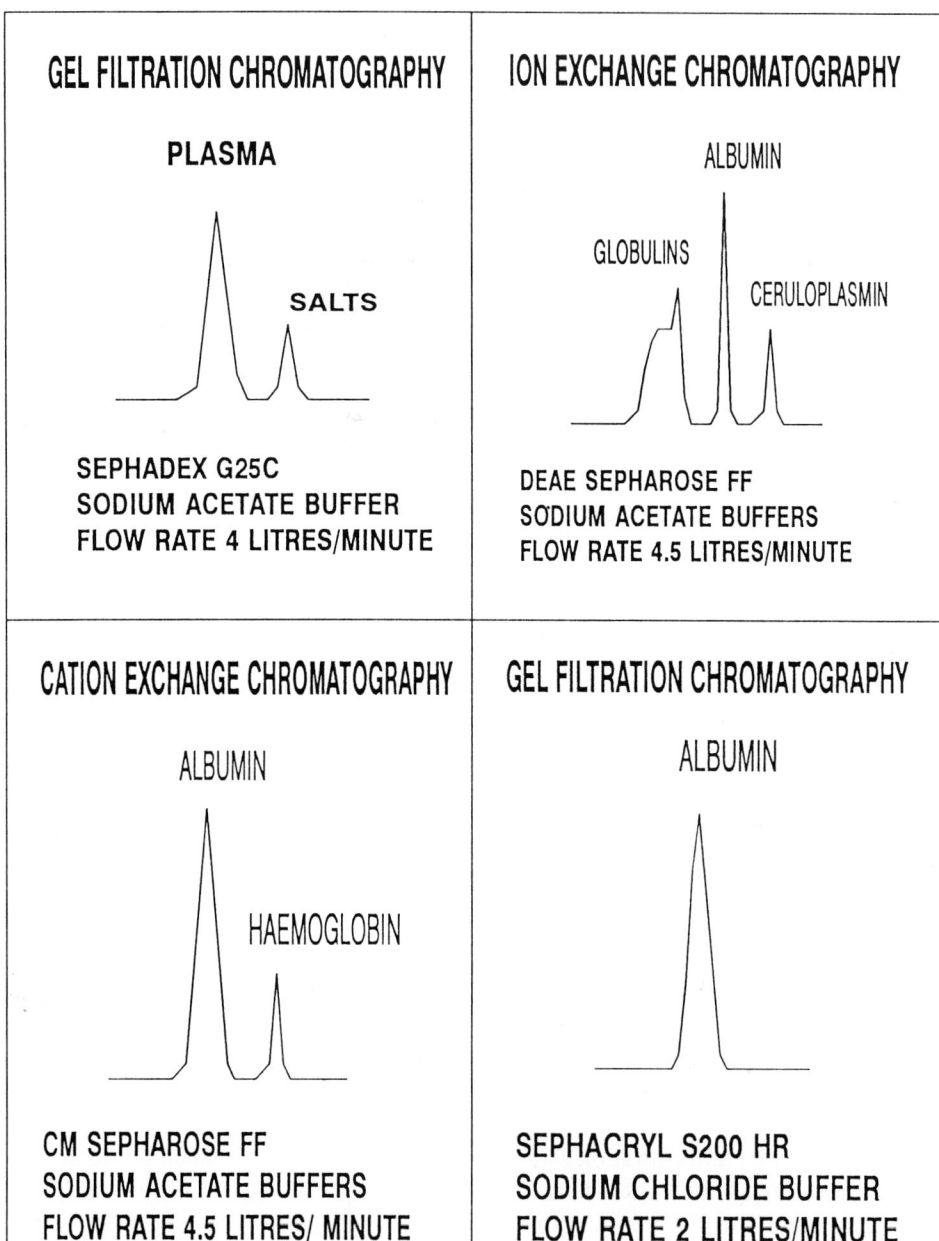

WATER PRODUCTION

The production of sufficient quantities of water for injection necessitated the implementation of several upgrading stages. In the fractionation of 600*l* plasma, between 15,000 to 20,000 litres of sterile, pyrogen-free water per day is required. A Millipore Milli-RO Series 2000TS double pass RO system was installed to provide 1,000 litres of water per hour. A problem was encountered in the feedwater, in that levels of aluminium were high enough to cause fouling of the RO membranes. This problem was solved by the introduction of a sodium hydroxide dosing system prior to reverse osmosis. Sufficient quantities of high quality water with an endotoxin level of less than 0.250 Eu/ml is being produced.

Over the past 12 years, 130,000 units of 100 ml, 20 per cent (m/v) Human Serum Albumin have been issued for clinical use (with eight non-serious reactions reported to date).

Future plans include the installation of a computer-controlled production process and the preparation of a virus-inactivated intravenous gammaglobulin.

Description and assessment of an industrial chromatography unit for preparing human plasma albumin

J.-F. Stoltz[1,2], C. Geschier[1], L. Dumont[1], C. Rivat[2], M. Grandgeorge[3], J. Ribeyron[3], E. Boschetti[4], J. Liautaud[3] and F. Streiff[1]

[1]*Centre Régional de Transfusion Sanguine et Laboratoire d'Hémorhéologie-Hématologie, Faculté de Médecine, Brabois, 54500 Vandœuvre-lès-Nancy, France,* [2]*INSERM, CO 10, 54511 Vandœuvre-lès-Nancy, France,* [3]*Institut Mérieux, 69280 Marcy-l'Etoile, France,* [4]*Sepracor-IBF, 92390 Villeneuve-la-Garenne, France*

ABSTRACT

Almost all the human plasma albumin used in therapy (or in biology) is now prepared by methods based on the process described by Cohn et al. These techniques consist of using cold ethanol at various pH and ionic strengths to precipitate proteins. Recently, chromatographic purification techniques have been developed, mainly based on ion-exchange chromatography. In particular, a process using Spherodex and Spherosil ion-exchangers (Sepracor-IBF, Villeneuve la Garenne, France) has been developed for purifying human placental albumin and human plasma albumin. Undenatured, very high purity albumin can be produced with this process. The trials described in this paper were undertaken at the Centre Régional de Transfusion Sanguine in Nancy (Regional Blood Transfusion Centre) in partnership with the Institut Mérieux (Marcy l'Etoile, France) with a view to developing an automated industrial chromatography unit for processing 350 to 400 litres of plasma per cycle.

INTRODUCTION

The first industrial process for purifying plasma albumin was developed by Cohn et al. (1946). The technique is based on achieving protein precipitation by adding ethanol and by varying the pH and plasma temperature. This standard procedure, or the existing variations on this technique, do, however, have the drawback of partially denaturing the proteins. Other methods have therefore been suggested : ether, ammonium sulfate, octanoic acid, rivanol, heat coagulation, etc... Nevertheless, the Cohn's technique still remains the most widely used process for industrial scale plasma fractionation. More recently, however, the use of chromatographic techniques have made it possible to extract very high purity proteins on an industrial scale. As early as 1981, the firms Sepracor-IBF (Villeneuve la Garenne, France) and LKB-Pharmacia (Uppsala, Sweden) offered human albumin purification procedures using ion exchange chromatography. The same year, Institut Mérieux in Marcy l'Etoile, France (Tayot et al., 1980, 1981) offered a new placental albumin purification procedure based on using microparticles of silica for the ion exchange supports (Spherosil/Spherodex supports). In partnership with the firm Rhône-Poulenc, this procedure was later adapted for extracting and purifying plasma albumin (Dromard et al., 1985; Tayot et al., 1980). The Regional Blood Centre in Nancy (France) took over the process and adapted it for purifying human plasma albumin on a pilot scale. The feasibility and reproducibility trials carried out over the past five years have been highly successful (Stoltz et al., 1987, 1989, 1991). An automated industrial purification unit has now been developed jointly by the Nancy Blood Centre, Institut Mérieux and Sepracor-IBF and is capable of processing 350 to 400 litres of plasma per cycle.

Unit operations are managed by a logic controller with a programme for sequencing the various stages and controlling the parameters that has been fully checked for validity. The process provides very high purity albumin (>99 %). The product undergoes several successive sterilizing filtration procedures and the storage tanks and piping are submitted to stages of chemical or steam sterilization in order to guarantee that the unit remains totally free from contamination.

Moreover, the whole procedure has been validated for virus inactivation with hepatitis B virus, poliomyelitis virus and particularly, human acquired immunodeficiency virus (see paper published in this volume, Stoltz et al.). The results indicate that the viral safety of the albumin produced using this procedure is equivalent to that of the albumin obtained with the standard Cohn's technique.

MATERIALS AND METHODS

1. Description of the chromatography unit

The process involves three stages of ion exchange using chromatographic supports provided by the firm Sepracor-IBF (Villeneuve la Garenne, France) : DEAE-Spherodex R LS, QMA-Spherosil R LS and COOH-Spherodex R LS (photo 1). These supports have all received FDA approval.

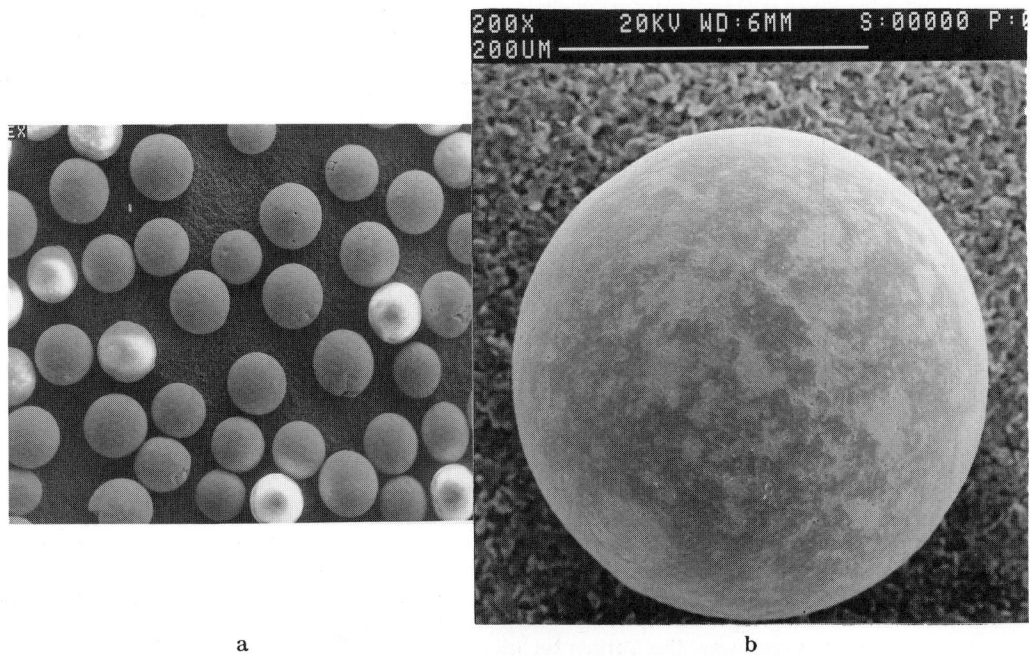

Photo 1 (a et b) : *Scanning microscopy of Spherodex support*

The circuit is fed by triple-case diaphragm pumps. The buffers and washing solutions are injected onto the columns after passing through ultrafilters (with a threshold level of 10000 Da) and/or a plate microfilter (0.2 µm). Pressure levels are checked at the entrance to each column. A UV absorptionmeter (280 nm) and a recorder both placed at the end of the circuit detect the different eluted protein solutions as they flow past. One cycle of the upscaled chromatographic technique is capable of processing approximately 350 to 400 litres of plasma supernatant II+III fractions obtained using the Cohn/Nietschmann method (photo 2).

The three stages of the chromatographic procedure can function completely independently on the industrial unit. The equipment used for each stage consists of : a heat controlled, stainless steel storage tank, a triple-case pump (Braun-Luebbe), a 0.2 µm filter (Millipore), a chromatographic column (Sepracor-IBF) and a heat controlled, stainless steel retrieval tank (Photo 3).

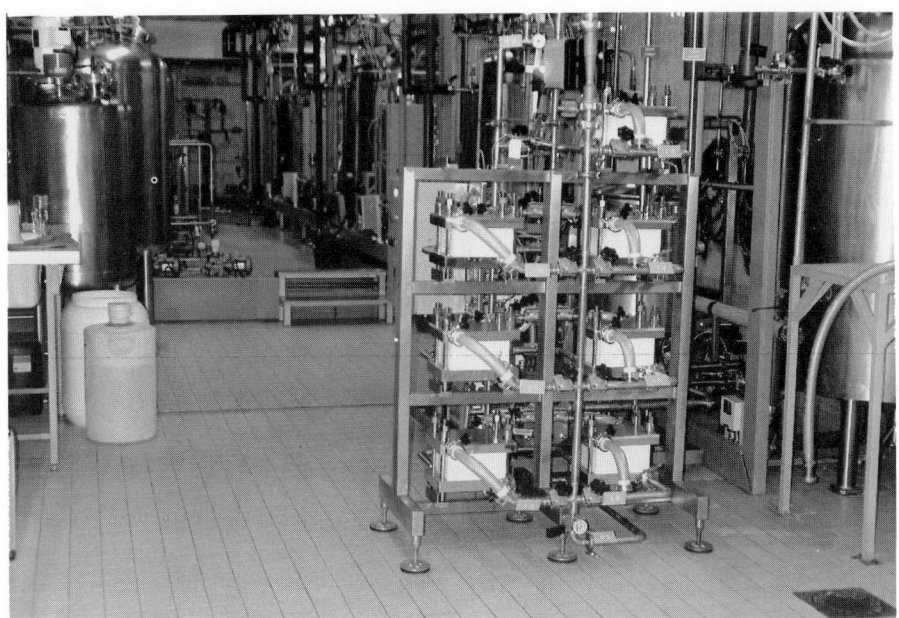

Photo 2 : *General view of the chromatography unit with ultrafiltration unit just upstream from column 1. The buffer preparation unit is situated to the left of the photograph.*

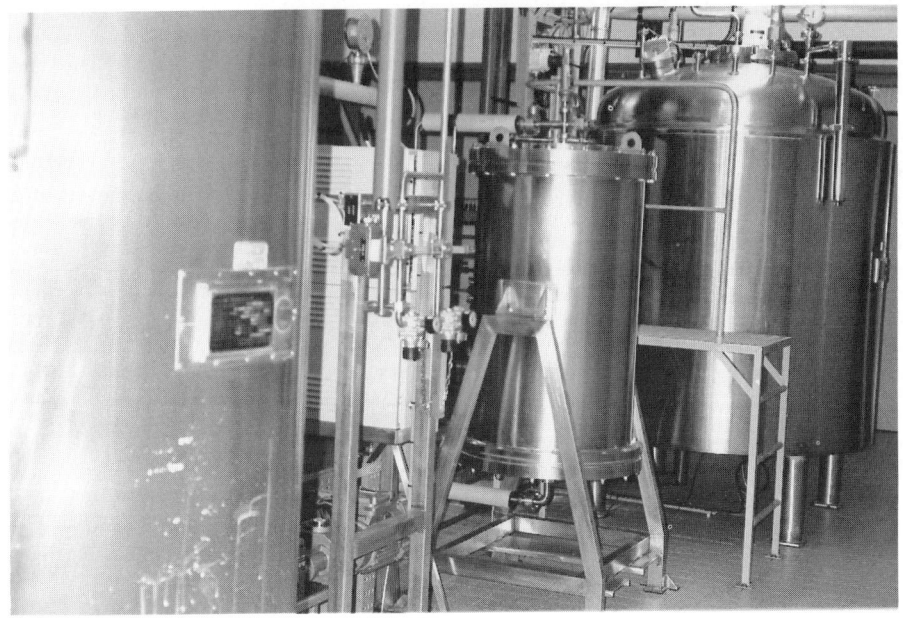

Photo 3 : *General view of column 3 (COOH-Spherodex) and the storage and retrieval tanks.*

A logic controller (CGEE Alsthom, C350) takes charge of the various stages and supervises the control parameters. The parameters are computered for each stage controlled by the PLC :
- ultrafiltration of plasma supernatant II+III prior to injection onto the first column,

- each stage of the chromatographic procedure,
- preparing buffers with ultrafiltration,
- washing/sterilization

The full cycle is continuously monitored on a synoptic screen (Sycolor, 8800 series) which provides a diagrammatic representation of the unit. If the event of a default that might jeopardize batch quality and safety of the equipment, the cycle stops automatically and the fault is typed out on the screen and on one of the four printers connected to the logic controller. Depending on requirements, the unit can function either automatically, semi-automatically or manually. Static and dynamic trials have been successfully undertaken to validate the computer programmes and the various sensing devices in the unit.

2. Operating procedure for the chromatography unit

2.1. On-line buffer dilution

Highly concentrated buffers, used for equilibration, elution and washing are prepared in sufficient quantities for approximately 10 to 12 cycles and kept in storage tanks. The buffers are subsequently diluted 10 to 100-fold in order to obtain the required concentration. The "on-line dilution" process is used for diluting buffer solutions. A feed pump sends a given amount of the concentrated buffer into the circuit at a predefined flow-rate. The triple-case pump that controls the overall flow-rate in the unit enforces a flow-rate above that of the feed pump supplying the buffer. The difference in volume resulting from the difference in flow-rates is compensated by the direct admission of water. The water sucked into the circuit is used to dilute the buffer, which consequently reaches the entrance to the columns at the required concentration.

2.2. Chromatographic procedure for purifying albumin

The industrial unit is capable of processing 350 to 400 litres of the starting plasma per cycle. For the first six batches only 300 litres of plasma were used on average per cycle. The plasma is first fractionated to stage II+III using the Cohn method when it contains on average 9.1 kg of albumin. The supernatant II+III is then diafiltered at constant volume against 5 volumes of water on 56 polysulfone 10000 D cassettes Photo 1). This procedure eliminates the ethanol and salts contained in the albumin solution (Martinache and Hénon, 1980). The diafiltered supernatant II+III is stored in a sterile, heat regulated tank at 4°C and then adjusted to pH 5.25, 0.70 mS/cm before being injected onto the first column.

Column 1 (220 l of DEAE-Spherodex LS) is first equilibrated with a 0.1 M phosphate buffer at pH 6.0, 6.6 mS/cm, in order to rapidly equilibrate and saturate the active areas of the chromatographic support. Final equilibration is achieved with a 0.01 M phosphate buffer at pH 5.25, 0.70 mS/cm. The equilibrated supernatant is injected onto the column at the flow-rate of 310 litres/hour, through two successive 0.2 µm filters, which guarantee fully sterile conditions throughout. If the first filter becomes clogged, the albumin solution is injected onto the second filter via a by-pass system to ensure that the sterility of the procedure is not interrupted. Throughout the chromatographic cycle, flow-rate, protein conductivity and elution (UV at 280 nm) are measured and recorded continuously.

Immunoglobulins and transferrin in particular pass through the first column without being bound. Albumin along with alpha- and beta-globulins are bound on the support. The column is rinced with the equilibrating buffer and the retained fraction is eluted with a 0.025 M sodium acetate buffer at pH 4.7, 1.0 mS/cm. The eluted protein solution is then retrieved in the second sterile, heat controlled tank at 4°C. At this stage the albumin is already 95 % pure, as the immunoglobulins, alpha-1-antitrypsin, haptoglobin, ceruloplasmin and polymers have mainly been removed. An average of 500 l of albumin fraction containing 8.4 kg of albumin is retrieved at the end of the first stage. The column is then washed using a cycle that is identical for the other two stages. This cycle consists of successively injecting the following solutions : 1 M NaCl, 0.1 M HCl and ethanol/0.5 M acetic acid (at a ratio of 60/40).

Column 2 contains 125 litres of QMA-Spherosil LS gel. Rapid equilibration is carried out first with a 0.05 M sodium acetate buffer at pH 5.5, 3.3 mS/cm. The column is then equilibrated with a 0.025 M sodium acetate buffer at pH 4.7, 1.0 mS/cm.

The albumin solution is adjusted to the values of the equilibrating buffer solution before it is injected onto the column at a flow-rate of 215 litres/hour. The control parameters are identical to those applied during the first stage. The albumin and alpha-1-globulins pass through the column without being bound. 800 litres of the fraction containing approximately 8.0 kg of albumin are stored in tank number 3. At this stage, the albumin solution is over 98% pure as the bile pigments and pyrogenic substances have been almost totally eliminated. The gel is then washed according to the procedure described above.

Direct equilibration of column 3 (280 litres of COOH-Spherodex LS) is carried out using a 0.05 M sodium acetate buffer at pH 5.5, 3.3 mS/cm. The albumin solution is adjusted to the same values and injected onto the column. The albumin flows through the column without being bound and comes out over 99 % pure. Tank number 4 contains an albumin solution of approximately 7.5 g/l. The albumin solution is then ultrafiltered against water and concentrated at the protein level required (40 or 200 g/l) (Photo 4). The chromatographic albumin is adjusted, stabilized, filtered and subjected to the legal controls.

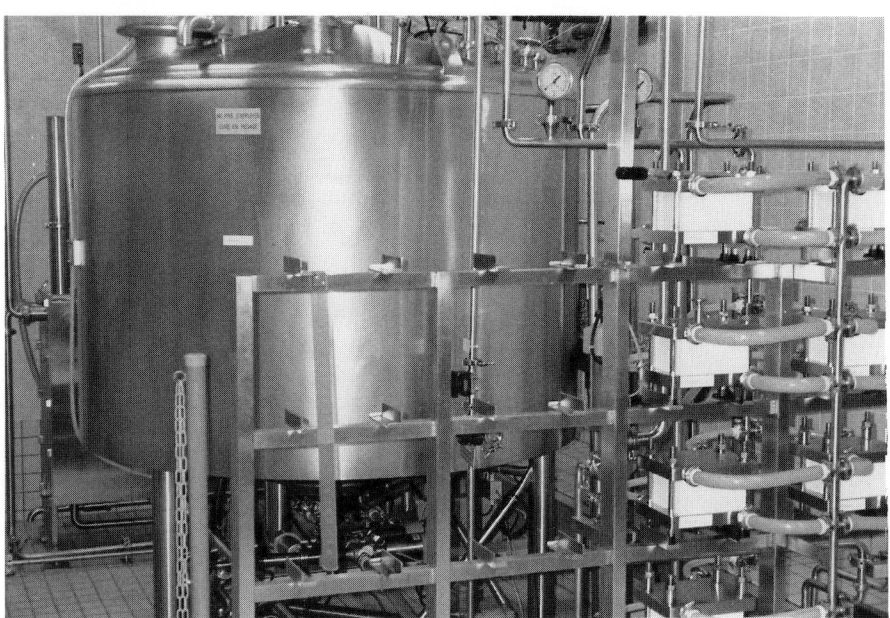

Photo 4 : *Final ultrafiltration unit place dowstream from column 3. This unit is capable of processing 2500 litres of albumin solution after passing through the last ion exchanger.*

2.3. Washing, sterilizing and gel regeneration

At the end of each stage of chromatography, the piping and tanks are washed and sterilized with a washing system incorporated in the unit (CIP). Several cycles consisting of injections of cold water, hot water, sodium chloride, nitric acid and hot distilled water guarantee complete cleansing of the storage tanks and connecting pipes. The circuit is sterilized by injecting steam at 125°C for 40 minutes.

During the final washing cycle, the chromatographic gels and the piping system in the unit are sanitized and any pyrogens removed chemically with the ethanol/acid mixture. They are kept in this solution until the following production cycle. These procedures have all been validated and confirmed during the pilot trials. During the process, the whole unit is kept sterile by filtering the diluted buffer solutions on 0.22 µm filters and by microfiltration of the buffers or the albumin prior to entering each column. Microfilter sterility is guaranteed by storing the system in 1.5 to 2 % formol.

RESULTS - OUTPUT

Overall albumin output for 6 batches of 300 litres of plasma was 74 %, i.e. 24.9 g/l. These values are higher than the results obtained on the pilot plant (Stoltz et al., 1987), when output was only 68 %. Further improvement on these figures should be possible by increasing the amount of supernatant II+III used at the start of the procedure to 350 or 400 litres, which should provide 27 to 28 g of albumin per litre of the starting plasma.

Throughout the cycle, the albumin and the buffer solutions are ultrafiltered and filtered several times under sterile conditions (4 for albumin and 2 for the buffer solutions). The storage tanks and piping are sterilized either with steam or chemicals between each stage of the procedure. These precautions guarantee that both the plant and, consequently, the fractionated albumin remain permanently sterile. As each stage of chromatography eliminates pyrogenic substances, polymers and hemoglobin, the end product results in a very high purity albumin solution (>99 %) corroborating the results obtained on the pilot plant. Table 1 gives the results of the main values that were checked.

The other parameters that were controlled all comply with the standards laid down by the European Pharmacopoeia, Edition II, 1990.

Table 1 : *Mean values obtained over 6 batches of 300 litres of starting plasma*

	Pharmacopoeia standard	Mean values
Purity	> 0.95	> 0.99
Polymers	< 5.00 %	0.10
Hb	A < 0.15	0.0
Aluminium	< 200 µg/l	20.00
Ethanol	< 0.30 g/l	0
Ag Hbs	negative	negative
Ac HIV	negative	negative
Pyrogen (3 rabbits)	non pyrogen T < 1.15°C	non pyrogen T < 0.1°C

CONCLUSIONS

The assessment of the pilot scale chromatographic procedure for purifying human albumin confirmed the optimal conditions for using Spherosil and Spherodex supports. The overall output for the first six batches of fractionated albumin supplied an average of 74% (24.9 g/l of the starting plasma). This figure could most probably be improved by using 350 to 400 litre-batches of the starting material. After passing through the second column albumin purity is already 98% and after the last column is above 99%. The results obtained during these trials are an improvement on the values registered during the manual pilot study, mainly due to scaling up and automating the process, which have provided the procedure with increased reliability and reproducibility.

Moreover, with this chromatographic purification technique it is possible not only to obtain very high purity albumin, but also to recover protein sub-fractions that may be of therapeutic or biological value (immunoglobulins, transferrin, alpha-1-antitrypsin, transthyretin...). These proteins can subsequently be purified using other chromatographic procedures.

REFERENCES

Cohn, E.J., Strong, L.E., Hugues, W.L., Mulfor, D.J., Ashworth, J.J., Melin, M., Trylor, H.L. (1946): Preparation and properties of serum and plasma proteins IV : a system for the preparation into fractions of proteins and lipoprotein components of biological tissues and fluids. *J. Amer. Chem. Soc.* 68, 459-476.

Dromard, A., Exertier, M., Rollin, C., Tayot, J.L., Tardy, M. (1984): Procédé de fractionnement de plasma. *Brevet Rhône-Poulenc, Institut Mérieux. Demande Europe N°84400602-3*.

Martinache, L., Henon, M.P. (1980): Concentration and desalting by ultrafiltration. In *Methods of plasma protein fractionation*, ed. J.M. Curling, pp. 223-235. Acad. Press.

Stoltz, J.F., Rivat, C., Geschier, C., Colosetti, P., Sertillanges, P., Tondon, J., Regnault, V. (1987): Purification chromatographique de l'albumine humaine à l'échelle pilote. *Biosciences* 6, 103-106.

Stoltz, J.F., Rivat, C., Geschier, C., Colosetti, P., Sertillanges, P. (1989): Chromatographic purification of human albumin. Technical and economic aspects. In *Biotechnologie de purification des Protéines,*. eds J.F. Stoltz et C. Rivat, colloque INSERM, vol. 175, 191-200. Paris, Editions INSERM.

Stoltz, J.F., Rivat, C., Geschier, C., Colosetti, P., Dumont, L. (1991): Chromatographic purification of human albumin for clinical uses. *Pharm. Tech. Int.* 3, 60-65.

Tayot, J.L., Tardy, M., Gattel, P. (1980): Ion exchange and affinity chromatography on silica derivatives. In *Methods of plasma protein fractionation*, ed. J.M. Curling, pp. 149-160. Acad. Press.

Tayot, J.L., Grandgeorge, M., Blanc, P., Gattel, P., Tardy, M., Paturel, J., Pla, J., Debrus, A., Liautaud, J., Plan, R., Peyron, L. (1981): Chromatographie industrielle, production et qualité de l'albumine humaine d'origine placentaire. In *Coopération internationale et dérivés sanguins*, pp. 47-58. Fondation Marcel Mérieux, Talloires (France).

Résumé

La quasi totalité de l'albumine humaine utilisée en thérapeutique (ou en biologie) est actuellement préparée par des méthodes dérivées du procédé initial dit de Cohn. Ces différentes techniques consistent à précipiter les protéines à basses températures en présence d'alcool, à pH et forces ioniques variables. Récemment, des alternatives à ces techniques ont été proposées par utilisation de supports chromatographiques d'échange d'ions. En particulier, un procédé à base de support de silice, utilisé initialement pour le placenta, (échangeurs d'ions Sphérosil-Sphérodex, Sepracor-IBF, France) a été proposé pour l'albumine plasmatique. L'installation industrielle, décrite dans ce travail, a été réalisée au Centre Régional de Transfusion de Nancy (France) en liaison avec l'Institut Mérieux (Marcy l'Etoile, France) et permet de traiter 350 à 400 litres de plasma par cycle. L'albumine obtenue est de haute pureté (>99 %) avec un rendement de l'ordre de 27 à 28 grammes par litre de plasma départ.

Combined Cohn/chromatography purification process for the manufacturing of high purity human albumin from plasma

J.-L. Véron, P. Gattel, J. Pla, P. Fournier and M. Grandgeorge

Pasteur Mérieux Sérums et Vaccins, 1541, avenue Marcel Mérieux, 69280 Marcy-l'Étoile, France

ABSTRACT

Cohn's alcohol fractionation method is still today the most widely used process to purify human albumin from plasma. Pasteurized Cohn's albumin is considered as clinically safe with regard to the risk of blood-borne virus transmission. Current such albumin preparations have an electrophoretic purity of $\approx$ 97 - 98% and contain 2 - 5% high molecular weight aggregates (partially heat denatured impurities bound to albumin). We now have developed a new manufacturing process which adds to Cohn's fractionation a 2 steps column chromatography purification using Spherosil^R gels. Cohn's supernatant IV or precipitate V obtained from 420 l plasma was successively processed on a 125 l DEAE-Spherodex^R column and a 50 l QMA-Spherosil^R column. The purified albumin was finally concentrated, stabilized and pasteurized as usual. The overall yield of chromatography was 91%. Final albumin was 100% pure by cellulose acetate electrophoresis. No contaminant was detected by two-dimensional crossed immunoelectrophoresis. Gel filtration on G 200 and HPLC on TSK 4000 showed practically no high molecular weight aggregate. Furthermore, chromatography purification *per se* demonstrated varying efficacy to remove viruses, from 0 (poliovirus) to 7.7 log 10 (HIV-1).

INTRODUCTION

Several chromatographic processes to purify human albumin from plasma have already been described : some of them add one or two chromatographic steps to the Cohn's ethanol procedure (Pharmacia, 1976 ; Matsuoka & Shodai, 1989), others start directly by chromatography from desalted plasma (Curling, 1980 ; Fourcart *et al.*, 1982), or from various intermediate stages in the ethanol process (Fisher *et al.*, 1980 ; Dromard *et al.*, 1984). All these processes are mainly based on ion exchange chromatography, but affinity chromatography may also be a good alternative (Saint-Blancard *et al.*, 1982).
However, these processes generally require high quantities of chromatographic media, particularly when they start from the first steps of Cohn's method, and are thus not well adapted to industrial development mainly for economical reasons. Another drawback is that albumin obtained in some of these processes still contains polymers/aggregates which have been suspected of causing adverse reactions in patients.
This paper describes a new combined Cohn/Chromatography purification process to purify human albumin whose main advantages are :
- Use of high capacity silica based chromatographic media, well adapted to industrial scale processing.
- High albumin yield and obtention of a high purity, aggregate free product.
- Improved viral safety as compared to classical Cohn's pasteurized albumin.

MATERIAL AND METHOD

Cohn/Chromatography purification process (Grandgeorge *et al.*, 1991)
As shown on Fig. 1, cryo-poor-plasma was first processed according to Cohn's method 6 (Cohn *et al.*, 1946) until Fraction V paste (Fr. V).

Fr. V paste was then dissolved in pyrogen free demineralized water (10 liters/kg Fr. V) with a final resistivity value of > 700 Ω cm. Optionally, precipitation V was omitted : in that case, supernatant IV was directly concentrated and diafiltered in order to remove alcohol and adjust resistivity.

Then, pH was adjusted at 5.25 and the solution was sterile filtered. The albumin solution (solubilized Fr. V or diafiltered supernatant IV) was filtered onto a DEAE-Spherodex^R column (IBF-Sepracor) previously equilibrated with 10mM, pH 5.25 phosphate buffer. Non adsorbed proteins were washed out with phosphate buffer and thereafter, bound albumin was eluted with 25mM, pH 4.7, Na-acetate buffer. At this step, the volume of chromatography gel used was ≥ 10 ml/g albumin.

Albumin solution was then directly passed through a QMA-Spherosil^R column (IBF-Sepracor) previously equilibrated with 25mM, pH 4.7, Na-acetate buffer. Albumin was recovered in the filtrate. At this step, the volume of chromatography gel used was ≥ 4 ml/g albumin. Regeneration cycles were identical for the two columns, i.e 1 M NaCl, 0.1N HCl, and a 60% ethanol - 0.5 N acetic acid solution.

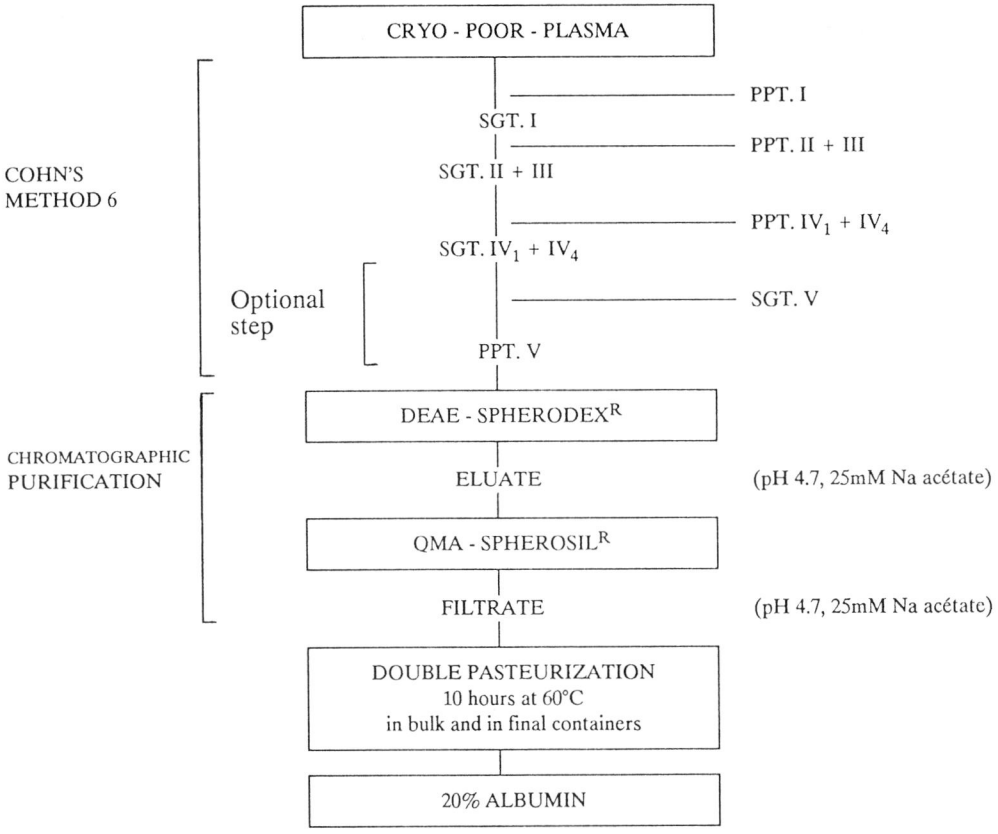

Fig. 1 Cohn/Chromatography process for human albumin manufacture

QMA-Spherosil filtrate was concentrated to 200 g/l by ultrafiltration and sterile filtered after addition of the stabilizers, Na-caprylate (2.7 g/l), N-acetyltryptophane (4 g/l) and Tween 80 (15 mg/l) (Grandgeorge & Fournier, 1989). Albumin solution was finally pasteurized (10 hours at +60°C), first in bulk, then in final containers after dispensing.

Batches were produced in a chromatography facility with the capacity to process the equivalent of 420 liters plasma (resp. 40 kg Fr. V precipitate). Chromatography columns used were 1 x 125 l (100 x 40 cm - h x d) DEAE-Spherodex and 1 x 50 l (71 x 30 cm - h x d) QMA-Spherosil glass columns (Biopass).

Standard Cohn's albumin

A standard commercial 20 % albumin produced by the Cohn's method was used for comparison in the following electrophoretic and size-exclusion chromatography analysis.

Electrophoretic analysis
Cellulose acetate electrophoresis were carried out on Cellogel^R strips (Sebia) in pH 9.2 tris-veronal buffer (200 V - 30 mn) ; staining was done with amidoschwarz 10B ; analysis were performed at protein concentrations of 2 % and 20 % ; strips were scanned on a Preference Ecran densitometer (Sebia).
Two-dimensional crossed immunoelectrophoresis were performed on 1.5 % agarose plates in pH 8.6 veronal buffer, against anti-human rabbit immune serum (Sebia) at a protein concentration of 100 g/l. Plates were stained with amidoschwarz 10B.

Size exclusion chromatography
Testing for polymers and aggregates was done by chromatography on Sephadex G200 (Pharmacia) in a pH 7.0, 0.4 M NaCl, 50mM phosphate buffer. Peaks were detected by 280 nm UV absorption. HPLC analysis was also performed on a TSKG 4000 SW column (300 x 7.5 mm, Hewlett Packard) using the same phosphate buffer. Peaks detection was done at 280 nm or by refractometry.

Other analysis
Aluminium was titrated by atomic absorption spectrophotometry (Faculté de Pharmacie, Lyon). Other quality control analysis were performed according to the European Pharmacopeia.

Viral validation of the manufacturing process
All the manufacturing steps, except Fr. V precipitation which is optional in the process, were investigated by spiking experiments for their capacity to eliminate and/or inactivate viruses, in accordance with viral validation recommendations of the CEC Note for guidance III/8115 189 - EN. Viruses used were relevant HBV and HIV1, and model viruses : Poliovirus (Sabin 2), Avian Reovirus (Van der Heide) and Sindbis virus (ATCC AR 39).

RESULTS

Albumin recovery and purification during chromatographic steps.
The overall albumin recovery during the chromatographic steps, i.e from Fr. V solution to QMA-Spherosil filtrate, was 91 % $\pm$ 6 (mean $\pm$ SD, n = 38 batches) of the initial total proteins. Essentially all protein loss (9 %) occured during the first DEAE-Spherodex step. During this step, the electrophoretic purity as measured by cellulose acetate electrophoresis at 2 % raised from 98 % to 100 %.
Electrophoretic purity improvement during the QMA-Spherosil step was only evidenced on overloaded acetate strips (20 % prot.). Moreover, this step was important to remove hydrophobic impurities as shown by the decrease of pigment absorption : $DO_{403nm - 1\%}$ from 0.040 down to 0.015.

Quality control on final product.
Table 1 summarizes the main purity characteristics of Cohn/Chromatography albumin compared to classical Cohn's albumin. All lots analysed were manufactured from the optional Fr. V precipitation step.
Cellulose acetate electrophoresis demonstrated the high purity of Cohn/Chromatography albumin since, even when performed at 20 %, no contaminant was detected. On the contrary, Cohn's albumin disclosed 2.7 % and 4.1 % α-globulins impurities at 2 % and 20 % protein concentration respectively.
Two-dimensional crossed immunoelectrophoresis (Fig. 2) also detected no contaminant in Cohn/Chromatography albumin, but 7 impurities peaks (some faint) were observed with classical Cohn's albumin.
High molecular weight species measured by Sephadex G200 were 0.24 % $\pm$ 0.29 (mean $\pm$ SD, n = 15) in Cohn/Chromatography albumin. On the contrary, 9.38 % polymers/aggregates were measured in Cohn's albumin : if we calculate this percentage as recommended by the European Pharmacopeia, i.e by nitrogen titration after mineralization, polymers/aggregates were somewhat lower : about 3.7 %.
By size exclusion HPLC on TSKG 4000 SW column and UV detection (Fig. 3) no polymer was detected in Cohn/Chromatography albumin but 7.4 % high molecular weight species were found in Cohn's albumin. By refractometry detection, this figure was lower (3.0 %). It is noteworthy that high molecular weight compounds found in Cohn's albumin eluted near the exclusion volume which corresponds to very high molecular weights, ranging from 1 to 7 x 10^6 daltons.

Viral validation of the purification process
Results of spiking experiments with relevant and model viruses are given in Table 2. Cumulative reduction factors obtained with relevant viruses (whole process except precipitation V) were : >22 $\log_{10}$ HIV-1, >5.58 DNA HBV and >5.04 DNA-polymerase HBV. When model poliovirus was not applicable due to the presence of high poliovirus antibodies titers (step I and step II + III), we used Avian Reovirus. For these 2 viruses, cumulative reduction factors obtained were : >8.8 $\log_{10}$ poliovirus (without precipitations I and II + III) and >9.55 $\log_{10}$ avian Reovirus (without chromatographic steps).

Table 1. Quality control of Cohn/Chromatography albumin versus Cohn's albumin

	Cohn/Chromatography (mean of 15 lots)	Cohn's albumin
- % purity (cell. acetate electrophoresis at 2 % protein)	100	97.3
- % purity (cell. acetate electrophoresis at 20 % protein)	100	95.9
- Two-dimensional crossed immuno-electrophoresis	no contaminant	7 contaminants
- % polymers / aggregates (280nm)		
. G 200 (mean ± SD)	0.24 ± 0.29	9.38
. HPLC TSKG 4000 SW	0 (all batches)	7.40
- Aluminium (μg/l)	≤ 20	300 (manufactured 1989, analysed 1990)

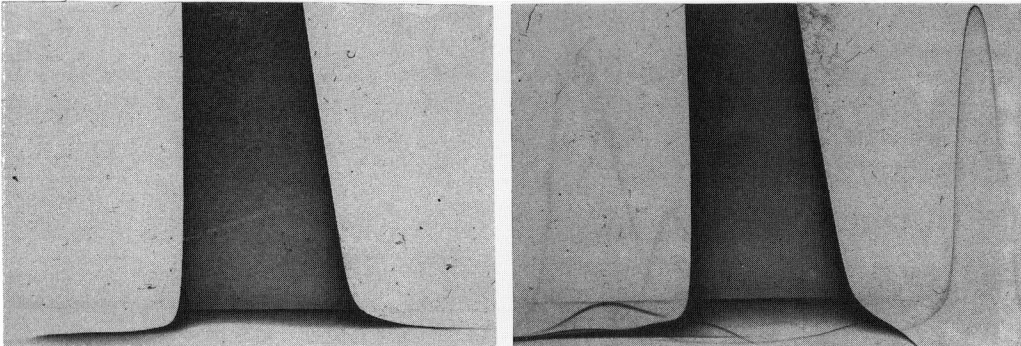

Fig.2 Two-dimensional crossed immunoelectrophoresis of Cohn/Chromatography albumin (left) and Cohn's albumin (right), against anti-human rabbit immune serum.

Two manufacturing steps proved to be of particular importance for viral safety :
- Step IV_1 + IV_4 was very effective in eliminating viruses and virus markers in the precipitate, either under native form (case of Poliovirus and Avian Reovirus) or fully inactivated (case of HIV-1).
- Pasteurization 10 hours at +60°C demonstrated a great efficacy in inactivating viruses, since reduction factors were obtained after only one hour of pasteurization. Sindbis virus which is used as a model for hepatitis C virus, was the most resistant to heat denaturation since some residual infectivity was found after 10 hours at +60°C.

The two chromatographic steps, despite a good efficacy in eliminating HIV-1 and HBV markers, were of no effect on Poliovirus.

A

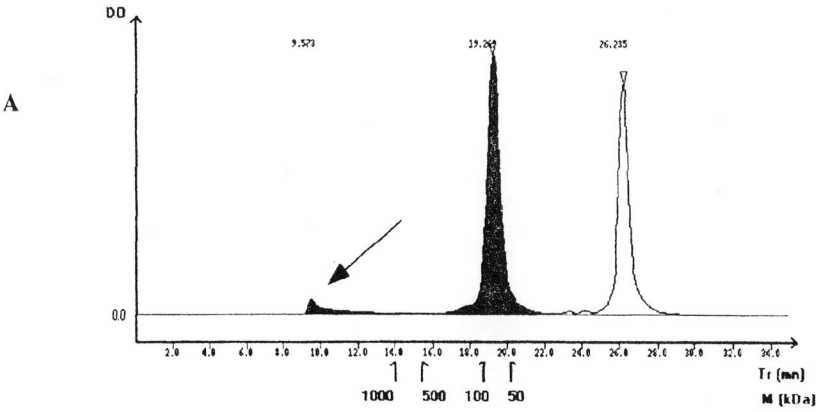

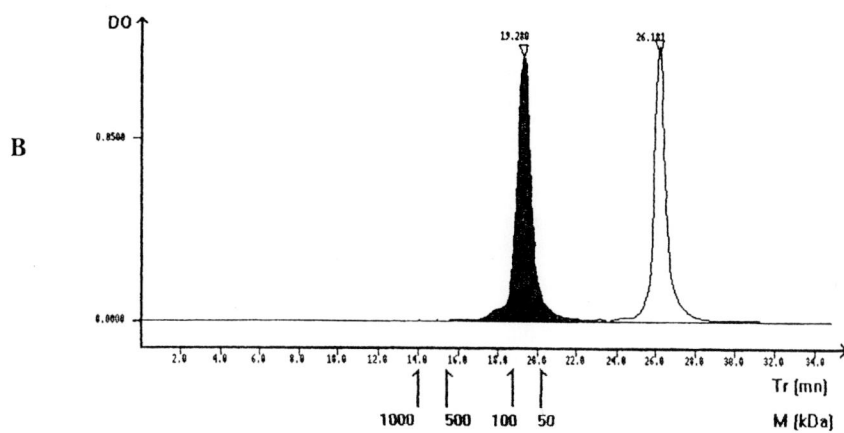

Fig.3 Size exclusion HPLC on TSKG 4000 SW. (A) Cohn's albumin, (B) Cohn/chromato albumin

Table 2. Virus reduction factors obtained in spiking experiments (in $\log_{10}$)   ND : Not Done

Manufacturing steps	HIV-1	HBV DNA	HBV DNA-polymerase	Poliovirus Sabin 2	Avian Reovirus	Sindbis virus
Precipitation I	2.0	0.17	0.56	ND	0	ND
Precipitation II + III	> 3.0	0.25	0.11	ND	0.9	ND
Precipitation IV$_1$ + IV$_4$	> 4.6	> 2.32	> 1.27	3.1	3.6	ND
DEAE-Spherodex	3.5	1.43	> 0.71	0	ND	ND
QMA-Spherosil	4.2	1.11	> 0.90	0	ND	ND
Pasteurization	> 4.7	0.3	1.49	> 5.7	> 5.05	4.2
OVERALL REDUCTION	> 22	> 5.58	5.04	> 8.8	> 9.55	4.2

DISCUSSION - CONCLUSION

A chromatographic process using Spherosils^R to purify human albumin from plasma had already been described before by Rhône Poulenc/Institut Mérieux (Dromard et al., 1984 ; Tayot et al., 1987) and further developed by CRTS of Nancy (Stoltz et al., 1987) : this process had only one optional alcohol precipitation step (I + II + III) but three chromatographic steps. The new Cohn/Chromatography process we described here has 3 important advantages as compared to the former process :
- Only two chromatographic steps are necessary, instead of three previously, to obtain pure albumin in two-dimensional crossed immunoelectrophoresis (no contaminant) and Sephadex G200 analysis (absence of polymers / aggregates).
- Amounts of gels in the new process are 2 times lower for DEAE-Spherodex and 3 times lower for QMA-Spherosil as compared to the former process. COOH-Spherodex step is omitted in the new process.
- Preserving the whole Cohn's method, and especially IV1 + IV4 precipitation step as demonstrated by our spiking experiments, is an important advantage for the viral safety of this new manufacturing process.

More generally, albumin manufactured by Cohn's method associated with pasteurization, has been recognized as clinically safe for more than 45 years regarding virus transmission ; nevertheless, we showed that the 2 more chromatographic steps after the Cohn's process further increased the safety towards the risk of HIV-1 and HBV transmission.

One main feature of this Cohn/Chromatography albumin is the absence of polymers/aggregates. Polymers/aggregates usually found in Cohn's albumin solutions are very high molecular weight species of more than 1×10^6 daltons (TSK 4000 HPLC analysis). These species contain only 30-50% albumin and are formed by disulfide bonds between albumin and the small amounts of denatured impurity globulins (haptoglobin, transferrin) during the pasteurization step. These polymers or aggregates are suspected of causing adverse reactions in patients, but there is no clear proof of this suspicion (Dengler et al., 1989). When a patient undergoes a double plasmapheresis, i.e 5 liters of 50 g/l albumin solution, the amount of denatured proteins infused could be as high as 7.5 g (if the level of polymers/aggregates is 3% of total albumin) ; This could lead to adverse reactions due to the activation/blockade of the reticuloendothelial system or non specific activation of complement. Potential immunogenicity of these aggregates might also cause adverse reactions (Finlayson, 1980).

Comparative clinical studies performed with a high purity, polymers/aggregates free albumin obtained from placentas, showed better tolerance of this product as compared to classical Cohn's albumin (Grandgeorge, 1988). Thus, we hope that the present Cohn/Chromatography albumin will also demonstrate an improved clinical tolerance.

REFERENCES

Cohn, E.J., Strong, L.E., Hughes, W.L. (1946) : Preparation and properties of serum and plasma protein. A system for the separation into fractions of the protein and lipoprotein components of biological tissues and fluids. J. Am. Chem. Soc. 68 : 459 - 475.

Curling, J.M. (1980) : Albumin Purification by Ion Exchange Chromatography. In : Methods of plasma protein fractionation. Academic Press, pp. 77 - 91.

Dengler, T., Stöcker, U., Kellner, S., Fürst, G. (1989) : Chemical and immunochemical characterization of polymers or aggregates in preparations of human serum albumin. Infusionstherapie. 16 : 160 - 164.

Dromard, M., Exertier, M., Rollin, C., Tayot, J.L., Tardy, M. (1984) : Procédé de fractionnement du plasma. Brevet Rhône Poulenc - Institut Mérieux. Demande Europe n° 84400602-3.

Finlayson, J.S. (1980) : Albumin products. In Seminars in Thrombosis and Hemostasis. VI (2) : 85-120.

Fourcart, J., Saint-Blancard, J., Girot, P., Boschetti, E. (1982) : Preparation de l'albumine et des immunoglobulines G par fractionnement chromatographique direct du plasma humain sur DEAE et CM-Trisacryl M. Revue Française de Transfusion et immuno-hématologie. XXV (1) : 7 - 17.

Grandgeorge, M. (1988) : Purification and quality control of human albumin at Institut Merieux. Proceedings of the symposium on biotechnology for blood derivatives, Bangkok. Chulalongkorn University Printing House (3205-269/500) (4).

Grandgeorge, M., Fournier, P. (1989) : Procédé de stabilisation des solutions d'albumine humaine et solutions obtenues. Brevet Institut Mérieux - Demande Europe n° 89400947.1

Grandgeorge, M., Véron, J.L., Fournier, P. (1991) : Procédé pour isoler de l'albumine humaine. Brevet Institut Mérieux - Demande Europe n° 91403570.4.

Matsuoka, Y., Shodai, O. (1989) : Albumin preparation and process for preparing the same. Green Cross Corporation. European patent application n°0367 220.

Pharmacia Fine Chemicals. (1976) : Procédé pour isoler de l'albumine à partir de produits provenant du sang. Brevet français n° 2327 256.

Saint-Blancard, J., Kirzin, J.M., Riberon, P., Petit, F., Fourcart, J., Girot, P., Boschetti, E. (1982) : A simple and rapide procedure for large scale preparation of IgG and albumin from human plasma by ion exchange and affinity chromatography. Affinity Chromatography and Related Techniques, pp. 305 - 312. Amsterdam : Elsevier.

Stoltz, J.F., Rivat, C., Geschier, C., Colosetti, P., Sertillanges, P., Tondon, J., Regnault, V. (1987) : Purification chromatographique de l'albumine plasmatique humaine à l'échelle pilote. BIO-SCIENCES. 6 (4) : 103 -106.

Tayot, J.L., Tardy, M., Gattel, P., Cueille, G., Liautaud, J. (1987) : Large scale use of Spherosil ion exchangers in plasma fractionation. Develop. biol. Standard. 67 : 15 - 24.

Résumé

La technique de Cohn est toujours très largement utilisée pour purifier l'albumine plasmatique humaine : cette albumine pasteurisée est considérée comme sûre vis-à-vis du risque de transmission virale. Les albumines issues de ce procédé présentent une pureté électrophorétique voisine de 97 - 98 % et contiennent 2 - 5 % de polymères/agrégats (en partie des impuretés liées à l'albumine après dénaturation à la pasteurisation).

Le nouveau procédé de fabrication décrit ici rajoute au fractionnement de Cohn, deux étapes de purification par chromatographie sur supports Spherosil^R. Le surnageant IV de Cohn ou la fraction V provenant de 420 l de plasma sont successivement traités sur une colonne de 125 l de DEAE-Spherodex^R et une colonne de 50 l de QMA - Spherosil^R. L'albumine purifiée est concentrée, stabilisée et pasteurisée 10h à +60°C. Le rendement global de la chromatographie est de 91%. L'albumine finale présente une pureté de 100% en électrophorèse sur acétate de cellulose. Aucun contaminant n'est visible en cross-immunoélectrophorèse. Une absence de polymères/agrégats est constatée en gel filtration sur G200 et en HPLC sur colonne TSK 4000.

De plus, les étapes de chromatographie ajoutent au procédé de Cohn, déjà considéré comme sûr, une efficacité supplémentaire pour éliminer VIH-1 et VHB.

Membrane based pseudobioaffinity chromatography of placental IgG using immobilized L-histidine

Sivanadane Mandjiny and M.A. Vijayalakshmi

Laboratoire de Technologie des Séparations, Université de Technologie de Compiègne, B.P. 649, Compiègne, France

SUMMARY

Histidine has already been reported as a pseudobiospecific affinity ligand for the purification of immunoglobulin G (IgG) using conventional chromatographic matrices such as Sepharose and silica. We now report the coupling of histidine to three different membrane based matrices namely Immunodyne (PAL), silica and nylon-methacrylate composite membranes. The chromatographic profile, elution volume and the cycle time of adsorption and desorption are comparable with those of protein A liganded commercial membrane for the purification of IgG from human placenta. The adsorption isotherm of IgG on these histidyl membranes have been determined to calculate the equilibrium dissociation constant K_D. For the commercial protein A liganded membrane K_D is determined to be 5.0×10^{-5} M and for histidyl membranes are of the order of 3.3×10^{-5} to 14×10^{-5} M. Adsorption capacity of IgG determined experimentally is found to vary with different flux.

INTRODUCTION

Affinity chromatography is essentially an adsorption method which exploits recognition between an immobilized ligand and the molecule to be separated. Adsorption to the ligand represents one separation step (in which all non-adsorbed molecules are removed) and desorption (elution) from the ligand a second step. A new dimension added to the concept of affinity chromatography is the use of pseudobiospecific ligands such as single amino acids, reactive dyes and metal ions (Vijayalakshmi,1989). Previous work from our laboratory has shown the versatility of a pseudobiospecific ligand, L-histidine, which has been successfully utilised to purify several proteins including IgG (Kanoun et al., 1986).

Adsorbents based on porous beads can impose severe limitations on the ligand accessibility due to diffusion. Moreover, the compressibility of soft beads such as agarose during scale up operations could be a drawback. To overcome these difficulties, porous polymer matrices in the form of flat membranes or in the form of hollow fibers have been introduced recently.These membranes have high surface area, low pressure drop, high mechanical strength and good convective flow characteristics which greatly shorten the process time (Brandt et al., 1988). In addition, they can handle large volume of an unclarified solution in a short time. Therefore, it would be of interest to combine the advantage of selectivity of an affinity ligand along with the high throughput of a membrane-based system.

In this study, we have coupled histidine, a pseudobiospecific ligand, to three different membrane matrices having different functional groups.Chromatography was done with IgG from human placenta and the results were compared with those obtained with a protein-A liganded commercial membrane, in terms of capacity and the affinity constants for the same area. Repeatability, storage stability, and pH tolerance of these pseudo affinity membranes were examined.

MATERIALS AND METHODS

Underivatised Immunodyne (PAL),silica and the protein A-liganded Nygene membranes were kindly supplied by PAL Biosupport, NJ, U.S.A., FMC Bioproducts, ME, U.S.A., Nygene Corporation, N.Y., U.S.A., respectively. Underivatised Nylon methacrylate composite membrane was supplied by Dr.Müller-Schulte, Aachen, Germany. L-Histidine and IgG from different source like dog, horse, sheep, cow, rabit, monkey, rat, goat and pig were obtained from Sigma, Saint Louis, U.S.A. Epichlorohydrin and sodium borohydride were purchased from Merck (Darmstadt, F.R.G). Purified IgG preparation from human placenta (batch N°.88G5390) containing protein 163 g/l, glycine 20 g/l, NaCl 1 g/l and traces of IgA < 3% was a kind gift from Dr. Grand George of Institut Merieux, France.

Preparation of histidyl-nylon methacrylate composite membrane

The Nylon - methacrylate composite membrane was prepared according to method described in (Müller-Schulte et al., 1991). The membrane contains free hydroxyl groups on the surface. Coupling procedure of histidine to this membrane is similar to that of coupling histidine to Sepharose ® 4B as described in (Kanoun et al., 1986). 1.5 g of this membrane (6.4 cm X 6.4 cm) was taken in a flask and then 755 µl of 2N NaOH was added drop by drop over the surface of the membrane. Simultaneously 76 µl of epichlorohydrin and 4 mg of $NaBH_4$ were added very slowly with gentle agitation. Again after 10 minutes 755 µl of 2N NaOH was added dropwise along with 380 µl of epichlorohydrin and the membrane was shaken in a water bath at 25°C for 18 hours. The activated membrane was then washed with water and the coupling of L-histidine was done by plunging the membrane into a 2M sodium carbonate solution containing 20% dissolved L-histidine with shaking laterally at 65°C for 24 hours. The amount of ligand (L-histidine) bound to the membrane was determined to be 21µmoles/g (0.77 µmoles/cm^2) from the difference in the concentration of L-histidine measured before and after coupling. The concentration of L-histidine was measured optically at 220 nm. The schematic diagram of the histidyl-methacrylate composite membrane is shown in Fig. 1(a).

Preparation of histidyl-silica membrane

As per the manufacturer's note, the membrane was supplied in the form of a preset module which was already activated with glutaraldehyde. L-Histidine was coupled to free aldehyde group as per instructions supplied by manufacturer for protein coupling. Tube connection was made with the membrane module (diameter 4.7cm) similar to that of a chromatographic setup and the flow rate was adjusted to 6 ml/min. with distilled water. By this process the air bubbles were completely removed. Subsequently the membrane was equilibrated with 10mM diethylamine buffer, pH 10.93 for 20 minutes and then a 5% histidine solution prepared in the same buffer was passed through the membrane and recycled for 1 hour. All steps were carried out at room temperature. Then the membrane was washed with diethylamine buffer without L-histidine for 20 min. to remove the uncoupled amino acid. Unreacted free aldehyde groups were blocked with Tris.HCl buffer, 0.5M, pH 7.6 for 20 min. and then saturated with 0.01 M phosphate buffer, pH 8.0 containing 2 mg/ml $NaBH_4$. Finally the membrane was equilibrated with 25mM Tris-HCl, pH 7.4, a starting buffer in chromatographic experiments. The schematic diagram of the histidyl-silica membrane is shown in Fig.1(b).

Preparation of histidyl Immunodyne (PAL) membrane

Since the surface of this membrane has already been preactivated for protein coupling, the coupling procedure of histidine was similar to that of a protein.

Briefly, the membrane (8.7 cm X 8.7 cm, approx. 1.2 g) was treated with 5% L-histidine solution in 0.1M phosphate buffer, pH 7.8, in a petri dish at room temperature for 24 hours. After that the membrane was washed thoroughly with water and then with Tris.HCl buffer, 25 mM, pH 7.4.

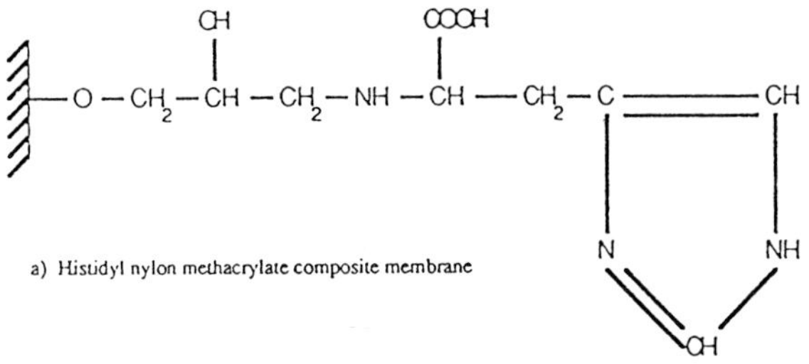

a) Histidyl nylon methacrylate composite membrane

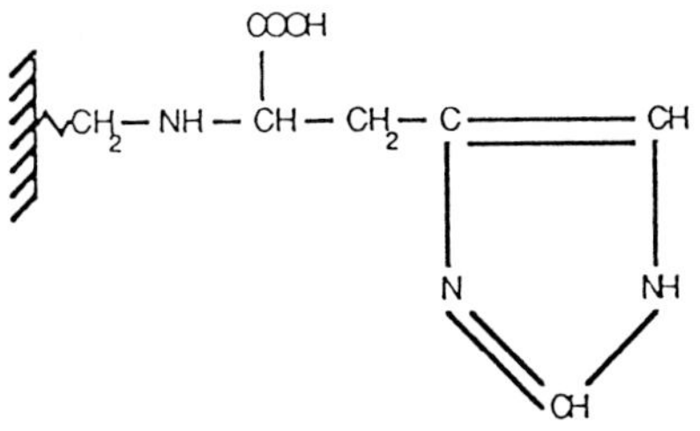

1b) Histidyl silica membrane

Fig.1 Schematic diagram of histidyl membranes
(a) Histidyl nylon-methacrylate composite membrane, (b) Histidyl silica membrane.

CHROMATOGRAPHY

Dynamic mode

In the dynamic mode, the histidyl nylon-methacrylate composite and histidyl Immunodyne (PAL) membranes were cut into circles of 4.6 cm. diameter and fixed into a commercially available filter module. The outlet of the module is directly connected to a pump, UV detector and then to a fraction collector. Initially, the membrane was equilibrated with the adsorption buffer Tris.HCl, 25 mM, pH 7.4, and an IgG solution of known concentration was injected into the module. Later on the membrane was washed with the same buffer to remove the loosely bound protein. The capacity of the membrane at that concentration was determined by eluting the adsorbed protein with the same starting buffer containing 0.2 M NaCl and 0.4 M NaCl. At the end of the cycle the membrane was washed well with NaOH, 0.05 M, and subsequently with the equilibrating buffer. The same experiment was repeated at different concentrations of IgG to measure the adsorption isotherm. Silica and protein A liganded Nygene membranes were run like a chromatographic column as they were supplied already in a sealed module. For protein A liganded Nygene membrane, conditions of adsorption and desorption of IgG were as per the manufacturer's instructions. In this case, the adsorption was done with PBS (Phosphate Buffered Saline) buffer, 0.15 M, pH 7.2 and desorption was with glycine-HCl buffer, 0.1 M, pH 2.5. After elution of bound protein the membrane was cleansed with Tris.HCl, 0.5 M, pH 9.6 and equilibrated with the starting buffer. All these experiments were carried out at 4°C.

Chromatography of IgG from different sources

Chromatography was performed as explained above but here the IgG sources are different like rat, pig, dog, monkey, cow, goat, sheep, horse and rat. Membrane used for this study was histidyl nylon-methacrylate composite. Flow rate was maintained at 144 ml/h. 5 mg of IgG of each source was injected. The percentage retention of IgG was determined by eluting the retained protein with the equilibrating buffer containing 0.2 M NaCl.

Chromatography of the serum IgG on histidyl-nylon methacrylate composite membrane

Human blood serum containing approx. 1.9 mg total protein was injected. Flow rate was maintained at 138 ml/h. After sufficient washing with the equilibrating buffer Tris.Hcl, 25 mM, pH 7.4, retained protein was eluted with the same buffer containing 0.2 M NaCl to check the selectivity of the membrane.

Effect of IgG concentration on adsorption

To see the impact of dilution on retention of IgG on histidyl-nylon methacrylate composite membrane, 6.6 mg of human placental IgG was dissolved in different volume from 1 ml to 25 ml and injected to the membrane. The amount of retained protein was determined after elution with the equilibrating buffer containing 0.2 M NaCl. Flow rate was maintained at 144 ml/h.

Adsorption Isotherm

For all the four membranes, namely, histidyl nylon-methacrylate composite, histidyl Immunodyne (PAL), histidyl silica and protein A liganded membranes the adsorption isotherms were measured at different concentrations of IgG. The capacity of the membrane at each concentration was defined as the amount of protein adsorbed per unit surface (cm^2) of the membrane. The equilibrium association/dissociation constants of human placental IgG and histidine immobilised on these four different membranes were calculated according to the equation 1 (Tsuchida et al., 1989; Sakai et al., 1989).

$$Q_a = \frac{Q_x K_a [C]}{1 + K_a [C]} \qquad \text{eq.(1)}$$

where [C]   —   Concentration of the protein (mg/ml)
Q_a —   Amount of protein adsorbed by the membrane (mg) (or) capacity of the membrane at conc.[C] (mg/cm^2)
Q_x —   Maximum protein adsorption by the membrane (mg) (or) maximum capacity of the membrane (mg/cm^2)
K_a —   Equilibrium association constant (ml/mg or M^{-1})

Effect of adsorption rate at different flow rates

The experiment was carried out as mentioned in dynamic mode except that for a fixed concentration of protein (6.6 mg IgG dissolved in 1ml), flow rate (Q,ml/min.) was varied and the capacity of the membrane ie., the quantity of protein retained per unit area as (mg/cm^2) was determined. The aim of this experiment was to ascertain whether the adsorption rate is a function of flow rate; the adsorption rate was calculated as follows:

$$\text{Adsorption rate (mg/cm}^2\text{/min.)} = \frac{\text{Amount of protein retained per unit area of the membrane (mg/cm}^2\text{)}}{\text{Time of adsorption (min.)}}$$

The concentration of IgG was maintained at 6.6 mg/ml and the flow rate was varied from 2.4 ml/min. to 6.3 ml/min. At all flow rates only 1 ml of the protein solution was injected. Time of adsorption was calculated as the ratio of volume of protein solution to flow rate ($t_{adsorption} = V/Q$; V in ml, Q in ml/min.).

To find a relation between the flow rate and the adsorption rate (AR), the flow rate is converted to flux (U) and plotted: ln (AR) against ln (U).

RESULTS

The chromatographic profiles of the four membranes, namely, histidyl nylon-methacrylate composite membrane, histidyl- Immunodyne (PAL) membrane, histidyl silica membrane and protein A-liganded nylon membrane are shown in Fig. 2. For the same amount of IgG injected i.e., 6.6 mg., the elution volume was measured as 27.6 ml, 23.0 ml, 58.0 ml and 33.6 ml for the histidyl nylon methacrylate composite, histidyl Immunodyne (PAL), histidyl silica and protein A liganded Nygene membranes, respectively. At the end of each chromatographic run the membranes were washed with NaOH, 0.05 M, to remove any strongly adsorbed protein, and thus to clean the membrane. Washing with NaOH, 0.05 M, did not cause any apparent problem. The results were reproducible even after one year, showing that all histidyl membranes are highly stable; this was not the case, though, with protein A liganded Nygene membrane. All histidyl membranes are also stable with respect to high pH.

Fig.3 represents the percentage retention of IgG from different sources. The data obtained suggest the differences in binding strength of those IgG towards the ligand. The selectivity of the membrane towards IgG was revealed by the chromatogram of the crude human serum. Fig.4 shows that the eluted peak with 0.2M NaCl was found to contain IgG. Fig.5 shows that the capacity of the membrane doesn't change much at different dilution. Even with many fold dilution of pure IgG, approx.the same amount was retained at 25 fold dilution.

Fig.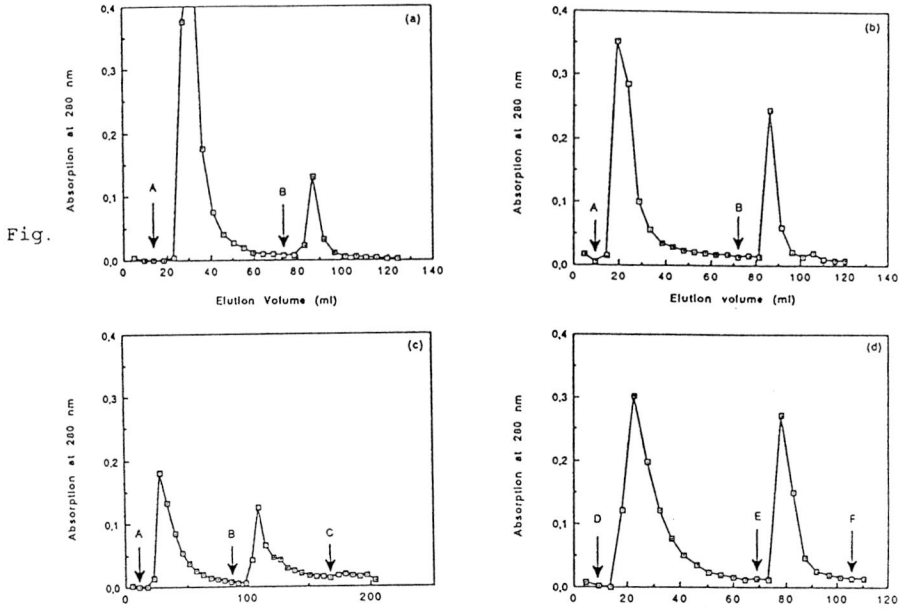

Fig.2 Chromatogram of human placental IgG on (a) histidyl nylon methacrylate composite membrane (b) histidyl Immunodyne (PAL) membrane (c) histidyl silica membrane and (d) protein A liganded Nygene membrane. 6.6 mg of IgG was loaded on these membranes. Flow rate: 138 ml/hr. Temp. 4°C, Fraction volume: 4.6 ml.
A - Injection of IgG in the equilibrating buffer, Tris.HCl buffer, 25 mM, pH 7.4.
B - Buffer A containing 0.2 M NaCl
C - Buffer A containing 0.4 M NaCl
D - Injection of IgG in the equilibrating buffer, PBS (Phosphate Buffered Saline) buffer, 0.15 M, pH 7.2
E - Glycine HCl, 0.1M, pH 2.5
F - Tris.HCl, 1M, pH 9.6

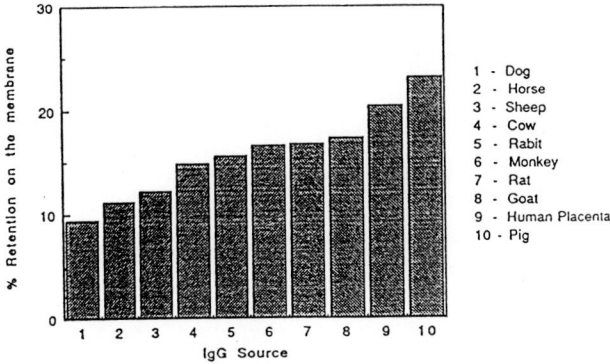

Fig.3 Histogram of IgG from different source.

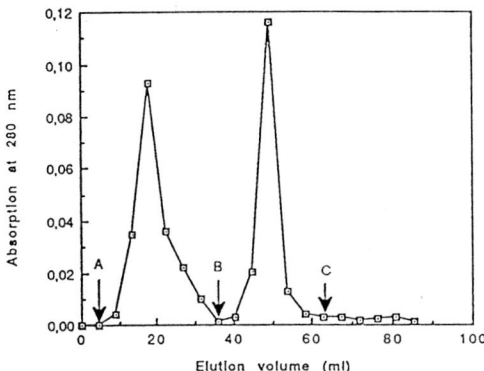

Fig.4 Chromatogram of human serum.
A - Injection of serum
B - Buffer A containing 0.2 M NaCl
C - Buffer A containing 0.4 M NaCl

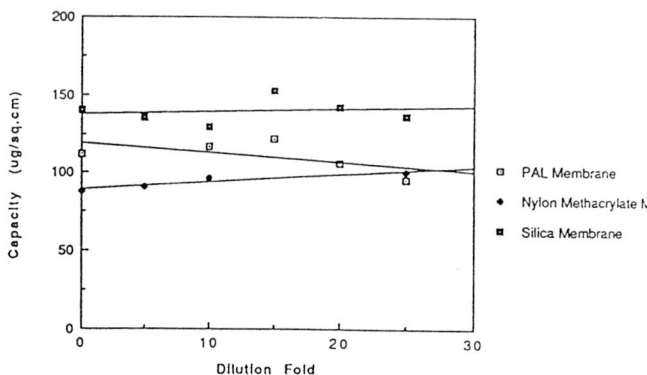

Fig.5 Effect of IgG dilution. (0 dilution represents 6.6 mg IgG in 1 ml buffer) (□) PAL membrane, (♦) Nylon methacrylate composite membrane, (■) silica membrane.

The adsorption isotherms were measured to determine the maximum adsorption capacity and equilibrium association constant for each membrane. Isotherms are shown in Fig.6 and the results obtained are summarised in Table 1.

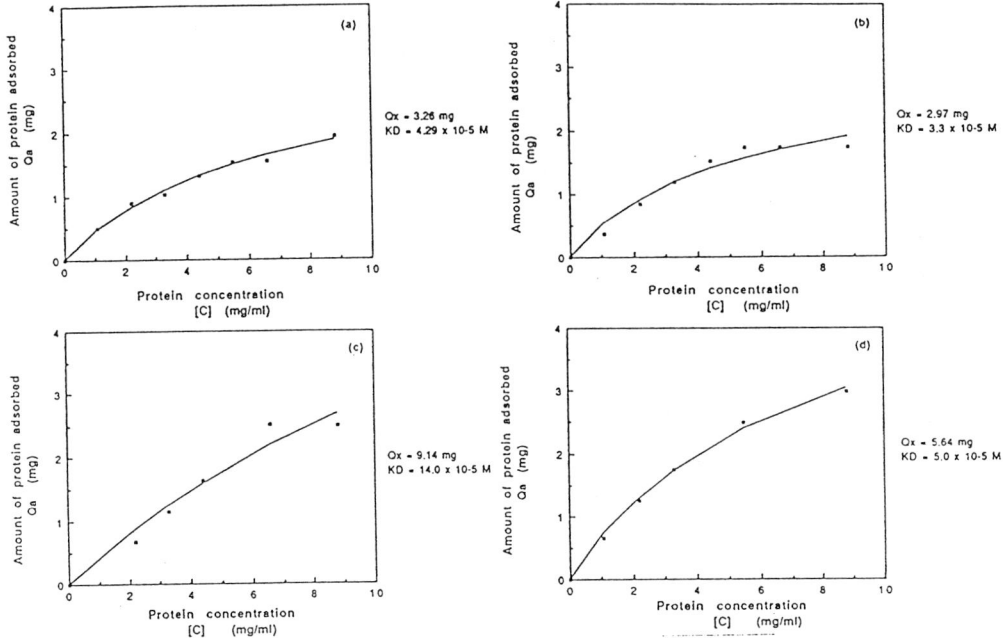

Fig.6   Adsorption isotherm of human placental IgG on different membranes. (a) nylon methacrylate composite membrane, (b) Immunodyne (PAL) membrane, (c) silica membrane, (d) Protein A liganded Nygene membrane. The conditions of adsorption and desorption for the individual membranes are described in Fig. 2. Flow rate: 138 ml/h.

Table 1. COMPARAISON OF MEMBRANES

No	Membrane	Specifications	Capacity ($\mu g/cm^2$)	Dissociation constant $K_D (M)$
1	Nylon Methacrylate	Ligand: L-Histidine Pore: Not determined Area : 16.6 cm^2	196	$4.3 \cdot 10^{-5}$
2	Immunodyne (PAL)	Ligand: L-Histidine Pore : 0.65 µm, Area : 16.6 cm^2	179	$3.3 \cdot 10^{-5}$
3	Silica (FMC)	Ligand: L-Histidine Pore : 1.00 µm Area : 17.3 cm^2	528	$14.0 \cdot 10^{-5}$
4	Nygene	Ligand: Protein A Pore : Not known Area : 17.3 cm^2	326	$5.0 \cdot 10^{-5}$

To see the effect of flux, experiments were conducted at different flux and amount of protein adsorbed per unit area of the membrane was measured. The results are presented in Fig.7. The effect of adsorption rate (AR) with different flux (U) was also calculated and the data are shown in Fig. 8. The empirical constants obtained from this relationship are presented in Table 2.

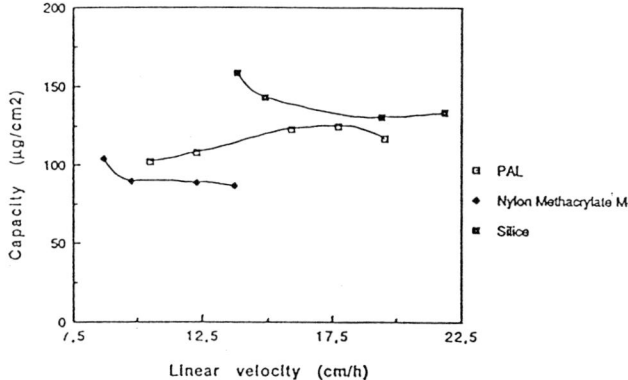

Fig.7 Flow behaviour of different membranes. (♦) nylon methacrylate composite membrane, (□) Immunodyne (PAL) membrane, (■) silica membrane. The conditions are as mentioned in Fig. 2. Amount of injected protein: 6.6 mg in 1 ml.

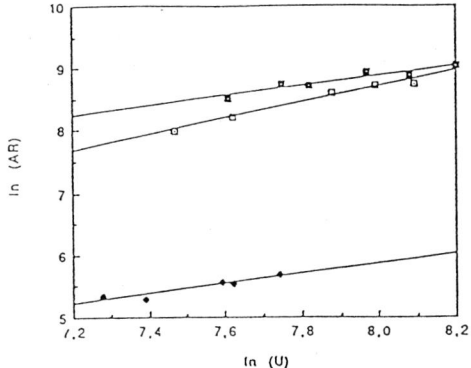

Fig.8 Effect of adsorption rate with different flux. (□) Immunodyne (PAL) membrane, (●) nylon-methacrylate composite membrane, (■) silica membrane.

Table 2. SUMMARY OF EMPIRICAL RELATIONSHIP FOR DIFFERENT MEMBRANES

S NO.	Membranes	Equation
1	Immunodyne	$AR = 0.2 (U)^{1.29}$
2	Nylon Methacrylate	$AR = 15.8 (U)^{0.69}$
3	Silica	$Ar = 10 (U)^{0.82}$

DISCUSSION

Although all four membranes retain IgG, the chromatographic profiles show differences in the size of the eluted peak, at the same concentration of injected protein. Fig. 2a and 2b, do not indicate significant difference in the elution volume whereas in the Fig. 2c the elution volume is more than two fold as for the same eluent (Tris-HCl, 25 mM, pH 7.4 + 0.2 M NaCl). This may be due to the surface area of a membrane because in the case of Immunodyne (PAL) membrane, pore size is 0.65 µm and in the case of silica membrane pore size is 1.0 µm. High pore size membranes have less surface area when compared to low pore size membranes, of course. Protein A liganded membrane is not comparable with the other membrane because the condition of adsorption and desorption are entirely different.

In general histidine demonstrats to be an effective ligand for IgG purification and as shown in Fig.3 histidine recognises IgG from different sources. The variation of the amount of protein retained by the membrane suggest the difference in affinity of these IgG towards the ligand. For the given chromatografical condition, the microenvironment of the ligand and that of the ligate favour the adsorption and the extent of adsorption differs from one source to the other. Adsorption takes place preferentialy at or around the isoelectric pH of the protein (Vijayalakshmi, 1989).

It is known that IgG binds to protein A and Kronvall et al.(1969) have demonstrated that protein A adsorbs specifically Fc part of IgG. Our result show that IgG binds to histidine. This mimetism of histidine to protein A has been assessed by El-Kak et al. (1992) that histidine binds Fc of human IgG with a weak affinity in a way similar to that of E domain of the N-terminal protein A.

The adsorption isotherms of IgG on different histidyl-membranes follow the Langmuir adsorption isotherm (Fig.6). The calculated equilibrium dissociation constants (K_D) shown in Table 1 are all of the same order of magnitude.

It is evident from Fig.7 that the capacity slightly decreases and then remains stationary with an increase in the flux for histidyl silica and histidyl nylon methacrylate composite membranes whereas for histidyl Immunodyne (PAL) membrane the capacity slightly increases and subsequently remains constant with an increase in the flux. The slight decrease in the capacity may be due to the contact time which is very high at the beginning and decreases with the increasing flux. Pressure drop, which we did not measure, is perhaps higher in the case of histidyl nylon methacrylate composite membrane than in the case of histidyl silica membrane. Pressure drop is inversely proportional to the pore size (Bean, 1972).

We have assumed that the adsorption rate changes with flux, U, empirically (Bowen & Hughes, 1990) in the following manner i.e., $AR = a(U)^b$ where a and b are empirical constants evaluated graphically from Fig.8 for three different membranes. From Fig.8 and Table 2, the adsorption rate for the membranes nylon methacrylate composite and silica are ten times more than that of Immunodyne (PAL) which indicate a high throughput for these membranes. This aspect combined with other advantages as discussed earlier confirms that histidyl nylon methacrylate composite is an excellent material for application as a pseudobiospecific membrane adsorbent. These membranes, including protein A liganded Nygene membrane, have high pH tolerance (~pH 10-11). After repeated washing of with NaOH, 0.05 M, these membranes are stable and the results are reproducible even after one year. Moreover, the time taken for one chromatographic cycle (Fig.2a to Fig.2d) is approximately 20-25 minutes which is comparatively faster than that for the particulate matrices.

CONCLUSION

This work shows that nylon methacrylate composite, silica and Immunodyne (PAL) membranes, coupled with L-histidine as ligand, are good alternatives to protein A coupled membranes which are conventionally used for the purification of IgG.

Cycle time of purification is about 20 min. which is very low by comparison with that of particulate matrices. This is due perhaps to high working flow rates. These histidine coupled membranes are highly stable in terms of reproducibility and have high pH tolerance.

ACKNOWLEDGEMENTS

Financial support by MRT, France and collaboration with Bertin & Co., France are kindly acknowledged. Mr.Müller Schulte, Aachen, Germany, is thankfully acknowledged for his nylon methacrylate composite membrane. Kind gift of IgG sample of human placenta from Institut Merieux, France, silica membrane from FMC Bioproducts, ME, U.S.A., and Immunodyne (PAL) membrane from PAL Biosupport, NJ, U.S.A., are also gratefully acknowledged. We gratefully acknowledge the most stimulating and fruitful discussions with Professor E.Sulkowski (Buffalo, NY) and Dr. H.Goubran Botros. Thanks to Miss.N. Barrast for typing this manuscript.

REFERENCES

Bean, C.P. (1972): In Membranes, macroscopic systems and models, vol 1, ed. G. Eisenman, pp. 92-100. New York: Marcel Dekker.
Bowen, W.R., and Hughes, D.T. (1990): Properties of microfiltration membranes. Part 2. Adsorption of bovine serum albumin at aluminium oxide membranes. J. Membrane Science, 51, 189-200.
Brandt, S., Goffe, R.A., Kessler, S.B., O'Connor, J.L., and Zale, S.E. (1988): Membrane - based affinity technology for commercial scale purifications. Bio/Technology, 6, 779 -782.
El-Kak, A., Manjiny, S., and Vijayalakshmi, M.A. (1992): Interaction of immunoglobulin G (IgG) with immobilised histidine: Mechanistic and kinetic aspects. J. Chromatogr., 604, 29-37.
Kanoun,S., Amourache, L., Krishnan,S., and Vijayalakshmi,M.A. (1986): A new support for the large scale purification of protein. J.Chromatogr. 376, 259-267.
Knonvall, G., Joslin, R.C.J., and Williams, R. (1969) : Differences in protein A activity among IgG subgroups. J. Immunol., 103, 828-830.
Müller-Schulte, D., Manjini, S., and Vijayalakshmi, M.A. (1991): Comparative affinity chromatographic studies using novel grafted polyamide and poly(vinyl alcohol) media. J. Chromatogr., 539, 307-314.
Sakai, K., Nagase, M., and Tsuda, S. (1989): Adsorption of β2-microglobulin on PMMA, PAN and cellulosic membranes. Chem. Eng. J., 42, B39-B45.
Tsuchida, T., Kimura, S., and Imanishi, Y. (1989): Adsorption of anti-human C-reactive protein immunoglobulin on phospholipid-coated microcapsules.J. Membrane Science, 45, 155-165.
Vijayalakshmi, M.A. (1989): Pseudobiospecific ligand affinity chromatography. Trends Biotechnol. 7,71-76.

Résumé

L'histidine a déjà été décrite comme un ligand d'affinité pseudobiospécifique pour la purification des immunoglobulines G (IgG) en utilisant des matrices conventionnelles comme le Sépharose®4B et la silice. Nous rapportons ici le couplage de l'histidine sur 3 matrices différentes, Immunodyne (PAL), silice et membrane composite de nylon-métacrylate. Le profil de chromatographie et le volume d'élution sont comparables avec ceux des membranes commerciales couplées avec la protéine A, pour la purification des IgG du placenta humain. L'isotherme d'adsorption des IgG sur ces membranes à histidine a été déterminé pour calculer la constante d'équilibre de dissociation (K_D). Le K_D a été déterminé à 5.10^{-5} M pour les membranes commerciales à protéine A, et de l'ordre de $3,3.10^{-5}$ à 14.10^{-5} M pour les membranes à histidyl. La capacité d'adsorption des IgG déterminée expérimentalement varie en fonction du flux.

Separation of immunoglobulins from human plasma by affinity membrane filtration

Gerd Birkenmeier and Holger Dietze

Institute of Biochemistry, University of Leipzig, Liebigstrasse, 16, 7010 Leipzig, Germany

INTRODUCTION

Purification of clinically high value products and recombinant proteins requires more economical processing of difficult fluids such as human plasma or cell culture fluid. Affinity filtration on microporous membranes has been developed to overcome the disadvantages of packed chromatographic beds. Potential limiting factors of separation in conventional particle-based methods are known to be associated with mass transfer, adsorption kinetics, volumetric throughput, and ligand utility. In membrane-based purification systems high flow rates can be applied due to the high porosity and high mass transfer capability. Short diffusional distances allow optimal utilization of the immobilized ligand which is situated at the inner surface of the membrane pores.

Various commercially available filtration membranes have been modified with affinity ligands to yield high binding selectivity. Dye-liganded membranes were found to be efficient to recover nucleotide-dependent enzymes from yeast extract (Champluvier & Kula, 1991; Champluvier & Kula, 1992). Antibody-coated filtration membranes were designed for effective capturing of recombinant antigens from culture fluids (Nachmann et al., 1992). A number of reports concern the purification of monoclonal antibodies applying protein A or G in conjunction with affinity filtration methods (Langlotz & Kroner, 1992; Bamford et al., 1992). In this study we present preliminary data on a new affinity filtration membrane applicable for binding of human immunoglobulins. The properties of this membrane, i.e. selectivity, capacity, and binding kinetics are described.

RESULTS AND DISCUSSION

Selectivity of the affinity filtration membrane

Nylon membranes (nominal pore size of 0.45 μm) were functionalized with a non-proteinogenous affinity ligand displaying affinity to human immunoglobulins (Birkenmeier, 1992). Analytical experiments were performed with 3 layers of filter discs (20-mm diameter) harboured in a filtration module yielding a total filtration area of 9.4 cm^2 and a membrane volume (mvol) of 0.15 ml (module I). Scaled-up experiments were conducted with a filtration device containing 5 layers of stacked membranes of 135-mm diameter having an effective filtration area of 715 cm^2 and a membrane volume of 11.4 ml (module II). Filtration was processed in the dead-end mode at various flow rates. Figure 1 illustrates the fractionation of whole human plasma by filtration on the immunoglobulin-sensitive affinity filtration membrane (Ig-s-AFM).

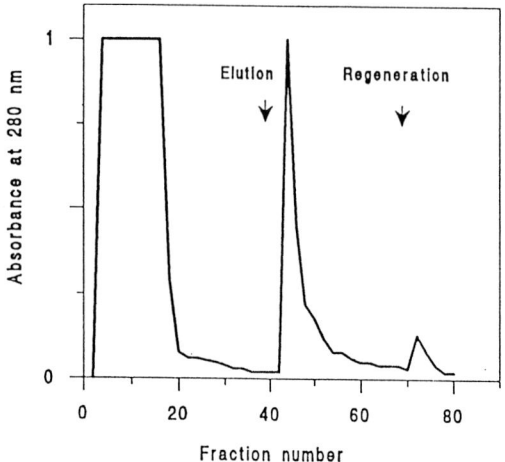

Fig. 1. Fractionation of human plasma by affinity filtration on the Ig-s-AFM.
0.5 ml human plasma dialysed against 10 mM sodium phosphate buffer, pH 7.0 was passed through the membrane module I at a flow rate of 3.3 mvol/min. After washing with buffer the bound proteins were eluted with 0.5 M NaCl. The membrane was regenerated by washing with 0.01 N NaOH.

The immunological analysis of main plasma proteins in the unbound and bound fractions revealed that abundantly occuring plasma proteins, i.e. albumin, transferrin, α1-proteinase inhibitor, α2-macroglobulin, haptoglobin, prealbumin, α1-acid glycoproteins and others, were not adsorbed. The bound proteins mainly comprised immunoglobulins. Their purity was analyzed by SDS electrophoresis as illustrated in Fig. 2. Refiltration of the bound and unbound fractions in separate experiments yielded single peaks in respective positions without further fractionation. Thus, the appearance of immunoglobulins in the unbound fraction is apparently not attributed to a protein overload.

Subclass specificity of the affinity membrane
As demonstrated in Table 1, the affinity membrane exhibits distinct specificity for IgG subclasses. The Ig-s-AFM preferentially binds IgG1 and IgG3, while IgG2 and IgG4 mainly constitute the immunoglobulins in the unbound fraction. Substantial amounts of IgA appeared in the breakthrough fraction while IgM was partially bound. It was found that the relative portions of bound and unbound IgA and IgM varied with plasma obtained from different individuals. The purity of immunoglobulins extracted by filtration on Ig-s-AFM was found to be almost comparable to the one of IgG purified by protein A-Sepharose as shown in Fig. 2.

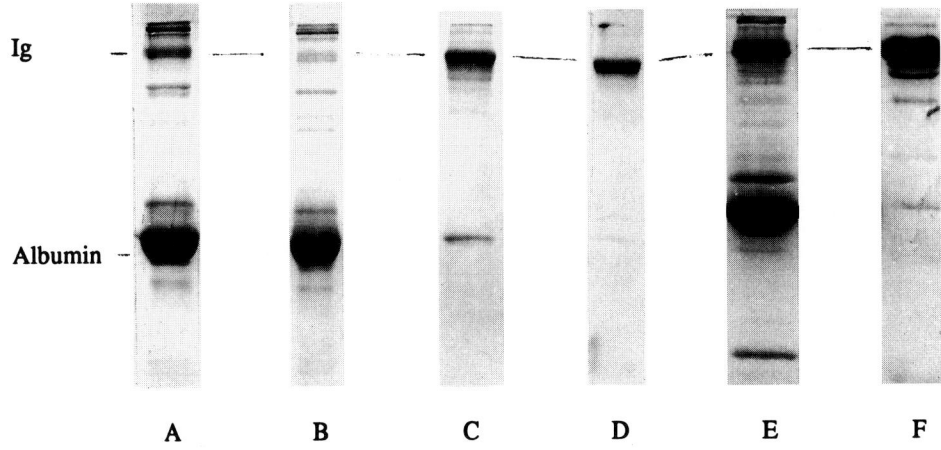

Fig. 2. SDS polyacrylamide gel (8%) electrophoresis under nonreducing conditions.
(A) human plasma, (B) unbound fraction from Fig. 1, (C) eluted fraction from Fig. 1, (D) immunoglobulins purified from human plasma by protein A-Sepharose, (E) paraproteinemia plasma, (F) eluted fraction after affinity filtration on Ig-s-AFM of (E).

In contrast to the Ig-s-AFM, immobilized protein A is known to lack affinity to human IgG3. As expected, a human monoclonal antibody (IgG1) present in plasma of a patient suffering from paraproteinemia is strongly bound to the affinity membrane (Fig. 2).
Interestingly, immunoglobulins from rabbit, mouse, and bovine were found to display negligible affinity to Ig-S-AFM.

Table 1
Subclass- and class-specific binding of immunoglobulins to the Ig-s-AFM

Ig / Fractions	IgG_1	IgG_2	IgG_3	IgG_4	IgM	IgA
Sample (mg)	1.58	0.69	0.08	0.36	0.32	0.69
Break-through (mg)	0.39	0.51	0.008	0.33	0.15	0.45
Elution (mg)	1.05	0.21	0.062	0.037	0.13	0.06

0.5 ml human plasma dialysied against 10 mM sodium phosphate buffer, pH 7.0 was passed through the membrane module I at a flow rate of 3.3 mvol/min. After intensive washing the elution was initiated by 0.5 M NaCl. The concentrations of the immunoglobulins in the unbound and bound fractions were determined immunologically.

Scale-up experiments

For scaling up the separation of immunoglobulins from human plasma the larger membrane device (module II) with a filtration area of 715 cm^2 was used. We have determined the throughput capability of the Ig-s-AFM membrane by examining the effect of plasma loading on the efficacy of immunoglobulin binding. Thus, plasma was passed through the membrane at three different flow rates, 65 ml/h, 300 ml/h, and 2100 ml/h which corresponds to 0.1, 0.44, and 3 membrane volume (mvol) per minute as indicated in Table 2. It is clearly shown that the flow rate has no significant impact on the amount and the relative distribution of the bound immunoglobulins. Even, a 36-times reduction of the fluid residence time (from 631 s to 19 s) does not effect the dynamic capacity of the membrane. It is interesting to note that highly diluted plasma containing IgG in a concentration of 50-100 µg/ml is as well affinity filtrated as undiluted plasma. Much higher flow rates could certainly be applied without changing the separation yield but pressure limitation in the device used made it difficult to test higher flow rates.

Table 2
Influence of the flow rate on the separation of immunoglobulins from human plasma

Flow rate	IgG_b (mg)	IgG_{nb} (mg)	IgA_b (mg)	IgA_{nb} (mg)	IgM_b (mg)	IgM_{nb} (mg)
0.065 l/h 0.1 mvol/min	172	216	6.1	45	15	15
0.3 l/h 0.44 mvol/min	188	178	5.4	52	19	13
2.1 l/h 3 mvol/min	186	174	4.4	59	14	11
2.1 l/h 3 mvol/min[a]	199	205	nd	nd	nd	nd

50 ml human plasma were affinity filtrated on 5 stacked membranes harboured in the module II. Loading, washing and elution (0.5 M NaCl) were performed at three different flow rates corresponding to 0.1, 0.44, and 3 membrane volume (mvol)/min, respectively.
[a] Plasma was 100-fold diluted before loading on the membranes.
b = bound; nb = not bound; nd = not determined.

The high throughput capability is one of the most important features of affinity filtration membranes. Due to minimized mass transfer resistance binding to the immobilized ligand seems to be limited only by the binding kinetic. It is expected that as long as the fluid residence time is much larger than the solute's diffusion time high flow rates can be applied without changing the yield of separation. This has been demonstrated for several model systems including antibody-antigen interactions, receptor-ligand interactions (Nachmann, 1992), and ligand-enzyme interactions (Champluvier & Kula, 1992).

Binding kinetics
Fig. 3 illustrates the adsorption characteristics of the Ig-s-AFM. The shape of the adsorption isotherm can be described by the Langmuir-equation:

$$Q_a = Q_x * K_a * [C]/(1 + K_a * [C])$$

where K_a is the association constant, Q_x is the maximum binding capacity of the membrane for IgG, and Q_a is the amount of bound protein in equilibrium with the protein concentration, [C], of the solution. A dissociation constant, K_d ($1/K_a$), of 4.6 µM and the maximum binding capacity of 1.42 mg/cm² were ascertained. When calculated on the basis of unit membrane volume the maximum binding capacity of the membrane corresponds to 89 mg/ml. In comparison to a protein A-membrane (K_d = 0.29 µM; Q_x = 4.74 mg/ml) as described by Langlotz and Kroner (1992) the affinity of IgG to the Ig-s-AFM was less but the binding capacity was found to be about 19-times higher. Is is to be expected, that the working capacity of the membrane will be less than the maximum capacity determined experimentally since processing of diluted rather than concentrated solutions are more common.

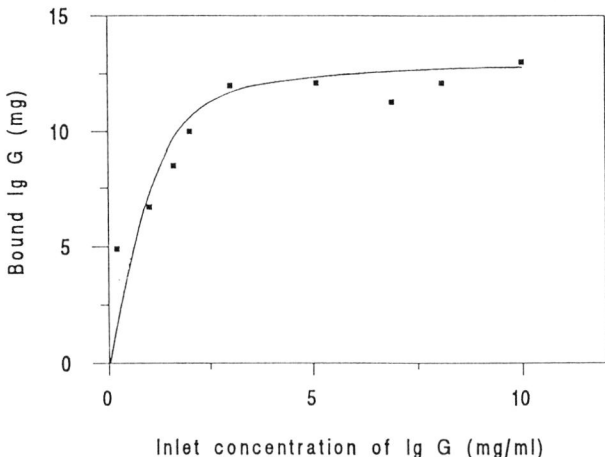

Fig. 3. Adsorption isotherm of IgG binding to the affinity membrane
Pure human IgG which has been further separated by pre-adsorption to the Ig-s-AFM was applied to the membrane module I until the effluent concentration was identical with the feed stream concentration. After washing the elution was accomplished by 0.5 M NaCl. A linear flow rate of 1.1 mvol/min was applied.

Membrane stability
No significant loss in binding capacity was observed after 30 cycles of immunoglobulin extraction from human plasma. Regeneration of the Ig-s-AFM membrane by washing with 0.01 N NaOH is usually sufficient to remove strongly bound material. The affinity membrane can resist much higher concentration of NaOH (1M) and even common organic solutions such as ethanol or aceton. The membrane can be autoclaved allowing purification of immunoglobulins under sterile conditions.

CONCLUSION

In the present preliminary report we offered a new affinity filtration membrane designed for binding of immunoglobulins from human plasma. With respect to the binding capacity the affinity membrane used is superior to protein A-membranes described in the literature. Elution of bound immunoglobulins is effected by sodium chloride and does not require harsh conditions as known for dissociation of protein A-immunoglobulin complexes. Owing to its subclass specificity the affinity filtration membrane can be applied for partial resolution of IgG subclasses. A further area of application of this membrane could be the purification of human monoclonal antibodies secreted by hybridoma cells. In that case membrane-based purification systems are ideally suited because of the high throughput capability allowing processing of large volumes in short times.

ACKNOWLEDGEMENT

H.D. was supported by the Axel Springer Foundation, Berlin. The authors are grateful to Prof. G. Kopperschläger for critical reading the manuscript and to E. Usbeck for the technical assistance.

REFERENCES

Bamford, C.H., Al-Lamee, K.G., Purbrick, M.D. & Wear, T.J. (1992): Studies of a novel membrane for affinity separations. I. Functionalisation and protein coupling. J. Chromatogr. 606, 19-31.

Birkenmeier, G. (1992): patent application.

Champluvier, B. & Kula, M.-R. (1992): Sequential membrane-based purification of proteins, applying the concept of multidimensional liquid chromatography (MDLC). Bioseparation 2, 343-351.

Champluvier, B. & Kula, M.-R. (1992): Dye-ligand membranes as selective adsorbents for rapid purification of enzymes: A case study. Biotechnol. Bioeng. 40, 33-40.

Langlotz, P. & Kroner, K.H. (1992): Surface-modified membranes as a matrix for protein purification. J. Chromatogr. 591, 107-113.

Nachmann, M. (1992): Kinetic aspects of membrane-based immunoaffinity chromatography. J. Chromatogr. 597, 167-172.

Nachmann, M., Azad, A.R.M. & Bailon, P. (1992): Membrane-based receptor affinity chromatography. J. Chromatogr. 597, 155-166.

Comparison of various chromatographic supports for purifying human plasmatic immunoglobulins from Cohn II+III fraction

N. Nourichafi, C. Geschier and J.-F. Stoltz

Centre régional de transfusion sanguine et laboratoire d'hématologie, Bâtiment E, Faculté de médecine Brabois, 54500 Vandœuvre-lès-Nancy, France

Summary

In order to define a protocol for the purification of human immunoglobulins using Cohn's II+III fraction, various chromatographic supports (DEAE Sepharose , DEAE Spherodex , DEAE Spherosil , DEAE Trisacryl and DEAE Trisacryl Plus) were tested in different types of buffer solutions (sodium acetate , sodium phosphate and Tris-HCl) .
Highly satisfactory results were obtained for all the supports with regard to extraction yield as compared with the Cohn's method . Highest yields were obtained with DEAE Spherodex and DEAE Trisacryl supports with a sodium-phosphate or Tris-HCl buffer . Futher it was possible to obtain with just one stage a 92% pure product with an average yield of 85-90% .
Dual stage purification on DEAE Spherodex followed by DEAE Trisacryl or on CM Trisacryl followed by DEAE Trisacryl supplied a 98% pure product with an average yield of 80-90% in the first case and 75-80% in the second case .

I-Introduction

Since the 1940s the preparation of plasmatic albumin or immunoglobulins is based mainly on the precipitation technique developed by Cohn and col (1946) . In the past decade chromatographic methods were developed for the fractionation of human proteins mainly for albumin and coagulation factors (Freisen and col (1985) , Bees and col (1989) , Berglof and col (1989) ...) . These methods are flexible , soft and non-denaturing for proteins separation . More recently an increasing number of immunoglobulins production procedure have been developed using different chromatographic medias , different buffer solutions and different starting materials (Jakab and col (1980) , Saint-Blancard and col (1981) , Fourcard and col (1982) , Friesen (1987) ...). In the present work we tested various commercially available chromatographic supports in three different types of buffer solutions to purify IgG from Cohn precipitate II+III.

II-Material and methods

Chromatographic purification of IgG was performed with different ion exchange medias : DEAE Sepharose Cl-6B (Pharmacia Uppsala,Sweden) ; DEAE Spherodex^{R}M ; DEAE Spherosil^{R}M ; DEAE Trisacryl Plus M and CM Trisacryl M (IBF-Sepracor , Villeneuve-la-Garenne , France) .
Cohn precipitate II+III (CRTS Nancy , France) has been used as starting material .
Chromatographic buffer solutions were prepared with sodium acetate , sodium phosphate , sodium chloride , Tris and hydrochloric acid (Prolabo , Paris , France) .

The study was carried out on laboratory scale columns to determine the suitability of various ion exchanger in different buffer solutions.

The sample prepared from Cohn precipitate II+III was diafiltered to pH and ionic strength of the first elution buffer and was applied to the anion exchanger which had been equilibrated with the same buffer. Fractionation was performed on a column packed with anion exchanger by stepwise elution with four buffers as shown in figure 1.

Acetate buffers were : (1) 0.07 M sodium acetate, pH 5.2 ; (2) 0.09 M sodium acetate, pH 4.7 ; (3) 0.4 M sodium acetate, pH 4 and (4) 0.4 M sodium acetate, 1 M sodium chloride, pH 5.2.

Phosphate buffers were : (1) 0.025 M sodium phosphate, pH 7.5 ; (2) 0.025 M sodium phosphate, 0.075 M sodium chloride, pH 7 ; (3) 0.025 M sodium phosphate, 0.15 M sodium chloride, pH 6 and (4) 0.1 M sodium phosphate, 1 M sodium chloride, pH 7.5.

Tris-HCl buffers were : (1) 0.025 M Tris-hydrochloric acid, 0.035 M sodium chloride, pH 8.8 (2) 0.025 M Tris-hydrochloric acid, 0.075 M sodium chloride, pH 8.5 ; (3) 0.025 M Tris-hydrochloric acid, 0.15 M sodium chloride, pH 7.5 and (4) 0.1 M Tris-hydrochloric acid, 1 M sodium chloride pH 8.8.

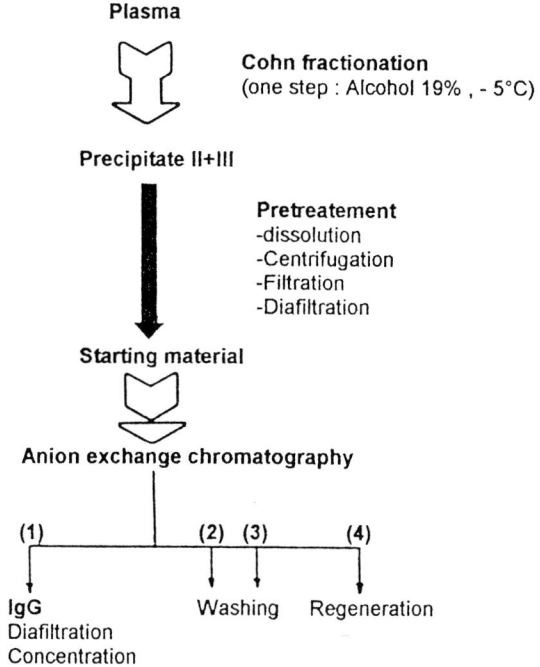

Figure 1 : Schematic representation of the one step anion exchange purification of IgG

Experiments with a two steps purification procedure were also realised :
a-Purification on DEAE Trisacryl and DEAE Spherodex :The IgG fraction eluted from the column of DEAE Trisacryl was applied to the column of DEAE Spherodex which had been equilibrated with the same elution buffer, then stepwise elution was done with four phosphate buffers as shown in figure 2. Buffers (1), (2), (3) and (4) were the same used in all the study.

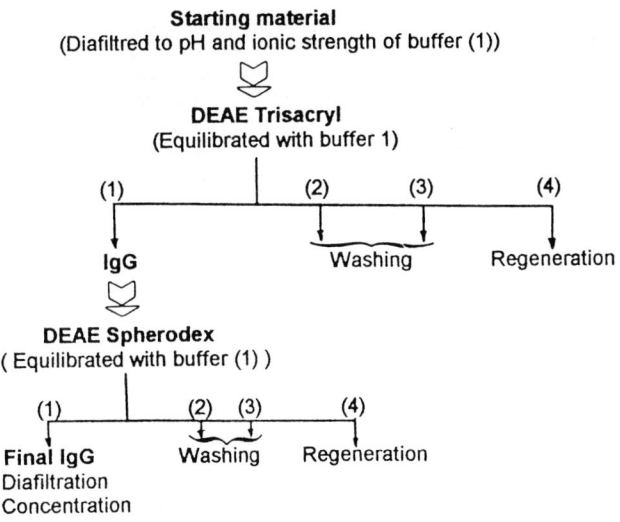

Figure 2 : Schematic representation of a two steps chromatographic purification of IgG (DEAE Trisacryl and DEAE Spherodex)

b-Purification on CM and DEAE Trisacryl : Sample was diafiltred to pH and ionic strength of buffer (5) 0.025 M sodium phosphate , pH 5.5 and was applied to the CM Trisacryl which had been equilibrated with the same buffer . At the elution two IgG fractions were collected : Fraction B eluted with buffer (1) contain mainly IgG and fraction C eluted with buffer (2) contain pure IgG . The fraction B was applied to the DEAE Trisacryl column which had been equilibrated with buffer (1) and elution stepwise was done as shown in figure 3 .

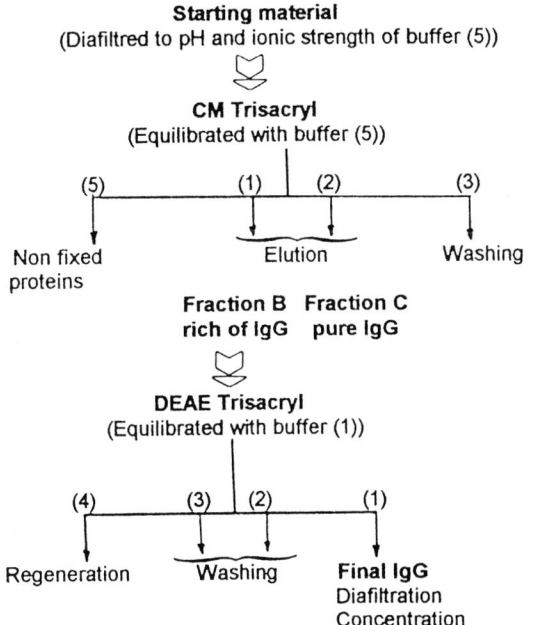

Figure 3 : Schematic representation of a two steps chromatographic purification of IgG (CM and DEAE Trisacryl)

Analytical methods
Protein concentrations were determined by the method of Bradford (1976).
IgG, IgA and IgM were determined by nephelometry (Beckman ICS Nephelometer).
The electrophoretic purity was determined by cellulose acetate membrane electrophoresis using veronal buffer, pH 8.6.
Immunoelectrophoresis was performed according to Grabar and Williams (1953) using immunoagar slides with veronal buffer, pH 8.6.

III-Results

- Purification with a one step procedure :
Experiences were done five times on 1 x 7 cm columns, three times on 2.5 x 11 cm columns and three times on 2.5 x 22 cm columns. Proteins concentration was 15 g/l and 30 mg of proteins were applied per 1 ml of gel. Results of this comparative study are summarised on table I which displays the average values of dilution factor (eluate volume/sample volume), purity and yield. Average values remain the same even if column size was changed.

Table I : Mean results obtained with one step methods.

Eluates	Buffers	Dilution factor	Ig/proteins %	Recovery %
DEAE Sepharose	Acetate	2.6	50	100
	Phosphate	2.4	85	96
	Tris-HCl	3	88	77
DEAE Spherodex	Acetate	2.6	86	98
	Phosphate	3	92	80
	Tris-HCl	2.7	92	83
DEAE Spherosil	Acetate	1.6	72	85
	Phosphate	2.8	92	86
	Tris-HCl	2	64	98
DEAE Trisacryl	Acetate	3	80	94
	Phosphate	2.4	92	96
	Tris-HCl	3	90	86
DEAE Trisacryl Plus	Acetate	1.6	88	96
	Phosphate	1.7	97	86
	Tris-HCl	2.5	98	83

The best yield was obtained with DEAE Trisacryl Plus in phosphate and tris-HCl buffers ; this results are confirmed by electrophoresis and immunoelectrophoresis figure 4 .

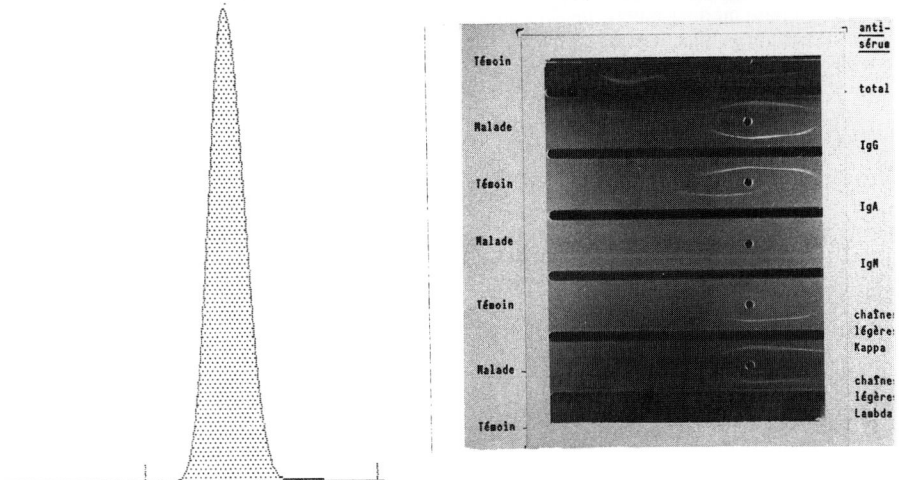

Figure 4: Electrophoresis and immunoelectrophoresis of IgG purified on DEAE Trisacryl Plus.

- Purification with two steps methods :
Experiments were performed three times on 2.5 x 11 cm columns and three times on 2.5 x 22 cm columns .Table II and table III summarised the average values obtain .

Table II : Purification with tow steps method on DEAE Trisacryl and DEAE Spherodex

Eluate	Dilution factor	Ig/proteins %	Ig recovery %
DEAE Spherodex	2.4	92	96
DEAE Trisacryl	3.5	98	95

Table III : Purification with tow steps method on CM and DEAE Trisacryl

Eluate		Dilution factor	Ig/proteins %	Recovery %
CM Trisacryl	B fraction	5.5	86	85
	C fraction	1	100	8
DEAE Trisacryl		5.8	98	83

211

IV : Conclusion

In summary, one stage purification of IgG on DEAE Trisacryl Plus with sodium phosphate or tris-HCl buffers gives a pure product (purity 98 %) with a good yield (90 %) in addition dilution factor was less 2 ; whereas the purification on two associated gels gives a product with the same purity with a yield lower , dilution factor was higher and time of production was longer .

References

Bees W.C.H. , Friesen A.D. and Janzen R.G. (1989) : Validation of a large scale column chromatographic process for production of albumin and intravenous immune globulin . In biotechnology of plasma proteins , Editions INSERM (Paris , France) J.F. Stoltz and C. Rivat ed 175 : 207-216 .

Berglof J.H and Eriksson S.E. (1989) : Plasma fractionation of albumin and IgG . In biotechnology of plasma proteins , Editions INSERM (Paris , France) J.F. Stoltz and C. Rivat ed 175 : 201- 206 .

Bradford M.M. (1976) : A rapid and sensitive method for the quantitation of microgram quantities of proteins utilizing the principle of protein dye binding . Anal. Biochem. ; 72 : 248-254 .

Cohn E.J. and al (1946) : Preparation and properties of serum and plasma protein . A system for the separation into fractions of protein and lipoprotein components of biological tissues and fluids . J. Am. Chem. Soc. ; 68 : 459-475 .

Fourcard J. , Saint-Blancard J. , Girot P. and Boschetti E. (1982) : Préparation de l'albumine et des immunoglobulines G par fractionnement direct du plasma humain sur DEAE et CM-Trisacryl . Revue française de transfusion et immunohématologie ; xxv , 1 : 7-17 .

Friesen A.D. (1987) : Chromatographic methods of fractionation . Develop.biol.Standard. 67 :3-13.

Friesen A.D., Bowman J.M.and Bees W.C.H. (1985) : Column ion exchange chromatographic production of human immune serum globulin for intravenous use . Vox sang. ; 48 : 201-212 .

Grabar P.and Williams C.A. (1953) : Méthode permettant l'étude conjuguée des propriétés éléctrophorétiques et immunochimiques d'un melange de protéines . Application au serum sanguin . Biochem. Biophys.Acta ; 10 : 193-194 .

Jakab M. , Vasileva R. and Hasko F. (1980) : Application of CM-Sephadex C-50 for the production of immunoglobulins . Journal of chromatography ; 201 : 281-286 .

Saint-Blancard J., Fourcard J. , Limonne F. , Girot P. and Boschetti E. (1981) : Nouveaux échangeurs d'ions Trisacryl : intérêt et application au fractionnement des protéines du plasma humain . Annales pharmaceutiques françaises ; 39 ; 5 : 403-409 .

Résumé

Comparaison de différents supports chromatographiques utilisables pour la purification des IgG plasmatiques humaines à partir de la fraction II+III de Cohn

Dans le cadre d'une étude sur la purification des immunoglobulines plasmatiques humaines à partir de la fraction II+III de Cohn , différents supports chromatographiques pour échange d'ions (DEAE Sepharose , DEAE Spherodex , DEAE Spherosil , DEAE Trisacryl et DEAE Trisacryl Plus) ont été testés avec différents tampon (acétate de sodium , phosphate de sodium et Tris-HCl) . Dans tous les cas les rendements et la pureté sont supérieurs à ceux obtenus avec le fractionnement de Cohn . Des produits de grande pureté sont obtenus avec les supports DEAE Spherodex et DEAE Trisacryl dans des tampons phosphate de sodium ou Tris-HCl . Il est par ailleurs possible d'obtenir en une seule étape un produit pur à 92% avec un rendement de 85 à 90% . La purification en deux étapes sur DEAE Spherodex suivi du DEAE Trisacryl ou encore sur CM Trisacryl suivi du DEAE Trisacryl donne un produit pur à 98% avec un rendement de 80 à 90% dans le premier cas et 75 à 80% dans le deuxième cas .

IV. Virus safety

IV. Sécurité virale

The regulation of medicinal products derived from human blood or plasma in the European Community

Patricia Brunko

Pharmaceuticals Unit, DG III/C/3, Commission of the European Communities, 200, rue de la Loi, 1049 Brussels, Belgium

Summary

In the interests of public health and in order to promote the free movement of medicinal products, a series of legislative measures has been adopted to harmonize the conditions of manufacture, testing and authorization of medicinal products in the European Community. Since the adoption of Directive 89/381/EEC, the scope of EC pharmaceutical legislation has been extended to cover medicinal products derived from human blood or plasma. These medicinal products are now subject to marketing authorization on the basis of strict criteria of quality, safety and efficacy. Moreover, Directive 89/381/EEC also presents an ethical dimension, in encouraging the Member States of the European Community to promote voluntary unpaid blood donation and the use of such donations for the manufacture of medicinal products.

Introduction

Since the adoption of the first pharmaceutical directive in 1965, the pharmaceutical legislation of the European Community has constantly pursued two objectives: the protection of public health and the free movement of products.

The first directive relating to medicinal products mentioned blood derivatives in the European definition of a medicinal product. However, in 1975, a series of medicinal products, including blood derivatives, were provisionally excluded from the scope of the directives on marketing authorization.

In December 1986, the Council gave the Commission a mandate to present proposals for the harmonization, before 1993, of the authorization for manufacturing and marketing of all categories of medicinal products still excluded from the scope of Community legislation.

Following in-depth consultation with representatives of European organizations, namely the Committee of experts on blood transfusion and immunohaematology of the Council of Europe and the Liaison Bureau of the Red Crosses, the Commission presented to the Council a proposal for a directive extending the scope of Community pharmaceutical legislation to medicinal products derived from human blood or plasma. The European Parliament adopted a favourable opinion on this proposal and thus the Council adopted Directive 89/381/EEC unanimously on 14 June 1989.. In adopting this Directive, the Council gave the Commission the mandate to adapt the current testing requirements of Directive 75/318/EEC to blood derivatives in cooperation with representatives of the member States within a Regulatory Committee. The technical directive was adopted by the Commission on 19 July 1991, following a unanimously favourable opinion of the representatives of the Member States (Directive 91/507/EEC).

Directive 89/381/EEC

Directive 89/381/EEC covers stable industrially prepared blood derivatives, intended for a large number of patients, namely albumin, coagulation factors and immunoglobulins. Whole blood, plasma and cellular components are excluded from the scope of the directive.

As a consequence of the inclusion of blood derivatives in Community pharmaceutical legislation, these products are now subject to its general provisions regarding manufacturing and marketing authorization. The principles of good manufacturing practice (GMP) laid down in Directive 91/356/EEC and detailed in a guide for manufacturers have become mandatory, as well as the tests in Directive 91/507/EEC aimed at demonstrating quality, safety and efficacy for the purpose of marketing authorization. The European format for the application file as well as the Community procedures for marketing authorization are applicable.

In addition to these general provisions, which are applicable to all medicinal products, Directive 89/381/EEC contains several elements which are specific to medicinal products derived from human blood or plasma. By virtue of Directive 89/381/EEC, the measures for selection and control of blood donors recommended by the Council of Europe and the World health Organization have become compulsory. The Member States must ensure that donation centres and donors are identifiable. They must also apply all the requirements of the directive to products from third countries. Moreover, for these particularly sensitive products, the Council has explicitly demanded the application of validated manufacturing and purification processes, in order to guarantee, insofar as the state of technology permits, the absence of specific viral contamination.

The objective of Community self-sufficiency in blood and blood derivatives by voluntary unpaid donations is clearly expressed in the text of the directive and the Member States have to inform the Commission on measures taken in this area.

For new medicinal products, the directive entered into force on 1 January 1992. For products already on the market, a transitional period of one year is provided, during which the Member States must proceed with the review of these produts. A coordinated exercise with regard to the review of safety and efficacy of the major blood derivatives was completed by the competent authorities of the Member States in October 1992 and this has led to the establishment of a series of "core" summaries of product characteristics.

The guidelines of the Committee for Proprietary Medicinal Products

The Committee for Proprietary Medicinal Products (CPMP) was set up in accordance with Directive 75/319/EEC, in order to facilitate the adoption by the Member States of common positions with regard to marketing authorizations. The Committee, composed of representatives from the authorities competent for marketing authorization of medicinal products, is called upon to give its opinion on applications for marketing authorization presented by virtue of the Community procedures. The Committee has also undertaken the task of harmonizing the details of quality, safety and efficacy testing by adopting guidelines intended for manufacturers. The Committee is assisted by groups of highly qualified experts designated by the Member States.

The guidelines reflect the consensus of the Member States on particular subjects and give the manufacturers all the information necessary to carry out tests which are recognized as valid by all the member States. In December 1991, the Committee adopted a guideline on medicinal products derived from human blood or plasma. The document emphasises the special aspects of manufacture and control of these products and elaborates on the requirements laid down in the directives. Additionally, the guideline on validation of virus inactivation and elimination procedures, adopted in February 1991, is applicable to blood derivatives; it gives a general framework for validation studies and the virological approach to be followed.

The promotion of voluntary unpaid blood donation

Directive 89/381/EEC states that 'Member States shall take the necessary measures to promote Community self-sufficiency in human blood or human plasma. For this purpose, they shall encourage the voluntary unpaid donation of blood and plasma and shall take the necessary measures to develop the production and use of products derived from human blood or human plasma coming from voluntary unpaid donations. They shall notify the Commission of such measures'.

Thus the directive does not question the ethical principle of unpaid blood donation. On the contrary, it has established this as an objective for the 12 member States of the Community. But, in addition to the directive, the general rules of the EC Treaty are applicable, namely with regard to free movement of products, public procurement and monopolies.

References

The Rules governing Medicinal Products in the European community

Volume I	The rules governing medicinal products for human use in the European Community EC Catalogue Nr. CO-71-91-631-EN-C
Volume II	Notice to applicants for marketing authorizations for medicinal product for human use in the Member States of the Europen Community EC Catalogue Nr. CB-55-89-293-EN-C
Volume III	Guidelines on the quality, safety and efficacy of medicinal products EC Catalogue Nr. CB-55-89-843-EN-C Addendum (July 1990) CB-59-90-936-EN-C Addendum (May 1992) in press
Volume IV	Good manufacturing practice for medicinal products EC Catalogue Nr. CO-71-91-760-EN-C

Résumé

Pour protéger la santé publique et promouvoir la libre circulation des médicaments, des mesures ont été prises en vue d'harmoniser les conditions de fabrication, d'essais et d'autorisation des médicaments dans la Communauté européenne. Depuis l'adoption de la directive 89/381/CEE, la législation pharmaceutique communautaire couvre également les médicaments dérivés du sang et du plasma humains. Par conséquent, ces médicaments sont maintenent soumis à autorisation de mise sur le marché sur la base des critères de qualité, sécurité et efficacité. En outre, en demandant aux Etats membres de prendre toutes les mesures utiles pour promouvoir le don volontaire et non rémunéré du sang et l'utilisation de tels dons pour la fabrication de médicaments, la directive 89/381/CEE présente également une dimension éthique.

Methods for inactivation of viruses in plasma products

Jean-Jacques Morgenthaler

Research Department, ZLB Central Laboratory, Blood Transfusion Service SRC, Wankdorfstrasse 10, 3000 Bern 22, Switzerland

ABSTRACT

The safety of blood and blood products may be increased by four different types of measures: (1) screening of the donors, (2) screening of the donations, (3) production steps that either remove or inactivate viruses, (4) identification of batches. Screening methods will not be discussed here; however, their importance in insuring that the virus load in the starting material be as low as possible cannot be overemphasized. Neither screening methods nor virus inactivation methods are infallible; it has been estimated that even with today's screening methods most large plasma pools are contaminated with one or several viruses which can potentially render the whole batch infectious. Both screening and virus inactivation must therefore be used in conjunction to insure the best possible safety of the final product. Methods for reducing the virus load in plasma products can be broadly categorized into (1) removal of infectious agents (2) physical treatments and (3) chemical treatments. Physical separation of viruses from the therapeutically useful fractions may happen in the course of the normal fractionation process. This has been shown, e.g., in the case of immunoglobulin preparations and during isolation of coagulation factor concentrates by affinity chromatography on monoclonal antibodies. The simplest physical treatment consists in heating the dry (lyophilized) final product. This was one of the first methods used for inactivating viruses. Unfortunately heating at temperatures of 60 to 68°C for 24 to 72 hours does not inactivate all viruses. It was shown, on the other hand, that a severe heat-treatment (80°C/72 hours) or pasteurization (heating of a protein solution at 60°C for 10 hours) both lead to virally safe products. Chemical treatment with a suitable combination of a solvent and a detergent was also shown to inactivate all enveloped viruses. Newer methods are still being developed. The aim of all virus inactivation methods has to be an optimum discrimination between viruses which have to be eliminated or destroyed and proteins which should not be damaged. In addition, an ideal method would not require the use of toxic chemicals which subsequently have to be removed from the proteins. Methods which might fulfil these requirements include filtration processes and photodynamic virus inactivation methods. The latter consist in addition of a suitable dye to a protein solution followed by illumination with light of appropriate wavelength. Many enveloped viruses can be inactivated by this method while proteins are left largely unharmed. Some of these methods may eventually be useful for inactivation of viruses in the presence of blood cells.

INTRODUCTION

It is now well known that blood and blood or plasma products can transmit a number of viruses (see Table 1). The most important of these viruses are the various hepatitis viruses and, because of the severity of the illness it causes, HIV.

Table 1. Viruses transmissible by blood and plasma/plasma derivatives.

Virus	transmission by blood	by plasma/ plasma derivatives
Hepatitis B virus (HBV)	+	+
Hepatitis D virus (HDV)	+	+
Hepatitis C virus (HCV)	+	+
Human immunodeficiency virus 1/2 (HIV 1/2)	+	+
Human T-cell lymphotropic virus I/II (HTLV-I/II)	+	-
Cytomegalo virus (CMV)	+	-
Epstein-Barr virus (EBV)	+	-
Parvovirus B 19 (B19)	+	+
Hepatitis A virus (HAV)	(+)	(+)

All the viruses listed in Table 1 except B19 and HAV are enveloped viruses. This is important to know because enveloped viruses are in general much easier to inactivate than non-enveloped viruses. All individual blood donations are now screened for a number of viral markers; inspite of this, large plasma pools are still contaminated with a number of viruses. This may be caused by lack of sensitivity of the assay, or by the fact that the assay detects antibodies against the virus and not the virus itself. Viruses may also remain undetected because the donor is in the window period or because there is no assay available at all for a particular virus. However, screening methods do help to reduce the virus load in a plasma pool and should always be used in conjunction with virus removal and/or inactivation during production of plasma products, since even the best virus inactivation methods might fail if the initial viral burden is too high.

METHODS FOR VIRUS INACTIVATION

Table 2 lists most methods that have been used so far for reducing the danger of virus transmission by plasma-derived products. The different methods are classified according to an operational definition. The table therefore does not indicate the mechanism(s) responsible for inactivation; in any event, the mechanism is unknown in most cases.

Table 2. Methods for reducing the infectivity of plasma-derived products

> removal of infectious agent(s)
>> chromatography
>>> hydrophobic interaction
>>> polyelectrolytes
>>> affinity chromatography
>> partitioning during fractionation
>> (ultra)filtration
>
> physical treatments
>> heat treatments
>>> dry
>>> dry, in solvents
>>> steam
>>> wet (pasteurization)
>> ionizing radiation
>> light (uv)
>
> biochemical and chemical methods
>> immune neutralization
>> ethanol
>> solvent/detergent treatment (S/D)
>> chemicals
>>> NA-breaking
>>> ozone
>>> anthraquinones
>
> combined physico-chemical methods
>> β-propiolactone/uv
>> other chemicals/uv
>> or chemicals/visible light (photodynamic treatment)

At least in theory every virus could be removed by passing the contaminated solution over a column with the appropriate immobilized antibody against a particular virus. The practical application of this principle would be extremely difficult since it would require antibodies against all the relevant viruses. Obviously this method is powerless against new and unknown viruses. A more important mechanism is the serendipitous loss of viruses during chromatography, particularly when coagulation factors are prepared by immuno affinity chromatography: viruses are not bound to the highly specific immobilized antibody and therefore pass through the column without being retained. Reduction factors of about 10^4 have been demonstrated for these procedures. Ion exchange chromatography, although not nearly as specific as immunoaffinity chromatography, has also been shown to substantially decrease the virus load during production of coagulation factor concentrates (Schwartz et al., 1991). If chromatographic purifications are optimized for the recovery of a particular plasma protein we would expect them to simultaneously discriminate against any virus that might be present, i.e., we may expect a reduction of virus burden for any kind of virus.

Well before the introduction of chromatographic methods plasma was fractionated by precipitation with ethanol in the cold. The path followed by viral markers during ethanol fractionation was already investigated over twenty years ago. Schroeder et al. (1970) for instance were able to show that HBsAg was absent from fraction II (the immunoglobulin fraction) when HBsAg positive plasma was fractionated according to Cohn/Oncley. Fraction V (albumin) on the other hand probably still contained some small amounts of HBsAg. Similar experiments were done later on by Wells et al. (1986) with HIV: they spiked with HIV, plasma and plasma fractions obtained by Cohn-Oncley fractionation at every step of the fractionation procedure immediately before phase separation and measured subsequently HIV antigen and virus titer both in the precipitate and the supernatant. By multiplying the clearance factors at every step they calculated an overall reduction of infectivity from plasma to fraction II in the order of 10^{15}. It should also be noted that the virus titers in the corresponding precipitate and supernatant did not always add up to the amount used for spiking the previous fraction; this most likely indicates at least partial inactivation of the virus by ethanol. More recently the FDA has also conducted experiments with HCV (Yei et al., 1992). The authors fractionated a plasma pool which consisted exclusively of anti-HCV-positive donations. Since it is not possible to grow and titrate HCV in vitro, they monitored HCV RNA with PCR at limiting dilution and were thus able to quantitate HCV RNA. Overall reduction of HCV from starting plasma to fraction II amounted to 4.7×10^4. Obviously this clearance factor is not sufficient to guarantee safety of immunoglobulins with respect to transmission of HCV. On the other hand long standing clinical experience has demonstrated absence of transmission of HCV by properly manufactured immunoglobulin preparations. Other mechanisms contribute to the inactivation of HCV during the preparation of immunoglobulin. They may include disruption of the virus by ethanol and by freezing and thawing and/or other chemical treatments. It should also be remembered that the assay detects RNA, which does not necessarily parallel virus titer.

Another method for physically removing viruses which became available recently is filtration with membranes that have pores of narrow size distribution. Separation of viruses from the protein solutions is based on true physical removal and not on adsorption processes. The procedure should therefore be applicable to all viruses, known and unknown. Upscaling should also be easy since modules of different size are available; this allows testing of the procedure in the laboratory and subsequent transfer to the pilot plant and production scale. However, small viruses and large proteins are similar in size. This method will therefore not be able to separate, e.g., parvovirus from von Willebrand factor aggregates.

Various kinds of heat treatments have been used successfully for the inactivation of viruses in plasma protein preparations. The obvious advantages of a heat-treatment - particularly of the lyophilized end product - are that no chemicals have to be added to the product and that there is no danger of downstream contamination. Inactivation of viruses by heat depends not only on the temperature used but also on the medium: inactivation procedes more rapidly at higher temperatures and in the liquid state than in the dry (lyophilized) state. Also, substances that are added in order to protect the proteins might inadvertently protect viruses (McDougal et al., 1986). While dry-heat treatments are usually carried out without stabilizers, pasteurization (i.e., heating the solution, usually at 60°C for a minimum of 10 hours) is normally done in the presence of stabilizers. These substances are commonly removed after the heat treatment. Recently, a high temperature/short time heat treatment was proposed which calls for increasing the temperature of a protein solution (without stabilizers) within about 100 ms with a microwave heater, keeping it at a set temperature for about 6 to 12 ms, then cooling it down within another 100 ms. The total treatment time is therefore <0.25 s. Charm et al. (1992) have shown that at holding temperatures in the order of 70°C several model viruses have higher inactivation rates than coagulation factors. It might therefore be possible to selectively inactivate viruses with this treatment without causing damage to proteins even in the absence of stabilizers. Future experiments will have to show if the method can be applied on a larger scale.

A disadvantage of most chemical virus inactivation methods is that chemicals generally have to be removed from the proteins after the virus inactivation. The acceptable level of contamination in the final product obviously depends on the toxicity of the chemicals used. A chemical virus inactivation method which is widely used nowadays relies on a combination of solvents and detergents to disrupt the lipid envelope of viruses; this method is dealt with in detail elsewhere in this volume. Another chemical method for inactivation of viruses consists in a treatment at pH4 with traces of pepsin. Originally introduced for inducing intravenous tolerance in immunoglobulin preparations, this treatment was shown to inactivate a number of viruses, including HIV (Reid et al., 1988; Kempf et al., 1991).

Photodynamic treatments, i.e., combinations of dyes and light have been known for a long time to inactivate viruses. During the last years several groups have attempted to adapt the method to the treatment of plasma proteins and even blood cells. The main problem is to find a dye which is sufficiently active but also reasonably non-toxic and has a suitable absorption spectrum, in other words which absorbs light in a region where the products that will be treated do not. Psoralenes (Alter et al., 1988), hematoporphyrins (Matthews et al., 1988), benzoporphyrins (Neyndorff et al., 1990), merocyanines (O'Brien et al., 1990), phenothiazines (Lambrecht et al., 1991) and phthalocyanines (Horowitz et al., 1991) have all been proposed for that purpose. The use of methylene blue and light to inactivate viruses in fresh frozen plasma is also discussed elsewhere in this volume.

What ultimately interests the patient who is treated with blood-derived products is the record these products have in the clinic. Several surveys may be found in the literature where the authors have attempted to summarize the performances and failures of the different methods (see, e.g., Bloom, 1991). These tables all vary in details since the criteria that the authors used for acceptability of a particular study are different. Additionally, some incidents are published more than once, while others may never be published at all. Nevertheless, some common points emerge from all those tables: (1) There are only few failures with HIV; most likely, some dry heat treated preparations (60°C/24h) transmitted HIV when they were prepared from unscreened donations. (2) There were also some failures with HBV early on; however, most patients are vaccinated nowadays and safety with respect to HBV transmission cannot be followed anymore. (3) Most failures seemed to occur with non-A, non-B hepatitis (HCV). (4) Dry-heat treatment does not guarantee safety unless it is carried out as so-called "severe dry-heat treatment" (80°C/72h, as described by Winkelmann et al., 1989). (5) Pasteurization as well as solvent/detergent treatment both have an excellent clinical record. The few problem cases with pasteurized products that have appeared in the literature could so far not be linked with the product with any degree of certainty.

CONCLUSIONS

In summary, plasma protein solutions are now much safer with respect to transmission of viruses than they were in the past. We should remember however that absolute safety is an unattainable goal. Introduction of additional measures to inactivate viruses may indeed increase safety with regard to transmission of viruses. On the other hand this may also decrease the overall safety of plasma derived products because of the addition of chemicals, potential damage to proteins, increased chance of clerical errors, etc. The aim of all virus inactivation methods therefore remains to obtain products with *optimum overall safety*, not with *absolute viral safety*.

REFERENCES

Alter, H.J., Morel, P.A., Dorman, B.P., Smith, G.C., Creagan, R.P., Wiesenhahn, G.P., Corash, L., Popper, H. & Eichberg, J.W. (1988): Photochemical decontamination of blood components containing hepatitis B and non-A, non-B virus. *Lancet* II, 1446-1450.

Bloom, A.L. (1991): Progress in the clinical management of haemophilia. *Thromb. Haemost.* 66, 166-177.

Charm, S.E., Landau, S., Williams, B., Horowitz, B., Prince, A.M. & Pascual, D. (1992): High-temperature short-time heat inactivation of HIV and other viruses in human blood plasma. *Vox Sang.* 62, 12-20.

Horowitz, B., Williams, B., Rywkin, S., Prince, A.M., Pascual, D., Geacintov, N. & Valinsky, J. (1991): Inactivation of viruses in blood with aluminium phthalocyanine derivatives. *Transfusion* 31, 102-108.

Kempf, C., Jentsch, P., Poirier, B. Barré-Sinoussi, F., Morgenthaler, J.-J., Morell, A. & Germann, D. (1991): Virus inactivation during production of intravenous immunoglobulin. *Transfusion* 31, 423-427.

Lambrecht, B., Mohr, H., Knüver-Hopf, J. & Schmitt, H. (1991): Photoinactivation of viruses in human fresh plasma by phenothiazine dyes in combination with visible light. *Vox Sang.* 60, 207-213.

Matthews, J.L., Newman, J.T., Sogandares-Bernal, F., Judy, M.M., Skiles, H., Leveson, J.E., Marengo-Rowe, A.J. & Chanh, T.C. (1988): Photodynamic therapy of viral contaminants with potential for blood banking applications. *Transfusion* 28, 81-83.

McDougal, J.S., Martin, L.S., Cort, S.P., Mozen, M., Heldebrant, C.M. & Evatt, B.L. (1985): Thermal inactivation of the acquired immunodeficiency syndrome virus, human T lymphotropic virus-III/lymphadenopathy-associated virus, with special reference to antihemophilic factor. *J. Clin. Invest.* 76, 875-877.

Neyndorff, H.C., Bartel, D.L., Tufaro, F. & Levy, J.G. (1990): Development of a model to demonstrate photosensitizer-mediated viral inactivation in blood. *Transfusion* 30, 485-490.

O'Brien, J.M., Montgomery, R.R., Burns, W.H., Gaffney, D.K. & Sieber, F. (1990): Evaluation of merocyanine-540 - sensitized photoirradiation as a means to inactivate enveloped viruses in blood products. *J. Lab. Clin. Med.* 116, 439-447.

Reid, K.G., Cuthbertson, B., Jones, A.D.L. & McIntosh, R.V. (1988): Potential contribution of mild pepsin treatment at pH4 to the viral safety of human immunoglobulin products. *Vox Sang.* 55, 75-80.

Schroeder, D.D. & Mozen, M.M. (1970): Australia antigen: distribution during Cohn ethanol fractionation of human plasma. *Science* 168, 1462-1464.

Schwarz, T.F., Roggendorf, M., Hottentrager, B., Stolz, W. & Schwinn, H. (1991): Removal of parvovirus-B19 from contaminated factor-VIII during fractionation. *J. Med. Virol.* 35, 28-31.

Wells, M.A., Wittek, A.E., Epstein, J.S., Marcus-Sekura, C., Daniel, S., Tankersley, D.L., Preston, M.S. & Quinnan, G.V. (1986): Inactivation and partition of human T-cell lymphotrophic virus, type III, during ethanol fractionation of plasma. *Transfusion* 26, 310-213.

Winkelmann, L., Feldman, P.A. & Evans, D.R. (1989): Severe heat treatment of lyophilised coagulation factors. In *Virus Inactivation in Plasma Products; Curr. Stud. Hematol. Blood Transfus.* 56, ed. J.-J. Morgenthaler, pp. 55-69. Basel: Karger.

Yei, S., Yu, M.W. & Tankersley, D.L. (1992): Partitioning of hepatitis C virus during Cohn-Oncley fractionation of plasma. *Transfusion* (in press).

Résumé

La sécurité du sang et des produits sanguins peut être augmentée par quatre différents types de mesures:(1) criblage des donneurs,(2) criblage des dons,(3) étapes de production qui éliminent ou inactivent les virus,(4) identification des méthodes de criblage ne seront pas discutées ici.Ni les méthodes de criblage ni les méthodes d'inactivation des virus ne sont infaillibles;il a été estimé que même avec les méthodes de criblage actuelles, la plupart des grands pools de plasma sont contaminés avec un ou plusieurs virus qui peuvent rendre potentiellement infectieux le lot entier.Le criblage et l'inactivation des virus doivent donc être utilisés l'un et l'autre pour garantir le mieux possible la sécurité du produit final.

Les méthodes pour réduire le taux en virus des produits du plasma peuvent être définies en trois catégories:(1) l'élimination des agents infectieux,(2) les traitements physiques,(3) les traitements chimiques.L'élimination physique des virus des fractions thérapeutiques peut intervenir au cours du processus normal de fractionnement.Ceci a été montré,par exemple, dans le cas des préparations d'immunoglobulines et au cours de l'isolement des concentrés de facteurs de coagulation par chromatographie d'affinité sur anticorps monoclonaux. Le traitement le plus simple consiste à chauffer le produit lyophilisé.Le chauffage fut une des premières méthodes d'inactivation des virus.Malheureusement,le chauffage à des températures de 60 à 68°C pendant 24 à 72 heures ne permet pas d'inactiver tous les virus.Par ailleurs, il a été montré qu'un chauffage important (80°C,72 h) ou une pasteurisation(chauffage d'une protéine en solution 10h,60°C) permettent d'obtenir des produits viralement sûrs.Les traitements chimiques avec l'association d'un solvant et d'un détergent permettent d'inactiver tous les virus enveloppés.Des méthodes plus récentes sont en cours de développement.Le but de toutes les méthodes est d'obtenir que les virus soient éliminés ou détruits et que les protéines ne soient pas endommagées.De plus, la méthode idéale ne devrait pas utiliser de substances toxiques qui devraient être éliminées des protéines. Les méthodes qui pourraient être retenues incluent les procédés de filtration et les méthodes d'inactivation photodynamique des virus.Ces dernières consistent en l'addition d'un colorant à une solution protéique suivie d'une illumination à une longueur d'onde appropriée.Beaucoup de virus enveloppés peuvent être inactivés par cette méthode qui ne détériore pas les protéines.Quelques unes de ces méthodes peuvent être employées pour l'inactivation des virus en présence de cellules sanguines.

Biological products and viral safety

Florian Horaud

Laboratoire de Virologie Médicale, Institut Pasteur, 25, rue du Docteur-Roux, 75724 Paris Cedex 15, France

INTRODUCTION

The term biologicals emerged in the early history of microbiology (1) and was extended later to cover all medicinal products having a natural substance as source material. At the present time the term biologicals is currently used to indicate products obtained from i) micro-organisms (like bacterial or viral vaccines), ii) medicinal molecules (non self replicating agents) derived from bacteria, yeast or animal cells in culture, naturally expressed or obtained by r-DNA technology (like MAb, cytokines, hormones, etc.) and iii) products isolated from human or animal tissues or fluids (like hormones, blood derivatives etc.). The meaning of the term biologicals also implies the notion of *drug or medicine* since there is a process capable of transforming the source material (bacteria, viruses, tissue culture fluid, organs, plasma, etc.) in a medicinal substance. This process is favourable not only for the purification of the targeted molecule but also for the elimination of microbial contaminants.

The history of biologicals probably started some thousands of years ago when, in connection with religious or tribal customs, products derived from human and animal tissues and fluids were used for medical purposes. It is also probable that these habits long contributed to the propagation of some diseases. An example illustrating this was the spread, by ritual cannibalism, of Kuru disease in New Guinea (2).

VACCINES

The problem of the risks associated with the use of biologicals is best illustrated by the history of vaccines and vaccination, because the danger inherent in using vaccines is included in the concept of their preparation. The great achievement of Pasteur was to demonstrate that a well identified human microbial pathogen, like rabies virus, can be converted into clinical drug possessing a specific prophylactic activity. Although vaccines were a major factor that contributed in the last century to the improvement of public health, they were until recently, frequently involved in severe clinical accidents (3). Viral vaccines are a unique category of biologicals because they alone are able to control viral diseases. Their efficacy has been well established and is well illustrated by the eradication of small-pox by vaccination with vaccinia virus, a "product" developed by Jenner at the end of the 18th century. However, despite of the successful use of viral vaccines, they were in many instances implicated, for various reasons, in adverse reactions some of which were very severe (4). In general the adverse reactions observed after the administration of viral vaccines in which the virus was incompletely inactivated and used as immunogen were dramatic: large numbers of vaccinees presented a disease related to those naturally induced by the virus used to make the vaccine. However such a correlation was not possible in the case of FMDV, when residual live virus was at the origin of some outbreaks, until a powerful investigation tool able to characterise viral genomes became available. Most of the accidents with viral vaccines are now only of historical interest, because many of them were generated by products manufactured with empirical methods and in rudimentary conditions. Generally, the frequency of accidents provoked by viral vaccines has diminished since 1) the improvements of the methods used for viral inactivation and purification, 2) the introduction of good manufacturing practices and rigorous regulatory policy and 3) the progress in the post clinical surveillance of adverse reaction after vaccine administration, allowing a better risk-benefit analysis.

However, since in many cases the vaccines use a virulent or a potential virulent agent as starting material, they should be still considered products presenting a considerable risk.

NEW BIOTECHNOLOGICAL PRODUCTS

In the last ten years new drugs obtained by application modern biotechnology have been prepared from tissue culture of animal cells containing infectious or non infectious viruses. For example, hybridoma cells contain murine retroviruses, while CHO cells used frequently in the production by r-DNA technology of proteins of medical interest, having endogenous retroviruses (5, 6, 7). Human MAb are frequently obtained after cell immortalization by EBV. The *evaluation of the risk associated with products derived from tissue culture is greatly facilitated by the existence of cell banks.* Products manufactured from such cells are now processed using methods able to eliminate and/or inactivate viruses. This problem has been under scrutiny since 1978, when the use of continuous cell lines for the manufacture of biologicals was considered for the first time (8). The clinical use of new biotechnological products, like MAb, hormones, cytokines, growth factors, etc. prepared from mammalian cells in culture seems to be safe because they have not been involved in virus transmission.

PRODUCTS DERIVED FROM HUMANS AND ANIMALS

This category of biologicals represents a very large class of medicinal products. Some of them have been used in traditional pharmacy for a long time, others are modern pharmaceuticals obtained by the use of modern technology.

The common risk raised by the drugs produced from animal and human tissues and fluids is the high variability of source material. In many cases, it is not feasible to test the starting material, and in others the value of the initial screening is debatable. Therefore the safety of some products is mainly dependent on the capacity of the production process to eliminate and/or inactivate viruses. The concept of viral validation emerged principally because of this situation and its rationale is that an experimental design simulating the industrial process and the worst circumstances of contamination with virus should be set-up and checked for viral clearance.

An important distinction should however be made between the pharmaceuticals derived from animals and those obtained from humans: the iatrogenic contamination of humans is much more likely from products obtained from human body, because there is no species barrier.

In the last 10 years, despite the significant improvements in techniques of protein purification and molecular separation the use of certain biologicals has been at the origin of severe clinical accidents involving contaminating viruses or other infectious agents, like those observed in the case of human extracted HgH that induced Creutzfeldt-Jakob Disease (CJD). Once this problem had been identified HgH accidents were avoided first by using a product that was validated for the elimination of infectious PrP and subsequently by introducing a hormone produced by r-DNA technology.

There is no doubt that the contamination of haemophiliacs with HIV by clotting concentrate preparations was by far the most dramatic accident reported in the recent years. At the origin of HIV contamination of transfused and/or haemophiliacs patients was a complex situation in which the emergence of a new virus infection surprised the scientific community. Although the time necessary to realise the reality and the scale of AIDS outbreak was relatively short, it was enough to generate one of the most tragic iatrogenic episodes in the history of biologicals. It should also be underlined that the considerable effort successfully and rapidly uncovered much scientific knowledge on the aethiological agent leading and to diagnostic tests for AIDS. This achievement created the necessary condition for the definition of a strategy for AIDS prevention.

The accidents in the last years associated with blood derivatives also showed that in some cases viruses present by small amounts in the source plasma are concentrated in the final products. Some categories of patient, like immunocompromised subjects can be infected with virus by products contaminated with small amounts of virus that would not be harmful to healthy subjects : this was the case for clotting factor concentrates that included AIDS haemophiliacs with high frequency. The problem of viruses contaminating blood is complicated by the fact that some of them are not cultivable in cell culture (e.g. Hepatitis B and Hepatitis C) or grow poorly (e.g. Hepatitis A) or may not have been identified. As soon as a test for the detection of HepCV was available, it was realised that it is frequently transmitted by transfusion and blood derivatives. Recently hepatitis A viruswas incriminated in the inductiçon of hepatitis following the administration of Factor VIII. The source of these accidents is still obnscure and more studies are necessary to clarify their origin. Assessment of the risk associated with the use of plasma derivatives should take in consideration the limit of sensitivity and the variability of the tests used to detect contamination of the donors. For all these reasons the capacity of a production process to remove and/or to destroy viruses should be demonstrated by validation studies and the limitations of viral validation data in ensuring safety should be noted. The elimination of the risk of viral infection from blood derivatives has been helped by the development of methods able to abolish viral infectivity with little or no interference with the biological activity of the product. However, viral inactivation procedures have limitations, since some of them are only active against enveloped viruses, while others have negative effects on the physico-chemical state of the active molecule (9).

Biologicals produced from animal fluids or tissues have not been involved in the transmission of viral diseases to humans. There are several possible explanations for this. First, viral zoonoses of domestic animals, from which the medicinal products are usually derived, are relatively infrequent. Viral zoonoses of wild or laboratory primates and rodents have however caused major outbreaks (10). There is no doubt that host range specificity of virus infection which is mediated mainly by viral receptors, creates a barrier to the spread to humans of various viral diseases including FMDV, pseudo rabies and other herpesviruses of cattle, pigs and birds, etc.. Moreover some non protein products (heparin, bone derivatives) derived from animals are the results of severe procedures which destroy viruses. Moreover, the long experience of human consumption of animals as food demonstrates clearly that the main danger in eating animal products is bacterial and not viral contamination. Nevertheless, because the potential transmission of viruses to humans via products derived from animals cannot be ruled out, we have to remain vigilant and require viral validation studies for this category of biologicals.

CONCLUDING REMARKS.

The assessment of the risks raised by the clinical use of biologicals is a complex problem because it requires a happy marriage between virological expertise and case by case examination of each product, taking into account risk-benefit analysis.

Experience of the accidents caused by using biological products suggests that the species origin and the nature of starting material play a key role in viral safety. This view is justified by the dramatic HIV and Hep CV contamination accidents following the use of blood derivatives, and the occurrence CJD among subjects that received natural HgH. The starting materials had a human origin in all the cases and the active substances were proteins. If the species origin and the nature of starting material of biological products are indeed the major sources of risk the clinical hazards raised by different categories of these medicinal substances could be classified. We therefore propose four classes of products:

Class 4

Products derived from human fluids and tissues: blood and plasma derivatives, placental derivatives, hormones and enzymes obtained from urine or organs, bone products, etc. This class of products represents the highest risk because i) there is no species barrier for viruses potentially present in the source material, (many of them like hepatitis B and C, HIV are human specific pathogens), and ii) numerous as yet unidentifed viruses may be present in human tissues and fluids (like non-A, non-B, non-C and non-E hepatitis viruses). *However the risk can be modulated by other factors Including: i) the capacity of the process used for their manufacture to eliminate and/or inactivate viruses, ii) the chemical nature of the active molecule, iii) whether the product is used chronically or episodically and iv) the immunological status of the patient.*

<u>Class 3</u>

This class is for *vaccines* since they are manufactured from identified human pathogens (inactivated vaccines) or potential pathogens (live vaccines). The process used in their production and control and a strict observance of Good Manufacturing Practices are central to ensuring their safety.

<u>Class 2</u>

Products derived from animal tissues or fluids can be contaminated by animal viruses present in the source material. The significant difference between the risks associated with animal derived products and biologicals from human origin is the species barrier (see above). The absence in the literature of reports on contamination of patients by products derived from animals can also be explained by the fact that this category of products are frequently non protein drugs (heparin, gangliosides, etc.) or are highly purified, like MAb obtained from ascites : Contrary to common belief mouse ascites is quite "clean" in terms of virus contamination, since ascites usually contains a significant quantity of various antibodies and cytokines with antiviral activity.

<u>Class 1</u>

This class of biologicals includes chemicals obtained by biotechnological methods produced by animal tissue culture technology, like human and murine monoclonal antibodies and proteins obtained by r-DNA technology (hormones, cytokines, growth factors, etc.) The risks specific to these products are significantly diminished by the existence of *cell banks* as starting material. This has allowed the use of a unique and consistent source material for many years. The viruses potentially contaminating the cell banks can be detected and characterised once for ever and an informed decision to accept or to reject the cell bank can be taken. *In the last 15 years products obtained by this methodology and used clinically on large scale, have never been involved in transmission of viruses to humans.* One explanation might be the high purity of these products and the careful validation studies performed to demonstrate viral clearance in spiking experiments. It should be underlined that safety of products obtained from tissue culture can be affected by the reagents used (as calf sera). For this reason the origin and the results of testing for bovine contaminants of foetal calf sera should be documented by producers.

Finally, the classification of risk factors, as suggested in this paper, should be not considered in a rigid way. It could be best used as a general guideline, facilitating the understanding of quality control requirements and the regulatory approach in view of the evaluation of viral safety of biologicals. Further readings of the proceedings of meeting held in the last years are recommended (11, 12, 13, 14).

References

1) Jeffcoate S. L. What is a biological ? *Biologicals* (1991) **19**, 139-142.

2) Gajdusek C.D. Subacute Spongiform Encephalopathies: Transmissible Cerebral Amyloidoses Caused by Unconventional Viruses in: *Fields Virology*, Second Ed. Ed. Fields B.N., Knipe D.M. *et al.* vol. 2, *pp:* 2289-2324. Raven Press, New York (1990).

3) Wilson G.S. (1967). The hazards of immunization. University of London. The Athlone Press, London.

4) Horaud F. Viral Safety of Biologicals. *Develop. biol. Standard.,* **75**, 3-7 (S. Karger, Basel 1991).

5) Lueders K.K. Genomic oragnization and expression of endogenous Retrovirus-like elements in cultured rodent cells. (1991) *Biologicals,* **19**, 1-7.

6) Emanoil-Ravier R.,Hojman F., Serevenay M., Lesser J., Bernardi A. and Peries J. Biological and molecular studies of endogenous retrovirus-like genes in Chinese hamster cell lines *Develop. biol. Standard.* **75**, 113-122 (Karger, Basel, 1991).

7) Anderson K.P., Yolanda S.L., Low M.A., Willimas S.R., Wurm F. and Dinowitz M. Defective endogenous retrovirus-like sequences and particles of Chinese hamster ovary cells. *Develop. biol. Standard.,* **75**, 123-132.(Karger, Basel, 1991).

8) Cell Substrates - Their use in the production of vaccines and other biologicals. *Advances in Exp Med. & Biol.* Ed. Petricciani J.C., Hopps H.E. and Chapple P.J. vol. 118, (Plenum Press, N.Y., 1979).

9) Morgenthaler J.J. Edit. Virus inactivation in Plasma Products. (Karger, Basel 1989).

10) Mahy B.W.J., Dikiewicz C., Fisher-Hoch S., Ostroff S., Tipple M., and Sanchez A. Virus Zoonoses and their Potential for Contamination of Cell Cultures. *Develop. biol. Standard.* **75**, 183-189. (Karger, Basel 1991).

11) Abnormal cells, new products and risk. *in vitro Celular & Developmental Biology* - Ed. Hopps H.E. & Petricciani J.C. Monograph 8 - Tissue Culture Assoc. USA (1985).

12) Continuous Cell Lines As Substrates of Biologicals. *Develop. biol. Standard.* **70** (Karger, Basel, 1988).

13) Virological Aspects of the Safety of Biological Products. *Develop. biol. Standard.* **75** (Karger, Basel, 1989).

14) Continuous Cell Lines -An International Workshop. *Develop. biol. Standard.* **76** (Karger, Basel, 1991).

Viral safety of solvent/detergent treated blood products

Bernard Horowitz, Alfred M. Prince, Marilyn S. Horowitz and Christine Watklevicz

New York Blood Center, 310 East 67th Street, New York, NY 10021, USA

Laboratory research commencing in 1982 led to licensure in the United States in 1985 of a solvent/detergent (SD) treated AHF concentrate. Licensure was based on (a) studies demonstrating the inactivation of several marker viruses [vesicular stomatitis virus (VSV), Sindbis virus, Sendai virus], human immunodeficiency virus (HIV), hepatitis B virus (HBV), and non-A, non-B hepatitis virus [NANBHV; now known principally to be hepatitis C virus (HCV)] added to AHF just prior to treatment, (b) the realization that the principal viruses of concern in a transfusion setting (e.g. HIV, HBV, NANBHV) were all lipid-enveloped, and (c) laboratory, preclinical and clinical evidence indicating that AHF and other proteins present in the preparation were unaffected. The applicability of the SD method to a wide range of products and preparations, high process recoveries, and a growing body of viral safety information linked with the failure of several other virus inactivation methods to eliminate hepatitis transmission fostered the adoption of SD technology by more than 50 organizations world-wide. SD mixtures are now used in the preparation of products as diverse as intermediate purity and monoclonal antibody purified AHF and other coagulation factor concentrates, fibrin glue, normal and hyperimmune IgG and IgM preparations including those derived from tissue culture, plasma for transfusion, and various diagnostic controls. Over 4 million doses of SD-treated products have been administered, and numerous laboratory and clinical studies designed to assess virus safety have been conducted. SD treatment has been shown to inactivate $\geq 10^{9.2}$ tissue culture infectious doses ($TCID_{50}$) of VSV, $\geq 10^{8.8}$ $TCID_{50}$ of Sindbis virus, $\geq 10^{6.0}$ $TCID_{50}$ of Sendai virus, $\geq 10^{7.3}$ duck infectious doses of duck HBV, $\geq 10^{11.0}$ $TCID_{50}$ of HIV-1, $\geq 10^{6.0}$ $TCID_{50}$ of HIV-2, $\geq 10^{6.0}$ chimpanzee infectious doses (CID_{50}) of HBV, $\geq 10^{5.0}$ CID_{50} of HCV, $\geq 10^{6.0}$ $TCID_{50}$ of cytomegalovirus, $\geq 10^{5.8}$ $TCID_{50}$ of herpes simplex virus type 1, $\geq 10^{4.0}$ $TCID_{50}$ of PI-1, $\geq 10^{6.0}$ $TCID_{50}$ of murine leukemia virus (Mov-3), $\geq 10^{4.0}$ $TCID_{50}$ of murine xenotropic virus, and $\geq 10^{2.0}$ $TCID_{50}$ of Rauscher murine leukemia ecotropic virus.

Evidence of Virus Safety in Formal Clinical Trials

Numerous clinical viral safety investigations have been carried out on SD treated products (Table I). In aggregate, 10.7 million units were infused, and 0/53, 0/427, and 0/455 of the patients developed signs of HBV, HCV, and HIV transmission, respectively. It is interesting to note that one center prepared an SD-AHF (intermediate purity) and a prothrombin complex concentrate (PCC) which was heated in the lyophilized state at 60°C for 72 hours from the same plasma pool. The SD-AHF proved to be safe; the heated PCC transmitted HBV and HCV[1]. This finding is all the more remarkable since these viruses are known to concentrate away from the PCC fraction and into the AHF fraction during cryoprecipitation, the AHF was subjected to little additional purification, and the PCC was chromatographically purified.

Routine Clinical Use

SD-treated products have been approved for routine use in numerous countries, including Argentina, Australia, Austria, Belgium, Canada, Czechoslovakia, Denmark, Finland, France, Germany, Israel Italy, Japan, Korea, the Netherlands, Norway, Poland, Portugal, Saudi Arabia, South Africa, Spain, Sweden, Switzerland, the United Kingdom, the United States, and Venezuela. Products which are approved and the approximate number of doses transfused following approval are given in Table IV. It should be noted that the 3.8 million doses of AHF transfused represents over 45,000 man-years of treatment, assuming an average infusion of 80,000 IU per man-year. Based on current usage patterns, approximately 2/3 of the AHF transfused in North America, western Europe, and Japan is SD-treated. Throughout this time period, not a single case of HBV, HCV, or HIV transmission has been reported. To place this in perspective, prior to 1985, based on studies in chimpanzees and on clinical studies of the first of the dry heat-treated AHF concentrates available in the U.S., essentially every vial contained HCV, and transmission of HIV and HBV occurred frequently.

Based on estimates of the viral load present in plasma pools and evidenced removal and inactivation during processing, we conclude that vials of modern plasma derived coagulation factor concentrates prepared with the SD method have less than 1 chance in 10^{16}, 10^{13}, and 10^6 of having HIV, HBV, or HCV present, respectively[2].

HIVIG

In response to the AIDS epidemic, we developed procedures for the manufacture of a hyperimmune anti-HIV immune globulin derived from individuals infected with HIV but without overt signs of disease. Because of the potential danger to fractionation technicians, the plasma was virally inactivated with TNBP at the time of pooling. Subsequently, the IgG was isolated by Cohn-Oncley cold ethanol fractionation, and was given a second treatment with SD to further assure safety to the recipient. As a safety test, both the virally inactivated plasma and the purified final product were injected into chimpanzees. Despite being prepared exclusively from high risk donors, neither sample resulted in the transmission of HIV or of hepatitis[3]. Moreover, the injected IgG exhibited a normal circulatory recovery and half-life. In a subsequent study, the prevention of HIV infection on challenge of an injected animal with 10 CID_{50} of HIV^4 (but not 200 CID_{50}) has fostered the evaluation of HIVIG, prepared using SD treatment, in the United States and Europe.

Introduction Into Manufacture

Given the reproducible and predictable viral killing achieved with numerous different protein preparations, the SD method can figuratively be considered as a cassette which can be inserted into virtually any purification scheme. While the method was developed for use with blood protein solutions, SD treatments have been applied successfully to animal sera for use in tissue culture, both IgG and IgM monoclonal antibodies, products of recombinant DNA technology (especially when cell culture derived), and to diagnostic reagents[5]. To provide assurance that virus kill occurs as expected, NYBC requires that the rate and extent of kill of VSV and Sindbis virus be measured in each preparation and the results compared with the kill achieved on treatment of the NYBC AHF concentrate. If the rate of kill is comparable, it is our belief that the safety exhibited by our AHF concentrate and by other SD treated AHF concentrates purified by a similar method would be exhibited by the new preparation. Of course, other factors are also important, e.g., whether the viral load in plasma used in the manufacture of the new preparation is substantially higher than previously encountered. Since our preparation was of low purity, and since cryoprecipitation serves to concentrate virus, most new preparations will have a lower viral load than was present in our original AHF concentrate.

SD-Plasma

At one time, the viral danger presented by coagulation factor concentrates greatly exceeded the danger from single donor products, e.g., fresh frozen plasma (FFP) or cryoprecipitate. With the development of powerful virus inactivation procedures, AHF concentrates and other virally inactivated plasma products are now safer than the individual donations from which they were derived. This safety has encouraged the development of SD-Plasma as a substitute for FFP[6]. Briefly, units of FFP are combined, thawed, treated with 1% TNBP and 1% Triton X-100 at 30°C for 4 hours, the reagents removed by hydrophobic chromatography, and the final product sterile filtered, frozen, and, optionally, lyophilized. Virus inactivation has been extensively validated. Under these conditions of SD treatment, the rate of VSV and Sindbis virus killing exceeds that observed with AHF concentrates, treated either with TNBP/cholate or TNBP/Tween. We have also shown that $\geq 10^6$ CID_{50} of HBV, $\geq 10^5$ CID_{50} of HCV, and $\geq 10^{7.2}$ $TCID_{50}$ of HIV are killed. Additionally, because of our interest in validating the duck HBV model (described above), we have shown that $\geq 10^{7.3}$ ID_{50} of DHBV are inactivated. Coagulation factor content is high and in the range expected for FFP, and clinical results are excellent[7,8,9]. SD-Plasma is now in routine usage in France and Germany, and a Product License Application will be submitted to the U.S. FDA shortly.

Non-Enveloped Viruses

The SD method does not inactivate non-enveloped viruses, and the foundation for use in a blood transfusion setting was the realization that the principal viruses of concern (HBV, all forms of NANBHV including HCV, all retroviruses including HIV) were all enveloped.

Several comments regarding HAV would appear to be in order since there have been several recent reports of hepatitis A amongst recipients of an ion exchange chromatography purified, SD-treated, AHF concentrate[10,11,12].

Hepatitis A virus is a small, protein coated virus closely resembling other picorna viruses. It is generally transmitted by the fecal-oral route and is highly prevalent in the developing world where ≥ 50% of the population may be infected in early childhood. In countries with advanced standards of hygiene, infections may occur at any time throughout life since most adults are not immune. In infancy, most infections are subclinical, while about 25-50% of infected adults develop overt hepatitis. The incidence of HAV infection in developed countries is highly variable depending on the occurrence of epidemics, but it has been rather stable overall in the United States in recent decades. The infection is in all cases self-limited, with viremia persisting for only a few days or weeks. Except in the rare case of fulminant infection, exposure is followed by complete recovery without chronic residua such as cirrhosis.

HAV transmission to blood recipients has occurred only rarely. For example, HAV transmission did not occur in any of the numerous, prospective studies of single donor products designed to monitor hepatitis transmission and conducted in the past 10-15 years (Table II). Moreover, HAV was not transmitted to chimpanzees in any of the evaluations assessing coagulation factor concentrates, including the challenge phase when animals received the non-virally inactivated control. Moreover, we are aware of only 1 case of HAV reported in any of the numerous, prospective safety trials conducted with any coagulation factor concentrate, independent of viral inactivation method used[13].

Regarding the recent HAV outbreaks, the first was associated with an SD-treated AHF concentrate manufactured at one site in Italy from U.S. commercial plasma. At least 41 cases of HA, widely dispersed throughout Italy, were described[35]. 38 (93%) involved icteric disease. Lot tracking indicated that if SD-AHF was the vector in all cases, at least 12 different lots of product were involved. The AHF production method used ion exchange chromatography in addition to SD treatment. Between batches, the column was regenerated and sanitized with NaOH. Interviews with and serological screening of fractionation employees ruled them out as a possible vector. Since the manufacturer of the implicated AHF supplied 90% of the AHF used in Italy, an epidemiological investigation which utilizes a control group matched for age and severity of clotting factor defect is extremely difficult. While a recently reported case-control study is compatible with the conclusion of product involvement[14], a measurement of seroprevalence of IgG anti-HAV amongst hemophiliacs in southern Italy showed that patients treated with SD-AHF, SD-treated prothrombin complex concentrate, or pasteurized factor AHF were essentially all identical (60-70% seropositive) and not different from the general population[15]. If product did serve as the rector of transmission, given the number of lots implicated and the use of U.S. plasma, it seems unlikely that plasma was the source. One reasonable alternative was the process water, which was derived from a local well and purified by reverse osmosis. Before use, it was neither distilled nor heated at 80°C. A study has been initiated with Dr. Robert Purcell and with the cooperation of the manufacturer to determine if infectious HAV or HAV genomic sequences could be found in some of the implicated lots of AHF. A preliminary report of the results was given recently. Although HAV was found to be present by PCR in at least one lot of product, infectious HAV was not found on injection of chimpanzees.[41] Preliminary sequence analysis indicates that this strain of HAV is homologous to strains more typically found in Italy than in the United States[16]

Perhaps stimulated by this initial Italian episode, more recent reports of HA amongst hemophiliacs in Germany, Ireland, and Belgium have appeared, and we must await a final assessment of the cause of these transmissions. However, it should be pointed out that at least in the case in Ireland, infections occurred simultaneously with a general community epidemic. There is no evidence of hepatitis A transmissions associated with product usage in the United States.

Of importance, Nowicki and the U.S. Transfusion Safety Group concluded that there were no product-related HAV infections amongst 141 seronegative study subjects who were treated with ≥50,000 IV of AHF or factor IX when followed for 4-5 years[19]. Although, eleven appeared to seroconvert, most were attributable to passive transfer of antibody from immunoglobulin injections. This finding is relevant since many received products subjected to virus inactivation by only the solvent/detergent procedure. Additionally HAV nucleic acid sequences, as measured by nested PCR, has been shown to be absent on examination of over 30 lots of AHF and factor IX concentrates, produced mostly in Europe (P.L. Yap, Personal Communication). Thus, there is increasing and substantial evidence that blood and blood products do not transmit HAV.

Conclusion

The SD method of virus inactivation has been validated extensively with regard to virus killing and protein compatibility. SD-treated products would appear to enjoy a high margin of safety with regard to all major blood-borne viruses, including HBV, HCV, and HIV. The SD method can be inserted readily into virtually any purification scheme, providing predictable and effective virus killing. The high specificity of reaction derives from its mechanism of action, being directed against the lipid coat of enveloped viruses. Non-enveloped viruses, should they be present, will not be inactivated; thus, protection against these viruses needs to come from other factors, e.g., donor selection, antibody neutralization, and/or complementary methods of viral removal and killing. Fortunately, in a transfusion setting and with products of cell culture, including monoclonal antibodies and recombinant DNA-derived products, non-enveloped viruses present little if any risk. Several recent outbreaks of hepatitis A in hemophiliacs in Europe treated with an AHF concentrate prepared using the SD method and the same ion exchange chromatographic system requires additional investigation as to source of virus and reasons for transmission. These cases stand in contrast to the absence of icteric hepatitis A transmission in the United States[17] or Japan[18] and to the historical hepatitis A safety exhibited by all blood products, including coagulation factor concentrates. Several epidemiological and biochemical investigations have been initiated and should be completed in the coming months. Initial information from these studies, thus far, confirm the absence of HAV and HAV transmission to hemophiliacs.

Acknowledgements

Special appreciation is given to the manufacturers of the AHF concentrates implicated with the outbreaks of hepatitis A, and to the academic and governmental investigators who are attempting to understand the cause of these outbreaks, for making their findings available to us.

TABLE II

ABSENCE OF HEPATITIS A TRANSMISSION ON TRANSFUSION OF BLOOD

Reference	Country	Number Patients	UNITS Transfused	PTH	NUMBER HA	NANBH	HB	CMV	EBV
Aach et al, 1981	United States	1,528	5,564	171	0	156	15		
Alter et al, 1981	United States	283	3,359	36	0	35			
Katchaki et al, 1981	Netherlands	380	740	15	0	13	0	1	1
Cossart et al, 1982	Australia	842	4,789	18	0	14	3	1	
Grillner et al, 1982	Sweden	74	814	15	0	14	0	1	
Collins et al, 1983	Great Britian	248	1,796	38	0	38	0	0	
Hernandez et al, 1983	Spain	230	936	40	0	29	10	1	
Tremulada et al, 1983	Italy	246	1,500	34	0	29	+	+	
Tur-Kaspa et al,1983	Israel	50	606	4	0	4	0		
Aynard, et al, 1986	France	64	447	5	0	4	0	1	
Colombo et al, 1987	Italy	676	4,813	96	0	92	3		
Sugg et al, 1988	Germany	417	2,270	16	0	15	1		
Widell et al, 1988	Sweden	742	3,342	19	0	14	0	5	
Sirchia et al, 1991	Italy	780	5,200	52	0	50	0	1	
	TOTAL	6,560	36,176	559	0	507	32	11	1

TABLE III

VIRAL SAFETY OF SOLVENT/DETERGENT-TREATED COAGULATION FACTORS

References	Concentrate	Total Units infused (approx.)	Positive/Total		
			HBV	NANBHV	HIV
Horowitz, M.S., et al. (1988) Horowitz, M.S., et al. (1990)	AHF	145,000	na	0/17	0/18
Guerois, C., et al. (1991)	AHF	ua	na	0/27	0/27
	FIX	ua	na	0/5	0/5
	AHF, FIX			0/4	
Brackman, H.-H. (1992)	AHF	ua	na	0/165	0/49
Gonzaga, A.L., (1991)	PCC	1,104,600	0/16	0/21	0/21
	AHF	5,476,000	0/16	0/22	0/12
Panicucci, F., et al. (1990)	AHF	1,371,600	na	0/23	0/40
Di Paolantonio, T., et al. (1992)	AHF	1,272,000	na	na	0/29
Mariani, G. (1992)	AHF	165,000	0/14	0/31	0/31
Gomperts, E. (1991)	AHF	ua	na	0/109	0/60
Perret, B.A., et al. (1989)	AHF	541,000	na	na	0/18
	PCC	265,000	na	na	0/8
Perret, B.A., et al. (1991)	AHF	158,600	na	na	0/6
Peerlinck, K., et al. (1991)	AHF	ua	0/3	0/7	0/19
		10,498,800	0/53	0/427	0/45

TABLE IV

REPORTED USAGE OF S/D-TREATED PRODUCTS
1985 - October, 1992

Product	Units	Doses (Approximate)
FVII	1.9 MU*	1,900
FVIIa	2.6 MU	2,600
FVIII	3,864 MU	3,864,000
FIX	187 MU	187,000
PPSB	69 MU	69,000
CPPA	10 MU	4,400
FIBRIN GLUE	75,931 mL	15,190
FIBRINOGEN	75,688 g	19,000
IMIG & IVIG	318,000 g	63,600
Mab IgM	2,697 units	2,697
PLASMA	7,707 units	1,926
		4,231,313

* Million Units

References

(1) Gonzaga A. personal communication.

(2) Horowitz, B. (1990). Blood protein derivative viral safety: observations and analysis. Yale J Biol Med, 63, 361.

(3) Prince, A.M., Horowitz, B., Baker, L. et al. (1988). Failure of a human immunodeficiency virus (HIV) immune globulin to protect chimpanzees against experimental challenge with HIV. Proc. Natl. Acad. Sci. USA 85, 6944.

(4) Prince, A.M., Reesink, H., Pascual, D., Horowitz, B., Hewlett, I., Murthy, K.K., Cobb, K.E. and Eichberg, J.W. (1991). Prevention of HIV infection by passive immunization with HIV immune globulin. AIDS Res and Hum Retrov 7, 971-973.

(5) Horowitz, M.S., Bolmer, S.D. and Horowitz, B. (1991). Elimination of disease-transmitting enveloped viruses from human blood plasma and mammalian cell culture products. Bioseparation 1:409-417.

(6) Horowitz, B., Bonomo, R., Prince, A.M., Chin, S.N., Brotman, B. and Shulman, R.W. (1992). Solvent/detergent-treated plasma: A virus inactivated substitute for fresh frozen plasma. BLOOD 79, 826-831.

(7) Vezon, G. (June 1992). Viral inactivation of frozen fresh plasma by solvent detergent. Transfusion Today.

(8) Inbal, A., Shaklai, M., Kornbrot, N., Brenner, B. and Epstein, O. Clinical and laboratory evaluation of the treatment of hereditary or acquired coagulation disorders with solvent/detergent treated plasma (Octaplas), Blood 78, 73 abs.

(9) Pehta, J., Sellers, P., Horowitz, M. and the S/D Plasma Study Group. Clinical studies with solvent detergent-treated plasma in patients with coagulation factor deficiencies. BLOOD 80:222A, suppl, 1992.

(10) Mannucci, P.M. (1992). Outbreak of hepatitis A among Italian patients with haemophilia. Lancet 339:819.

(11) Gerritzen, A., Schneweis, K.E., Brackmann, H-H., Oldenburg, J., Hanfland, P., Gerlich, W.H. and Caspari, G. (1992). Acute hepatitis A in Hemophiliacs. Lancet 340, 1231-1232.

(12) Normann, A., Graff, A., Gerritzen, A., Brackmann, H-H. and Flehmig, B. (1992). Detection of hepatitis A virus RNA in a commercially-available factor VIII preparation. The Lancet 340, 1232-1233.

(13) Mariani, G., DiPaolantonio, T., Baklaja, R., Mannucci, P.M. (1991). Prospective hepatitis C safety evaluation of a high-purity, solvent-detergent treated FVIII concnetrate, Blood 78:10 Abs.

(14) Mannucci, P.M. (1992). Preliminary report given at Virological Safety Aspects of Plasma Derivatives, Cannes, France.

(15) Scaraggi, F.A., Perricci, A., Petronelli, M., Lomuscio, S., Mitrio, V. De. and Schiraldi, O. (1992). Prevalence of serum IgG antibodies to hepatitis A virus in Italian haemophiliacs. The Lancet 339, 1486.

(16) Lemon, S. Personal Communication.

(17) Mosely, J.M. Personal communication.

(18) Sekiguchi, S. Personal communication.

Development and experience of a pasteurization process for pooled fresh frozen plasma

M. Burnouf-Radosevich, T. Burnouf and J.-J. Huart

Centre Régional de Transfusion Sanguine, 21, rue Camille Guérin, 59012 Lille Cedex, France

Abstract

The approach followed in the development of a pasteurization treatment (60°C, 10 hrs, liquid state) of fresh frozen plasma is presented. Apheresis plasma (100 donations or less) obtained from regular donors was thawed at 30°C, then mixed with stabilizers and subjected to pasteurization. Following cooling, the mixture was ultrafiltered to eliminate the stabilizers, sterile-filtered, dispensed into bottles, and frozen. Validations of the process revealed the inactivation of more than 4 to 6 logs of non-enveloped and enveloped viruses in less than 5 hours of heat-treatment, under conditions preserving 75 to 95% of the activity of coagulation factors including FI, FV, FVIII, FXI, and FXIII, and protease inhibitors. The APTT of the pasteurized plasma was within the normal range. Electrophoretic and chromatographic analyses, as well as preclinical studies in animals did not detect significant alterations (such as protein aggregation) or any hypotensive or thrombogenic side-effects. Thus, these results demonstrate that plasma can be pasteurized to improve its viral safety. However, as this pooled product will not be subjected to any fractionation step (which are known to contribute to viral elimination), additional viral safety precautions had to be taken in the selection of the donors, in the type of screening tests performed on each donation, and in the limitation of the batch size.

Introduction

In spite of improvement in screening tests used to detect markers of infectious viruses in blood and plasma donations, fresh frozen plasma (FFP) can still be involved in the transmission of serious diseases such as AIDS or hepatitis. As FFP still has a number of clinical applications, defining techniques to submit it to a viral inactivation treatment is important. Several approaches have been described recently. The solvent-detergent treatment has been applied to pooled plasma and has been found to have the capacity to inactivate several lipid-enveloped viruses, including the HIV and hepatitis B and C agents (Horowitz *et al.*, 1992). The process involves an incubation of plasma with 1% tri(n-butyl)phosphate (TnBP) and 1% triton X-100 at 30°C for at least 4 hours, followed by oil extraction to remove TnBP, and by chromatographic adsorption on a C18 packing material to adsorb triton X-100. Another method, designed to inactivate viruses in single plasma donations, consists of adding selected photosensitizers, such as methylene blue or toluidine blue, and exposing the plasma to light (Lambrecht *et al.*, 1991). In this method the virus sterilizing agents are not eliminated. Efficacy against several viruses, mainly enveloped viruses, has been found.

Pasteurization, a heat treatment at 60°C for 10 hours in the liquid state, has long been used successfully to inactivate viruses in purified plasma protein solutions, including albumin, factor VIII, antithrombin III, alpha 1-antitrypsin, and fibrinogen (Heimburger & Karges, 1989). However, pasteurizing whole human plasma has not yet been described, presumably because the highly complex composition of this material made it difficult to withstand such heat treatment. In this paper we present the data currently achieved in the application of our pasteurization process to pooled whole human plasma while explaining the reason for this choice of treatment and summarizing the viral validation experiments performed so far as well as the industrial approach followed to ensure convenient good manufacturing practices (GMP).

Viral safety of plasma derivatives

It has been clearly established that the viral safety of plasma-derived products results from a number of criteria: (a) efficient blood donor selection and viral screening of blood/plasma donations, (b) efficacy of viral inactivation treatment, (c) performance of the purification/fractionation process in eliminating infectious agents, and (d) good manufacturing practices to avoid deviations from an established and validated process or risks of downstream viral contamination (Burnouf, 1992). In the production of pooled virus-inactivated plasma, the absence of any purification/fractionation step made it necessary to increase the precautions taken at the blood donor selection level and to select the range of viral screening tests carefully. In addition, a careful choice of the viral inactivation method should be made so as to ensure a good efficacy against the major plasma-borne viruses known presently while at the same time providing a satisfactory margin of safety against other potential infectious agents.

Blood donor selection, viral screening tests, and batch size

Plasma used was collected from healthy, voluntary, unpaid, regular plasmapheresis donors. Each donation was tested for the absence of anti-HIV-1 and -2, anti-HCV, anti-HBc, anti-HTLV-1 and -2 antibodies, and HBsAg, and the level of transaminases had to be within normal values ($< N + 2.33$ SD). In addition, screening for Parvovirus B 19 antigen or by PCR was performed. To avoid additional (viral and immunological) risks associated with large plasma batches, the size of each batch was limited to 100 plasma donations, corresponding to about 60 liters of plasma.

Pasteurization process

Plasma was thawed at 30°C in a jacketed container to avoid the formation of a cryoprecipitate and then transferred to a tank where stabilizers were added to protect plasma proteins during pasteurization. The mixture was then transferred into a thermostated, double-jacketed pasteurization container to be heat-treated for 10 hours at 60°C under constant and gentle stirring. Following pasteurization, the mixture was cooled down and subjected to an ultrafiltration step using 10000-dalton cassettes to eliminate the stabilizers, concentrate the plasma to its initial volume, and formulate it prior to sterile filtration, filling into bottles, and freezing.

Viral validation

Viral validations, using infectivity assays, were performed by two independent virology laboratories, Institut Pasteur-Texcell (Paris, France) and Inveresk Research Incorporated (Edinburgh, Scotland) following current European regulations, as described in the Note for Guidance III/815/89-EN (CPMP guidelines, 1991).

Table. Viral inactivation during pasteurization of whole plasma

Virus	Envelope	Genome	Size (nm)	Viral reduction (log 10)	Duration
HIV-1	+	RNA	80-100	> 6.0	< 10 min
Pseudorabies	+	DNA	120-200	> 4.15	< 2 hrs
Sindbis	+	RNA	55-60	> 5.74	< 5 hrs
Vaccinia	+	DNA	400/200	> 4.3	< 1 hr
Parainfluenza 3	+	RNA	150-200	> 6.3	< 2 hrs
Polio Sabin	-	RNA	25-30	> 6.23	< 2 hrs
Reovirus 3	-	RNA	60-80	3.23	10 hrs

The Table indicates the viruses used for validating the pasteurization step. They include HIV-1, a relevant virus that can contaminate the starting plasma, and 6 other model viruses of different sizes and with distinct structures: enveloped or non-enveloped, with DNA or RNA genetic material. Among these, Sindbis virus is considered to be a convenient model for the hepatitis C virus due to structural homologies. The rate and extent of viral inactivation were high and rapid for 6 of the viruses studied (Appourchaux & Burnouf, 1992). For example, more than 6 logs of HIV-1 were inactivated in less than 10 minutes at 60°C, more than 4.3 logs of Vaccinia virus in less than 1 hour, more than 6.3 logs of Parainfluenza virus in less than 2 hours, more than 6.23 logs of Polio Sabin 1, a non-enveloped virus, in less than 2 hours, more than 4.15 logs of porcine Pseudorabies virus in less than 2 hours, and more than 5.74 logs of Sindbis virus in less than 5 hours. The inactivation of Reovirus type 3 was not complete: 3.2 logs were inactivated in the 10 hours period. It should be noted, however, that Reovirus type 3 is a highly resistant non-enveloped virus, which is considered to be more sensitive to physico-chemical treatment than animal parvoviruses. These results indicate that this pasteurization process , although it may show clear limitations for highly resistant non-enveloped viruses, has in our experience the potential of inactivating viruses at similar, and sometimes higher rate and extent than those found during pasteurization of plasma derivatives. This indicated that the presence of stabilizers and the relatively high protein content during pasteurization of whole plasma did not prohibit inactivation of significant doses of viruses, such as HIV-1, Sindbis virus, or Polio virus. The relative resistance of Reovirus type 3 fully supports our approach at optimizing the virological quality of the starting plasma by reinforcing the selection criteria of the donor population and the viral screening tests performed on each donation.

Biological characteristics

To maintain its physiological properties, plasma must not be significantly altered during the viral inactivation step. Biological activity of coagulation factors and protease inhibitors must be preserved. Also, the viral inactivation process must not induce activation of coagulation factors or other components and must provide a plasma that will be well tolerated in vivo.

The biological properties of pasteurized plasma have already been described elsewhere (Burnouf-Radosevich *et al.*, 1992)). The industrial processing of pasteurized plasma confirms the high recovery (95% or more) in total protein, due in part to the relative simplicity of the process which induced no major loss of product. The overall recovery in coagulation factor activity is 70 to 90% of that found in the starting plasma pool. The average activity in coagulation factors is comprised between 0.8 and 1 IU/ml for factors V, VIII, IX, XI, and XIII. Similarly, the content in clottable fibrinogen is generally between 2.2 and 2.5 g/l, indicating that the stabilizers selected are well suited to protect the activity of this thermosensitive protein. Recovery in plasma protease inhibitors, such as antithrombin III, alpha 1-antitrypsin, or C1-inhibitor, was close to 90%. The preservation of the biological activity of plasma proteins is well illustrated by the normal APTT value which expresses the overall clottability of plasma. This suggests that, in clinical applications, pasteurized plasma should play a normal physiological role. In addition, no thrombin, nor activated FIX or FX, nor kallikrein or prekallikrein activators could be found. Accordingly, the overall proteolytic activity, as determined by the S-2288 (Kabi) chromogenic substrate, was low and similar to that of the starting plasma, and no fibrinogen degradation products were detected.

One of the drawbacks that can be associated with the heating of protein solutions is the generation of aggregates. The absence of aggregates has been demonstrated by various methods including electrophoretic analyses in polyacrylamide gels; western blot analysis using specific antibodies directed against albumin, immunoglobulins, alpha 1-antitrypsin (the isoforms being previously separated by isoelectrofocusing), or haptoglobin; crossed immunoelectrophoresis; or size-exclusion chromatography.

Preclinical studies

Preclinical studies in animals have been conducted to check for the absence of side-effects associated with the infusion of pasteurized plasma. Infusion of plasma, pasteurized or not, at a dose of 4 ml/kg at 6 ml/min, did not induce hypotension or modifications of the cardiac rhythm in a rat model. No sign of toxicity in mice over an observation period of 7 days, was noticed after intravenous infusion of 25 ml/kg. The rabbit stasis model showed that the pasteurization process did not modify the thrombogenic potential of plasma. The injection of pasteurized plasma in rabbits did not induce detectable synthesis of neoantibodies over a nine-month follow-up period.

Good manufacturing practices

The viral safety of pasteurized plasma is dependent not only upon the efficacy of the viral inactivation process but also upon the respect of GMP at the production level. Following GMP is essential at all processing steps for controlling the pasteurization conditions and ensuring the absence of risks of virus overload prior to pasteurization or downstrean contamination following pasteurization. An overall computerized safety program allows optimal traceability at all of the processing steps and reduces human error.

The number and origin of each plasma donation comprising the pool is recorded by computerized optical reading of its bar-code, the system automatically limiting the number of donations to 100 per batch. A specific bar-code number is attributed to the plasma pool and is used, through optical reading, for characterizing the batch at all crucial steps of the process. The plasma is thawed at 30°C, then tranferred into a container only after computer-validated sterilization. The plasma weight is determined automatically, registered, and affiliated to the batch number. Stabilizers are added automatically after bar-code identification and in quantities depending upon the exact weight of plasma, as registered under its bar-code number. The stabilized plasma is then transferred to the pasteurization tank after validated sterilization, control of its integrity, and appropriate validation of the temperature probes. Temperature over the pasteurization cycle is recorded continuously at 4 points of the pasteurization system: product, atmosphere in the pasteurization unit (ensuring control of an even temperature in the tank), and inlet and outlet of the fluid in the double jacket. Similarly, a pressure detector verifies the integrity of the pasteurization tank. Treatment takes place under continuous controlled gentle stirring. Ultrafiltration, using an in-line cassette system, is started after appropriate sterilization and control of its integrity. Pasteurization, ultrafiltration, and subsequent processing (formulation, sterile filtration, filling) are performed in virus-secure areas equipped accordingly (air-lock systems, decontamination area, dedicated air-handling system, positive pressure, ...). Post-pasteurization reagents and water are sterilized to eliminate risks of bacterial (or viral) contamination. After filling, plasma is frozen and stored at - 35°C.

Conclusion

The development of a technique for subjecting whole human plasma to a liquid heat treatment at 60°C for 10 hours could represent a significant step in the improvement of the safety of fresh frozen plasma related to the risks of transmission of AIDS or hepatitis B or C. Pasteurization has the advantage of being a well-established viral inactivation procedure that has been applied to plasma derivatives for many years. This method is recognized as having the potential of inactivating a relatively broad range of viruses, both enveloped and non-enveloped. This could be of significant importance for such a pooled product which is not subjected to any fractionation/purification steps capable of eliminating viruses. This latter point also reinforces the necessity of carefully selecting and controlling the plasma donations as well as limiting the number (< 100) used to make the pool (Burnouf-Radosevich *et al.*, in press). Although in vitro data and preclinical studies in animals do not reveal any detectable alteration of the plasma upon pasteurization, only clinical experience will establish the safety and efficacy of this product.

References

Appourchaux, P. & Burnouf, T. (1992): Virus validation of a pasteurization treatment of therapeutic plasma. *Virological safety aspects of plasma derivatives*. IABS Congress, Cannes. Nov. 3-6.

Burnouf, T. (1992): Safety aspects in the manufacturing of plasma-derived coagulation factor concentrates. *Biologicals* 20, 91-100.

Burnouf-Radosevich, M., Burnouf T., & Huart, J.J. (1992): A pasteurized therapeutic plasma. *Infusionstherapie* 19, 91-94.

Burnouf-Radosevich, M., Burnouf T., & Huart J.J. (in press): Pasteurisation industrielle du plasma et critères de qualité. *Rev. Fr. Transf. Hémobiol.*

CPMP Guidelines - *Ad hoc* working party of biotechnology/ pharmacy (1991): Note for guidance ' Validation of virus removal and inactivation procedures (III/8115/89-EN). February 11-13.

Heimburger, N. & Karges, H.E. (1989): Strategies to produce virus-safe blood derivatives. In *Virus inactivation in plasma products*, ed. J-J Morgenthaler, pp. 23-33. Basel: Karger.

Horowitz, B., Bonomo R., Prince A.M., Chin S.N., Brotman B., & Shulman R.W. (1992): Solvent/detergent-treated plasma: A virus inactivated substitute for fresh frozen plasma. *Blood* 79, 826-831.

Lambrecht, B., Mohr, H., Knüver-Hopf, J., & Schmitt, H.(1991): Inactivation of viruses in human fresh frozen plasma by phenothiazine dyes in combination with visible light. *Vox. Sang.* 60, 207-213.

Résumé

Un procédé permettant de pasteuriser (10 heures à 60°C à l'état liquide) le plasma humain est décrit et analysé. Les unités de plasma, obtenues de donneurs réguliers de plasmaphérèse et soumises à des dépistages viraux (anti-VIH, anti-HCV, anti-HBc, anti-HTLV, antigènes HBs et Parvovirus B 19; dosage des transaminases) sont décongelées par lot maximum de 100, stabilisées, et pasteurisées en enceintes thermostatées et calorifugées. Après refroidissement, le mélange est dialysé pour éliminer les stabilisants, filtré stérilement, et réparti aseptiquement en flacons, puis congelé. Les épreuves de validation du procédé ont démontré une capacité d'inactivation de virus appartenant à différents groupes structuraux, enveloppés ou non enveloppés, à ADN ou à ARN. Les résultats d'activité biologique démontre une préservation satisfaisante des caractéristiques biologiques du plasma, telle que l'activité des facteurs de coagulation ou celle des inhibiteurs de protéases, et l'absence d'altérations biochimiques décelables par des techniques d'analyse *in vitro* ou lors de l'injection dans des modèles animaux. L'installation industrielle, automatisée et informatisée, ainsi que le déroulement des différentes étapes du procédé ont été conçus afin d'assurer une grande traçabilité et de respecter les bonnes pratiques de fabrication.

Optimization of parameters for photodynamic virus inactivation of human fresh plasma

H. Mohr and B. Lambrecht

DRK-Blutspendedienst Niedersachsen, Eldagsener Strasse 38, 3257 Springe 1, Germany

For virus inactivation single units of human fresh plasma at a volume of 250-300 ml in plastic containers may be photodynamically treated by illumination with light derived from fluorescent tubes in the presence of the phenothiazine dye methylene blue. The effective dye concentration is 1 µM, i.e. approx. 300 µg per litre of plasma. Besides the amount of photosensitizer used other critical parameters in the process are light intensity and illumination time. In the optimized procedure the plasma is illuminated at a light intensity of at least 50,000 Lux for 60 minutes. This destroys the infectivity of those viruses which are sensitive to photodynamic treatment whereas plasma proteins are only slightly influenced.

INTRODUCTION

Photodynamic virus inactivation offers the possibility to decontaminate plasma and eventually cellular blood products from single blood donations (Bull et al., 1992). We have developed a procedure to inactivate viruses in human fresh plasma, intended for therapeutical use by treating the plasma in its plastic bag with visible light in the presence of a small amount of a photoactive phenothiazine dye, e.g. methylene blue (MB). This reliably inactivates all lipid enveloped viruses tested so far (including HIV-1 and viruses similar to Hepatitis C virus) and also some non-enveloped viruses (Lambrecht et al., 1991; Mohr et al., 1992 a, b, c). Virus inactivation mainly depends on dye concentration, light intensity and illumination time. Because the procedure also affects the activities of plasma proteins it was necessary to find treatment conditions which allow effective virus kill but leaving the properties of plasma proteins largely uninfluenced.

MATERIALS AND METHODS

Photodynamic treatment of plasma

Human plasma was isolated from blood donations and kept frozen at $\leq -30\ °C$ until further use. MB was from Merck, Darmstadt (FRG). The plasma bags were from Baxter, Munich (FRG). For photodynamic treatment, the plasma in the presence of different concentrations of MB was illuminated on a light bank equipped with fluorescent tubes (TL-M 115 W/33 RS from Philips, Eindhoven (Netherlands)) for the times indicated. Further details of the procedure are described elsewhere (Mohr et al., 1992 b).

Virus cultivation and assays

The cultivation and assay of vesicular stomatitis virus (VSV) were previously described (Lambrecht et al., 1991). Virus titres are expressed as "Tissue culture infective doses" ($TCID_{50}$) according to Kaerber (1931) and Spearman (1908).

Determination of thrombin time (TT)

TT of plasma samples was measured by J.U. Wieding, University of Göttingen (FRG), using a routine assay.

RESULTS AND DISCUSSION

The virus inactivating properties of the phenothiazine dyes MB and toluidine blue (TB) in combination with visible light are well documented (Gerba et al., 1977; Hiatt et al., 1960; Schnipper et al., 1980; Wallis and Melnick, 1964). The use of these dyes for photodynamic decontamination of human plasma was proposed by Heinmets and his co-workers almost 40 years ago (Heinmets et al., 1955). They designed a procedure in which a photosensitizer containing plasma pool prepared from a number of blood donations was continuously passed through an illumination device. Our procedure is quite different: It uses single plasma units which are individually light treated in the presence of MB or TB (Lambrecht et al., 1991; Mohr et al., 1992 a, b , c). It is technically simple and avoids the potential risk of contaminating a whole plasma pool with a single unit containing a virus which is resistant to the inactivation procedure applied. We found that all enveloped viruses tested so far (including HIV-1 and 2 and some Toga viruses which might serve as models for Hepatitis C virus) were sensitive to photodynamic treatment. Among the non-enveloped viruses tested some were sensitive (e.g. SV40 and Calici virus), some were not (e.g. EMC and Polio virus).

The efficacy of the photodynamic procedure is mainly determined by three variables: The dye concentration used, the light intensity and the illumination time.

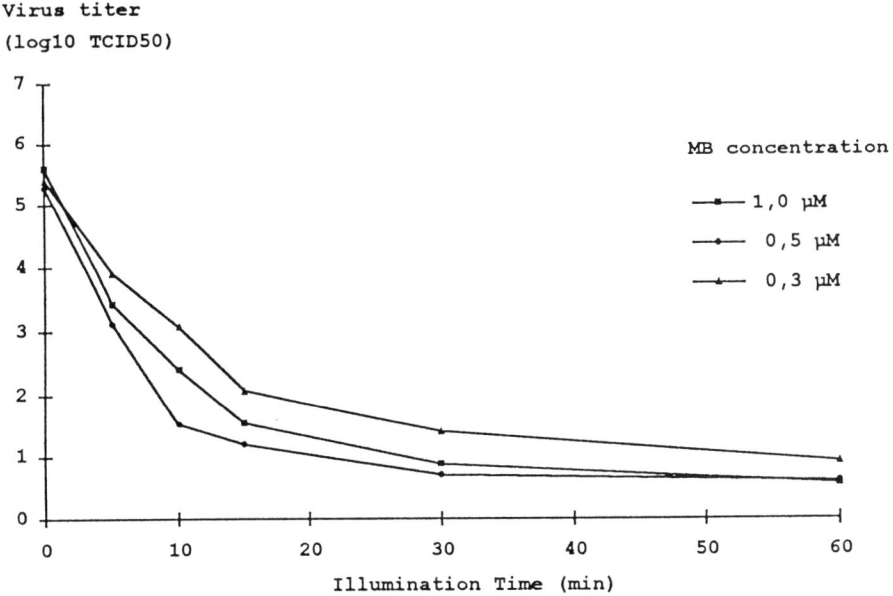

Fig. 1: Kinetics of the inactivation of VSV in human fresh plasma (300 ml in plasma bags) by photodynamic treatment in the presence of MB

In our process plasma units of 250-300 ml in plastic bags are illuminated on a light bank equipped with fluorescent tubes (Mohr et al., 1992 a, b, c). In small scale experiments a dye concentration of approx. 1 µM was required to reduce within 30 minutes the infectivity of plasma containing test viruses, which were sensitive to photodynamic treatment, below the detection limit of the assay systems applied (Lambrecht et al., 1991). That the same holds true under production conditions is shown in Fig. 1, in which the kinetics of the inactivation of VSV at plasma concentrations of MB between 0.3 and 1 µM are depicted. The concentration of the photosensitizer is also critical because photodynamic treatment additionally affects plasma proteins. As a consequence their activities are time dependently reduced, at 1 µM by approx. 20 % within 1 h (Mohr et al., 1992 a). Fig. 2 shows that on the other hand thrombin time, which is an indicator of clottability of the plasma, is prolonged. The same figure indicates that the increase in TT is directly dependent on the concentration of MB. At 1 µM and an illumination time of 1 h it was about 25 %. With regard to the applicability of the plasma for therapeutical purposes this seems to be tolerable.

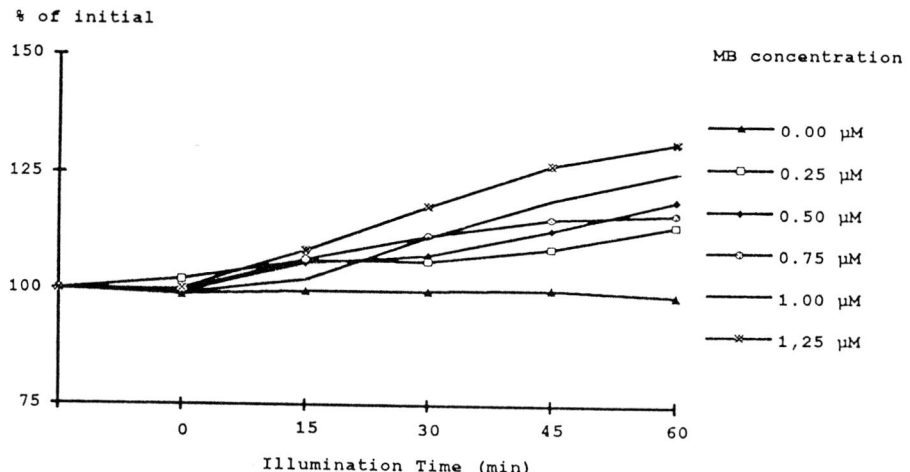

Fig.2 Photodynamic treatment of plasma with methylene blue. Influence of dye concentration and illumination time on thrombin time

Figure 3 shows the kinetics of VSV inactivation at light intensities between 30,000 and 70,000 Lux. The concentration of MB was 1 µM. It is obvious that at higher intensities the process is more efficient. At 30,000 and 40,000 Lux significant residual infectivity was observed even after 60 min of illumination, whereas above 50,000 Lux it was reduced to near or below the detection limit of the assay used within 30 min. Based on these results, photodynamic treatment of the plasma intended for therapeutical use is carried out at a minimal light intensity of 50,000 Lux.

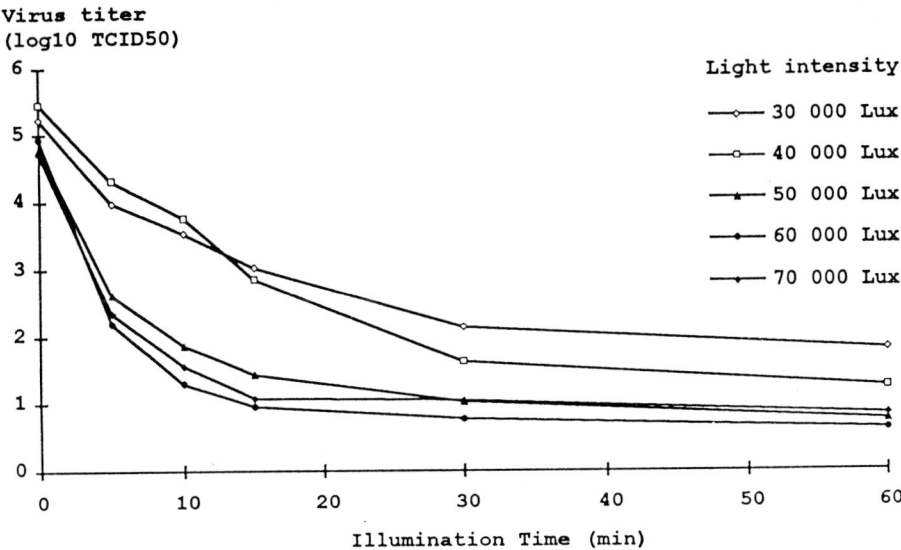

Fig. 3: Influence of light intensity on photodynamic inactivation of VSV in fresh plasma. Plasma volume was approx. 300 ml, MB concentration was 1 µM.

ACKNOWLEDGEMENTS

We thank J. U. Wieding for measuring the Thrombin time of plasma samples, Ch. Wittich for typing the manuscript and J. Linneweber for reviewing it.

REFERENCES

Bull, B.S., Orlic, D. & Bessis, M. (eds.) (1992): Photoinactivation of viruses and cells for medical applications. *Blood Cells* 18, pp. 3-162. Berlin, Heidelberg, New York: Springer International.

Gerba, C.P., Wallis, G. & Melnick, J.L. (1977): Application of photodynamic oxidation to the disinfection of tapwater, seawater, and sewage contaminated with poliovirus. *Photochem. Photobiol.* 26, 499-504.

Heinmets, F., Kingston, J.R. & Hiatt, C.W. (1955): Inactivation of viruses in plasma by photosensitized oxidation. Joint report of the Walter Reed Army Institute of Research Walter Reed Army Medical Center, Washington, D.C., with the Naval Medical Research Institute, Bethesda.

Hiatt, C.W., Kaufman, E. & Helprin, J.J. (1960): Inactivation of viruses by the photodynamic action of toluidine blue. *J. Immunol.* 84, 1480-484.

Kaerber, G. (1931): Beitrag zur kollektiven Behandlung pharmakologischer Reihenversuche. *Naunyn-Schmiedebergs Arch. Exp. Pathol. Pharmacol.* 162, 480-482.

Lambrecht, B., Mohr, H., Knüver-Hopf, J. & Schmitt, H. (1991): Photoinactivation of viruses in human fresh plasma by phenothiazine dyes in combination with visible light. *Vox Sang.* 60, 207-213.

Mohr, H., Lambrecht, B. & Knüver-Hopf, J. (1992 a): Virus inactivated single-donor fresh plasma preparations. *Infusionstherapie* 19, 79-83.

Mohr, H., Knüver-Hopf, J., Lambrecht, B., Scheidecker, H. & Schmitt, H. (1992 b): No evidence for neoantigens in human plasma after photochemical virus inactivation. *Ann. Hematol.* 65, 224-228.

Mohr, H., Pohl, U., Lambrecht, B. & Schmitt, H. (1992 c): Methylene blue-virus inactivated human plasma: Manufacturing and clinical experiences. *Infusionstherapie*, in press.

Schnipper, L.E., Lewin, A.A., Swartz, M. & Crumpacker, C.S. (1980): Mechanism of photodynamic inactivation of herpes simplex viruses. *J. Clin. Invest.* 65, 432-438.

Spearman, C. (1908): The method of "right and wrong cases" ("constant stimuli") without Gauss's formulae. *Br. J. Psychol.* 2, 277-282.

Wallis, C. & Melnick, J.L. (1964): Irreversible photosensitization of viruses. *Virology* 23, 520-527.

Intravenous immunoglobulin of high purity when production includes solvent/detergent treatment

Hannu Suomela and Eero Hämäläinen

Finnish Red Cross Blood Transfusion Service, Kivihaantie 7, 00310 Helsinki, Finland

Summary

A method has been developed for manufacturing an iv immunoglobulin preparation which is particularly pure IgG, contains an exceptionally low amount of IgA, and has no enzymatic contaminants. The content of monomer+dimer is > 95% and there are no aggregates. It contains antibodies and antitoxins in the concentrations that may be expected from its protein concentration. The IgG subclass distribution is normal, but the concentration of subclass 4 is lower than expected. The product has low anticomplementary activity and was well tolerated in a clinical trial.

Introduction

In recent years special attention has been paid to the viral safety of plasma products, since many preparations derived from plasma have transmitted hepatitis. Some intravenous immunoglobulin preparations have also been shown to transmit hepatitis (reviewed by Suomela (1993).

In order to improve the viral safety of our intravenous immunoglobulin preparation, we included in our production method the solvent/detergent (S/D) treatment outlined by the New York Blood Center (NYBC). In this paper we describe some properties of our product produced from freeze-dried Cohn fraction II, and also including mild pepsin degradation, S/D treatment, and chromatographic purification steps.

Purity

The major characteristic of our product is its high purity, judged by cellulose acetate electrophoresis to be >99%. The purity is demonstrated by Fig.1 (CA-electrophoresis) and Fig. 2 (immunoelectrophoresis).

Because of the chromatographic purification steps, the content of immunoglobulin A is exceptionally low, 1-3 mg /L in 6% solution. Immunoglobulin M is not detectable. The product is free from enzymatic contaminants such as plasmin, plasminogen, the prekallikein activator, and kallikrein.

Endotoxins, measured by the LAL test, are below 1.25 units/ml and the isoagglutinin titer (including IgG and IgM isoagglutinins) is < 1:32. S/D chemicals are not detectable in the final product. When the freeze-dried powder has been dissolved, the solution contains 60 g/L of protein at pH 6.5. The osmolality of the solution is 420 mOsm/kg. The high osmolality is mainly due to the sucrose content of 65 g/L.

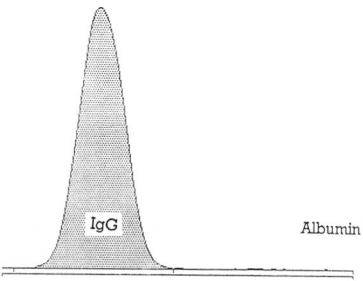

Fig. 1. Cellulose acetate electrophoresis of iv IgG FRC BTS

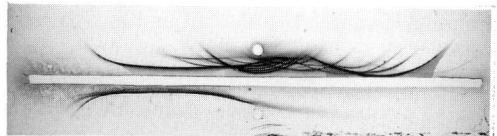

Fig. 2. Immunoelectrophoresis of iv IgG FRC BTS

Molecular size

We incubate the immunoglobulin solution with pepsin for 66 hours to improve its viral safety (Hämäläinen et al, 1992). This causes fragmentation of IgG. To remove the immunoglobulin fragments, the added pepsin and the solvent/detergent substances, we use chromatographic methods as final purification steps.
The final product is mainly monomeric and does not contain the IgG aggregates that are responsible for side effects in patients. The final product has been gel filtered with HPLC equipment under the conditions defined in the proposed monograph on intravenous immunoglobulin included in the European Pharmacopoeia (Ph. Eur., 1992). The elution curve demonstrates that there are no aggregates, but a minor dimer peak (<5 %) and a monomer peak which has a slight "shoulder" on the right side and a small amount of material in the elution volume of fragments (Fig. 3).
FPLC equipment provided with a Superose 12 column (Pharmacia, Sweden) likewise demonstrated the absence of aggregates. FPLC is not able to separate the dimers as a distinct peak; however, it separates the fragments as a small separate peak.

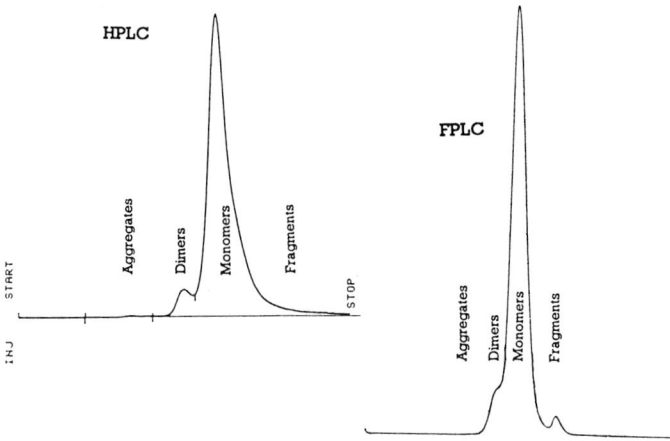

Fig. 3. Left panel: HPLC elution curve of iv IgG FRC BTS run in the conditions proposed by the working document of iv IgG of the European Pharmacopoeia (1992). The elution volumes of aggregates, dimers, monomers and fragments are marked as obtained in runs of the Ph. Eur. Reference Preparation. Right panel: FPLC run through a Superose 12 column with the same buffer as in the adjacent HPLC run.

Subclass distribution

It might be expected that the long production method, including chromatographic purification steps would alter the IgG subclass distribution. However, analyses demonstrate that the subclass distribution is normal, except that the relative content of subclass 4 is slightly lower than in normal plasma. This is not regarded as a drawback because no antigens are known that would cause a response in subclass 4 only. Table 1 represents the assay results obtained from two independent laboratories.

Table 1. Immunoglobulin G subclass distribution of iv IgG FRC BTS. Laboratory 1= Zentrallaboratorium Blutspendedienst SRK, Bern, Switzerland and Laboratory 2= Behringwerke AG, Marburg, Germany.

Lot number and laboratory	IgG 1	IgG 2	IgG 3	IgG 4
1434 1001				
Lab. 1	61.7	33.2	4.8	0.4
Lab. 2	56.0	38.0	5.4	0.7
1434 1002				
Lab. 1	64.6	30.1	4.5	0.8
Lab. 2	59.4	33.7	6.1	0.8
1434 1003				
Lab. 1	63.3	31.8	4.2	0.7
Lab. 2	54.5	38.6	5.9	0.9
WHO normal plasma	60-70	19-32	5-8	< 1-4

Contents of antibodies

Immunoglobulin G in our preparation (in solution) is concentrated 5- to 6-fold compared with plasma. If the immunoglobulin molecules are intact, the titers against both bacterial and viral antibodies should be 5- to 6-fold higher than those in plasma. The broad spectrum of antibodies assayed demonstrates titers 4- to 8-fold higher in the product than in plasma. This confirms that the IgG is intact and has retained its biological activity (Tables 2 and 3).

Table 2. Titers of viral antibodies of iv IgG FRC BTS.

Virus	Unit	Plasma	iv IgG
Adeno	titer	1:1280	1:5120
Cytomegalo	PEIE/ml		26
Hepatitis A	IU/ml		23
Hepatitis B anti-HBs	IU/ml		0.1
Morbilli	IU/ML	4	35
Parvo B19	titer	1:200	1:800
Polio 1	titer	1:320	1:3200
Polio 2	titer	1:1280	1:12800
Polio 3	titer	1:5120	1:12800
Rubella	EIA	1400	18600
Varic.-Zoster	CF-titer	1:8	1:128
Respir. syncyt.	titer	1:5120	1:20480

Table 3. Titers of bacterial antibodies and concentrations of antitoxins

Bacteria	Unit	Plasma	iv IgG
E coli Omp A	titer	1:<100	1:230
Hemoph. influenz.	ug/ml	5.4	25.7
Mycopl. pneumon.	titer	1:250	1:2700
Pneumoc. pneumolys.	titer	1:310	1:2440
Staphyl.staph.lys.	ug/ml	0.64	3.6
Streptoc. str. lys	IU/ml		480
Diphtheria	IU/ml		2.5
Tetanus	IU/ml	4	25

Anticomplementary activity

The anticomplemetary activity (ACA) of immunoglobulin G is usually removed from Cohn fraction II-based immunoglobulins by pepsin treatment at low pH. We have extended the pepsin treatment to 66 hours and during later production steps we carefully prevent the aggregation of IgG. The ACA in our product is exceptionally low.

Fig. 4 demonstates the levels of ACA in our products and compares them with those in licenced European and American preparations.

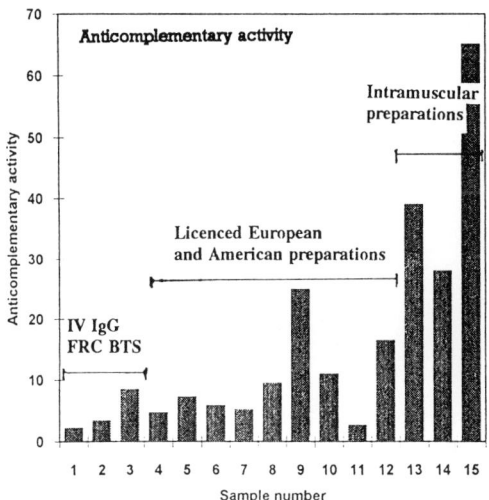

Figure 4. Anticomplementary activity in our product, in licenced European and American products, and in intramuscular preparations. Each of the preparations was assayed 20-30 times in the course of several months using a microtiter plate assay method (from Törmä et al, 1993).

Clinical trial

The clinical trial was run in 15 patients with hypogammaglobulinemia who were on regular substitution therapy with two licenced preparations. These patients received 43 infusions in seven hospitals. The side effects noticed were rare and mild (Ebeling F. et al, to be published).

REFERENCES

1. European Pharmacopoeia Commission (1992): Immunoglobulinum humanum normale ad usum intravenosum. Pharmeuropa: vol 3, No. 4, 259-267.

2. Hämäläinen, E. Suomela, H. and Ukkonen P. (1992): Virus Inactivation during Intravenous Immunoglobulin Production. Vox Sang. 63, 6-11.

3. Suomela, H. (1993): Inactivation of Viruses in Blood and Plasma Products. Trans. Med. Rev. 7, (1), 42-57.

4. Törmä, E., Suomela, H. and Hämäläinen, E. : Microtiter plate assay for measuring anticomplementary activity of immunoglobulins. Submitted for publication.

Study of the virus inactivation or elimination capacity of a chromatographic procedure for purifying human plasma albumin

J.-F. Stoltz[1,2], C. Rivat[2], M. Grandgeorge[3], C. Geschier[1], P. Sertillanges[2], J.-L. Véron[3], J. Liautaud[3] and L. Dumont[1]

[1]Centre Régional de Transfusion Sanguine et Laboratoire d'Hématologie, Brabois, 54500 Vandœuvre-lès-Nancy, France, [2]INSERM, CO 10, Brabois, 54511 Vandœuvre-lès-Nancy, France, [3]Institut Mérieux, 69280 Marcy-l'Étoile, France

ABSTRACT

Almost the whole of the human plasma albumin preparations intended for clinical or biological uses is at present fractionated by cold ethanol precipitation. However, ion-exchange chromatographic processes have been recently developed. The aim of this work was the evaluation of the viral inactivation efficacy of an automated industrial chromatographic process allowing fractionation of 350 to 400 l of plasma per cycle using the Spherodex-Spherosil gels. Three relevant viruses were selected for this validation study : hepatitis B virus (HBV), poliomyelitis virus and human immunodeficiency virus (HIV). In order to comply with EEC and FDA regulatory documents, significant amounts of the tested viruses were spiked into the different fractions obtained during the various purification steps and their removal or inactivation during the subsequent step were determined. Moreover, residual viral infectivity was checked on after elution and washing of the columns for each chromatographic step. Results have pointed out an overall reduction of : 4.4 $\log_{10}$ for HBV ; superior 10 $\log_{10}$ for the poliomyelitis virus ; superior 14 $\log_{10}$ for HIV. Moreover, no residual viral infectivities were detected after washing of the columns. This study showed that the viral safety of human albumin purified using the chromatographic Spherodex-Spherosil process should not be different from that of the classical Cohn's albumin.

INTRODUCTION

Almost all human plasmatic albumins used in therapy are now prepared by methods based on the process described by Cohn *et al.* (1946). Recently, chromatographic techniques have been developed, mainly based on ion-exchange chromatography. In particular, processes using Spherodex and Spherosil ion-exchangers (Sepracor-IBF, Villeneuve la Garenne, France) have been developed for purifying human albumin from placentas (Tayot *et al.*, 1981) or plasma (Stoltz *et al.*, 1987). Undenatured, very high purity albumin can be produced with these processes. The study described here was undertaken in 1989-1990 at the Regional Blood Transfusion Centre in Nancy in partnership with Institut Merieux (Marcy l'Etoile, France and IBF-Sepracor, Villeneuve la Garenne, France) with a view to develop an automated industrial chromatography unit for processing 350 to 400 litres of plasma per batch. This study focused on assessing the ability of the chromatographic fractionation procedure to inactivate or eliminate three different viruses.

MATERIALS AND METHODS

Chromatographic process : The experimental process and the plant are described in Stoltz *et al.* (1987-1991 and in these proceedings).

Choice of viruses : Three viruses were chosen for the validation study : hepatitis B (HBV), poliomyelitis (type I, Mahoney) and human immunodeficiency virus (HIV-1).

Objective of the procedure for validating virus inactivation

In accordance with the CEC directives, validation of the process was made on each step individually (CEC, 1991 ; Vicary et al. 1991). The source plasma was taken directly from a batch during a normal production cycle with the Cohn's method. The product then went through the 3 chromatography steps on a pilot plant. Each plasma fraction was subsequently spiked with the chosen virus. The fractionation stage requiring validation was then carried out in the laboratory under scale down conditions as similar as possible to actual production. The various products obtained at each step of fractionation were analyzed to assess virus removal (or infectivity) during processing. The sum of the removal/inactivation factors (in $\log_{10}$) of the fractionation procedure was made for each virus tested. This methodology was that adopted in 1986 by the Food and Drug Administration (FDA) for validating HIV-1 inactivation during plasma immunoglobulin production using the Cohn's method.

Simultaneously each chromatographic step was supplemented by : 1. a spontaneous inactivation control made up of the preparation (original product + added virus at room temperature) was maintained at the same temperature. In order to assess the source product's intrinsic inactivating capacity, the spontaneous inactivation control was assayed in parallel with the product that had undergone chromatography ; 2. an extra cycle using a product free from viral contamination was carried out after the chromatography columns had been regenerated, in order to assess possible persistance of the virus or virus markers on the chromatographic support (steps B', C' and D'). The detailed procedure for step A is given in Fig. 1 and steps B and B' in Fig. 2. The procedures for steps C and C', D and D' were the same as for steps B and B' respectively.

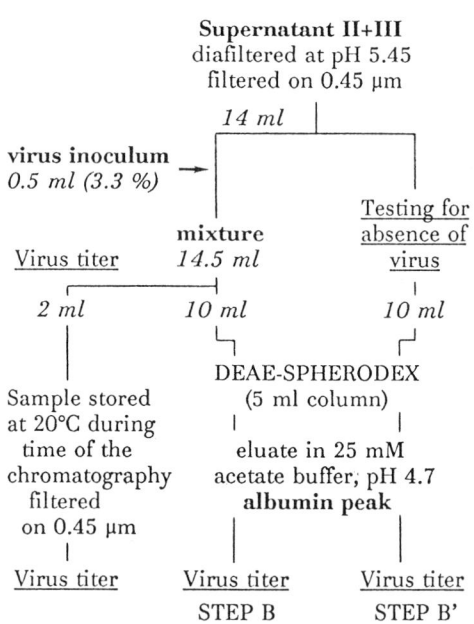

Fig. 1 : *Summary of the experimental procedure for step A (ethanol precipitation)*

Fig. 2 : *Experimental procedure for the validation of step B (and B') [for explanation see text]*

Assessing viral activities

a) HBV : As there is no *in vitro* system for measuring the infectivity of HBV, the virus was detected by biochemical markers. Three major HBV markers were used during this investigation :

* HBs antigen assay was carried out by radioimmunoassay (Abott's Ausria II kit) ;

* DNA polymerase activity was assessed by the difference between incorporating ^{3}H-thymidine with and without phosphonoformic acid (DNA polymerase of hepadnaviruses, contrary to bacterial and cellular DNA polymerase is inhibited by phosphonoformic acid) ;
* HBV-DNA assay was carried out either by molecular hybridization over a filter with a specific ^{32}P-labelled HBV-DNA probe, or by liquid phase molecular hybridization (Abott's Genostic'II kit).

b) Poliovirus : The infectivity of poliovirus was measured by studying the cytopathogenic effect of the virus on Hep II cells after 7 days culture on microplates.

c) HIV : HIV-1 infectivity was assessed by measuring the cytopathogenic effect of the CEM-ss cells cultured on microplates for 14 days. Work was carried out on locating another marker for HIV-1 : protein p24 which is a constituent of the "core" of HIV, and was assayed by an ELISA test (Dupont). With this protein the virus can be detected in fractions, even after it has lost infectivity.

RESULTS

Viral inactivation during a manufacturing cycle

The detailed results of HBV markers assays at each step of the albumin purification procedure are given in Table 1. Step A (ethanol precipitation) revealed high HBV solubility in alcohol. None of the precipitation or chromatography steps was capable of removing the markers completely. However, the presence of HBV markers in the final product does not imply infectivity of the end product. DNA polymerase was the most affected of the three markers, particularly during the last three steps (QMA, COOH and heating). It is the only marker that constitutes a functional test for HBV. The procedure's overall capacity for removing HBV infectivity was expressed as a reduction factor of 4.4 $\log_{10}$.

Table 1 : *HBV markers assays in each step of albumin purification process*

Step	Sample	HBs Ag (%)	DNA polymerase (%)	HBV DNA (%) hybridation on filter	HBV DNA (%) kit GENOSTIC
Step A ethanol precipitation	cryosupernatant + virus (t=0) SUPERNATANT precipitate	100 91.8 8.1	100 61.6 4.5	100 90 0.6	100 98 2
Step B DEAE-Spherodex chromatography	supernatant II+III + virus (t=0) control FRACTION D 1 M NaCl peak	100 97.7 78.4 24.0	100 67.2 38.7 7.3	100 50 48 46	100 45 42 27.5
Step C QMA-Spherosil chromatography	fraction D + virus (t=0) control FRACTION Q 1 M NaCl peak	100 100 71.6 10	100 56.6 5.7 1.1	100 100 40 10	100 100 27 7
Step D COOH-Spherodex chromatography	fraction Q control FRACTION C 1 M NaCl peak	100 100 34.3 45.7	100 88.9 8.6 63.9	100 50 38 80	100 100 26 64
Step E heating	albumin 4 % (t=0) 60°C, 1 h 60°C, 10 h	100 92 91	100 32.8 3.2	100 100 50	100 100 33.6
All steps		16	0.004	3	1
Elimination level ($\log_{10}$)		0.8	4.4	1.5	2.0

Table 2 summarizes the results for poliovirus inactivation during the fractionation procedure. The first four steps had little effect on inactivating the poliovirus. The results confirm the high resistance of this virus to alcohol, acidic pH and low ionic strengths. In contrast, heating is a very efficient barrier for poliovirus : after just one hour at 60°C the virus was no longer detectable. The results are summarized in Table 3. Results obtained with HIV-1 are given in Table 4. Four out of five steps were particularly effective for inactivating HIV-1, giving the whole procedure a very high safety level and an inactivating capacity of over 14 $\log_{10}$.

Table 2 : *Detection of poliovirus in each step during the purification process*

Step	initial mixture (theoretical)	time 0 titer	albumin containing fraction	static control	inactivation vs time 0
A	7.80	7.75	6.90		0.85
B	7.14	6.65	4.85	5.15	1.80
C	7.33	6.90	6.30	6.70	0.60
D	7.33	7.05	6.00	7.05	1.05
E 60°C, 1 h / 60°C, 10 h	7.80	8.55	<2.80*		>5.70
Total inactivation					>10

Virus titers were expressed as infectious doses/ml in $\log_{10}$
* undetectable virus

Table 3 : *Inactivation of three type of poliovirus during the pasteurisation step (E)*

	type I Mahoney	type II Mef I	Type III Saukett
Initial mixture	7.85	8.50	6.95
time 0	8.05	8.30	6.80
titer after 1 h at 60°C	2.75	2.60	<1.0*
titer after 10 h at 60°C	<1.0*	<1.0*	<1.0*

Virus titers were expressed as infectious doses/ml in $\log_{10}$
* undetectable virus, even after amplification test during 3 weeks on VERO cells.

Table 4 : *Detection of HIV-1 at each step during the albumin purification process*

Step	initial mixture (theoretical)	time 0 titer	albumin fraction	other fractions	static control	inactivation vs initial mixture*
A	4.40	4.6	<1.5	precipitate : <1.5		>2.9
B	4.80	3.5	<1.5	NaCl peak : 2.7	3.1	>3.3
C	4.95	3.1	<1.5	NaCl peak : <1.5	2.3	>3.45
D	4.95	3.7	3.8	NaCl peak : 2.6	>4.3	>1.15
E	5.25	4.8	<1.6			>3.65
					Total inactivation	>14.45

Virus titers were expressed as infectious doses/ml in $\log_{10}$
*Because the unstability of HIV-1 virus, inactivation levels were expressed as the difference between virus titers in initial mixture and in albumin containing fraction, respectively.

<u>Possible persistance of the viruses on the chromatographic columns following regeneration</u>

After elution of the albumin-containing fraction, each of the three ion exchangers was washed with the following successive solutions : 1 M NaCl, 0.1 M HCl and 60 % ethanol/0.5 M acetic acid. Additional cycles (steps B', C' and D') carried out on products that had not been spiked with viruses showed no residual viral infectivity for HIV-1 and poliovirus. Only small amounts of HBV-DNA still eluted in the albumin fraction of these blank cycles (without any HBs Ag or DNA-polymerase).

DISCUSSION - CONCLUSIONS

This study of virus removal and/or inactivation during a chromatographic purification procedure for plasma albumin was carried out with three model viruses. Hepatitis B virus (HBV) and acquired human immunodeficiency virus (HIV) were chosen because they are particularly associated with human blood. The poliomyelitis virus was chosen as a model because it is known for its high resistance to chemical denaturation.

These three viruses have very different structures. HIV is a RNA virus with a lipid envelope belonging to the retrovirus family. It is a relatively fragile virus and given the gravity and absence of any treatment for the diseases associated with this virus, an assurance of total inactivation is an absolute necessity. Four of the five fractionation steps have a very high capacity for inactivating HIV, and the procedure has an overall inactivating capacity of >14 $\log_{10}$. There is therefore no risk of HIV transmission in albumin produced under these conditions, since contamination of human blood does not exceed 2 $\log_{10}$ (Bossel, 1986). Moreover, it has been shown (Grandgeorge et Pelloquin, 1989) that heating of 20 % albumin totally inactivates HIV-1. Poliovirus is a non-enveloped RNA virus. It is extremely resistant to chemical denaturation. However, the overall inactivation capacity for the procedure was shown to be over 10 $\log_{10}$. The heat treatment is a very effective barrier. Heat treatment apparently causes denaturation of the capside proteins followed by RNA release (Breindl, 1971; Schaffer et Schwerdt, 1959). Some type I and II mutant viruses have been reported as being more resistant to heat denaturation (Fennell and Phillips, 1974; Medearis et al., 1960). One of the mutant viruses has even been described to resist during 1 hour at 75°C. However, no example of mutant poliovirus resistant to 10 hours at 60°C was described so far. HBV is an enveloped DNA virus which is particularly resistant to alcohol fractionation procedures. The traditional Cohn's method is not very effective for removing HBV. 21 % of the albumin batches produced with this method in the USA between 1957 and 1975 contained detectable amounts of HBs Ag (Hoofnagle et al., 1976). Moreover, in a study on the Cohn's method, Schroeder and Mozen (1970) carried out fractionation on HBV-contaminated plasma and the results of two experiments gave a residual load of 0 and 5 % of initial HBs Ag in the final albumin (fraction V). Trepo et al. (1980) in a similar experiment detected a residual level of 0.2 %. The overall reduction factor for HBs Ag obtained in the present study is somewhat lower than in the above mentioned studies, but the method adopted here was more severe, and involved a massive virus load at each step of the procedure. HBV lowering during the procedure is based on the succession of stages capable of reducing the virus load and on the heat treatment. The overall reduction figures were 0.8 $\log_{10}$ for HBs Ag, 1.5 to 2.0 $\log_{10}$ for HBV-DNA and 4.4 $\log_{10}$ for DNA polymerase activity. Final heat treatment for 10 hours at 60°C is known to reduce the infectivity of HBV-rich diluted serum in the chimpanzee by a factor of 4 $\log_{10}$ (Shikata et al., 1978). Heat treatment is necessary to remove infectivity in albumin produced by the tradional Cohn ethanol fractionation technique when starting from HBV-contaminated plasma (Hoofnagle et al., 1976; Gellis et al., 1948; Murray et al., 1953; Gerety and Aronson, 1982). For HBV, viral safety of the albumin produced by the present process depends primarily, as for the traditional Cohn's method, on the final pasteurization.

In conclusion, it can be consider that the viral safety of plasmatic albumin produced by means of this chromatographic Spherodex-Spherosil procedure should be similar to that of conventional pasteurized Cohn's plasmatic albumin.

REFERENCES

Bossel, J. (1986): Safety of therapeutic immune globulin preparations with respect to transmission of human T-lymphotropic virus type III lymphadenopathy associated virus infection. *Morbid Mortal Weekly Report* 35, 231-233.
Breindl, M. (1971): The structure of heated poliovirus particles. *J. Gen. Virol.* 11, 147-156.
Caliguiri, A., McSharry, J.J., Lawrence, G.W. (1980): Effect of arildone on modifications of poliovirus in vitro. *Virology* 105, 86-93.
CEC : Validation of virus removal and inactivation procedures (1991): *Notes Ad hoc working party on Biotechnology/Pharmacie.*

Cohn, E.J., Strong, L.E., Hugues, W.L., Mulfor, D.J., Ashworth, J.J., Melin, M., Trylor, H.L. (1946): Preparation and properties of serum and plasma proteins IV : a system for the preparation into fractions of protein and lipoprotein components of biological tissues and fluids. *J. Amer. Chem. Soc.* 68, 459-476.

Fennell, R., Phillips, B.A. (1974): Polypeptide composition of urea and heat-resistant mutants of poliovirus types 1 and 2. *J. of Virology* 14, 821-833.

Gellis, S., Neefe, J., Stokes, J., Strong, L., Janeway, C., Scatchard, G. (1948): Chemical, clinical and immunological studies on the products of human plasma fractionation XXXVI. *J. Clin. Invest.* 27, 239-244.

Gerety, R.J., Aronson, D.L. (1982): Plasma derivatives and viral hepatitis. *Transfusion* 22, 347-351.

Grandgeorge, M., Pelloquin, F. (1989): Inactivation of the human immunodeficiency viruses (HIV-1 and HIV-2) during the manufacturing of placental albumin and gammaglobulins. *Transfusion* 29, 629-634.

Hoofnagle, J.H., Barker, L.F., Thiel, J., Gerety, R.J. (1976): Hepatitis B virus and hepatitis B surface antigen in human albumin products. *Transfusion* 16, 141-147.

Hoofnagle, J.H., Gerety, R.J., Thiel, J., Barker, L.F.(1976): The prevalence of hepatitis B surface antigen in commercialy prepared plasma products. *J. Lab. Clin. Med.* 88, 102-113.

Medearis, D. Arnold, J., Enders, J. (1960): Survival of poliovirus at elevated temperatures (60°-75°C). *Proc. Soc. Exp. Biol.* 104, 419-423.

Murray, R., Diefenbach, W. (1953): Effect of heat on the agent of homologous serum hepatitis. *Proc Soc. Exp. Biol. Med.* 84, 230.

Schaffer, F.L., Schwerdt, C.R. (1959): Purification and properties of poliovirus. *Advances in Virus Research* 6, 159-199.

Schroeder, D.D., Mozen, M.M. (1970): Australia antigen : distribution during Cohn ethanol fractionation of human plasma. *Science* 168, 1462-1464.

Shikata, T., Karasawa, T., Abe, K., Takahashi, T., Mayumi, M., Oda, T. (1978): Incomplete inactivation of hepatitis B virus after heat treatment at 60°C for 10 days. *The Journal of Infectious Diseases* 138, 242-244.

Stoltz, J.F., Rivat, C., Geschier, C., Colosetti, P., Sertillanges, P., Tondon, J., Regnault, V. (1987): Purification chromatographique de l'albumine humaine à l'échelle pilote. *Biosciences* 6, 103-106.

Stoltz, J.F., Rivat, C., Geschier, C., Colosetti, P., Dumont, L. (1991): Chromatographic purification of human albumin for clinical uses. *Pharm. Tech. Int.* 3, 60-65.

Tayot, J.L., Grandgeorge, M., Blanc, P., Gattel, P., Tardy, M., Paturel, J., Pla, J., Debrus, A., Liautaud, J., Plan, R., Peyron, L. (1981): Chromatographie industrielle, production et qualité de l'albumine humaine d'origine placentaire. In *Coopération internationale et dérivés sanguins*, pp. 47-58. Fondation Marcel Mérieux, Talloires, France.

Trepo, C. Hantz, O., Jacquier, M.F., Nemoz, G., Cappel, R., Trepo, D. (1978): Different fates of hepatitis B virus markers during plasma fractionation. *Vox Sang.* 35, 143-148.

Vicary, G. (1990): Point to consider in the validation of purification procedures for removing and for inactivating viruses in biologicals. In *L'Europe du Médicament : Réalités et ambitions*, 4ème colloque DPh. M/INSERM, vol. 213, pp. 159-161. Paris, Editions INSERM.

Résumé

La quasi totalité des préparations d'albumine plasmatique humaine à usage thérapeutique sont actuellement préparées par précipitation à froid en présence d'alcool. Cependant, des supports chromatographiques ont été récemment proposés. Le but de ce travail était d'évaluer les capacités d'atténuation virale d'une chaîne chromatographique capable de traiter 350 à 400 l par cycle avec des supports à base de silice (Sphérodex-Sphérosil). Trois virus ont été testés dans cette étude : virus de l'hépatite B (HBV), virus de la poliomyélite et virus de l'immunodéficience humain (HIV). Les études ont été réalisées selon les recommandations de la CEE et de la FDA. Les résultats montrent une réduction de : 4,4 $\log_{10}$ pour l'HBV, de plus de 10 $\log_{10}$ pour le virus de la polio et 14 $\log_{10}$ pour le virus HIV. Par ailleurs, aucune infectivité résiduelle n'a été constatée après régénération et lavage des supports. Cette étude montre que la sécurité virale de l'albumine purifiée par ce procédé est au moins identique à celle obtenue par la méthode de Cohn.

V. Recombinant proteins

V. Protéines recombinantes

Comparison between proteins from plasma fractionation and recombinant proteins

C.V. Prowse

National Science Laboratory, Scottish National Blood Transfusion Service, Royal Infirmary, Edinburgh, EH3 9HB, United Kingdom

The potential impact of recombinant technology on the plasma fractionation industry may be initially considered by assessing for which products there is likely to be competition between plasma derived and recombinant products:

a. <u>Plasma products on which recombinant technology is unlikely to impinge</u>

   eg   normal immunoglobulin, coagulation factor IX

b. <u>Plasma products for which competition may arise from recombinant sources:</u>

   eg   coagulation factor VIII

c. <u>Recombinant products on which plasma-derived products are unlikely to impinge:</u>

   eg   Colony stimulating factors, plasminogen activator

In making a comparison of plasma-derived and recombinant therapeutic proteins (within the second category), one should first ask whether the biotechnologist is trying to copy nature. Assuming this is to be the case one may then ask various questions, relating to identity, purity, safety, supply and cost.

1. Identity

    There have been problems in this area, where biotechnology can only ever hope to match nature. Examples include the presence of additional amino acid residues in some growth hormone preparations, the inability of some monoclonal anti-Rhesus D antibodies to clear red cells, the rapid clearance of underglycosylated recombinant antitrypsin prepared from yeast and the problems associated with renaturation of recombinant proteins prepared in E coli. However none of these are insurmountable and it is certainly feasible to produce recombinant proteins indistinguishable from native products, although in some situations it may be necessary to make use of more costly mammalian cell culture. Two examples apparently showing the feasibility of copying nature are given by tissue plasminogen activator and coagulation factor VIII.

    Table 1. Two examples of failure to achieve identity with recombinant products

    a. Clearance of rhesus D red blood cells by human monoclonal antibodies (Thompson A et al, 1990).

Antibody	Percent cell survival at 3 hours
BRAD-3 (IgG3)	<10
FOG-1 (IgG1)	50

    b. Half life of human antitrypsin in mice (Mast A et al, 1990).

Plasma derived	150 min
Yeast recombinant (aglyosyl)	12 min

2. Purity

    As both plasma and recombinant proteins are initially obtained in solutions containing other products both require concentration (increased potency) and purification (increased specific activity) by downstream processing. For recombinant products it is usually necessary to achieve an essential pure product whereas, while possibly desirable, this is not the case for most plasma-derived products since any contaminating proteins are of human origin. Modern separation technology allows preparation of pure products, for instance coagulation factor IX, from either source, but this is achieved at a price. Plasma-derived products would therefore appear to be at an advantage.

Table 2. Purity required to achieve < 10ug extraneous protein for different product doses

Dose	Purity
10g (eg albumin)	99.999%
1 mg (eg factor VIII)	99%

However concerns over the effects of chronic infusion of extraneous protein on the immune system have been raised, for example, for coagulation factor VIII usage in haemophilia. Trials assessing the impact of different purity products have been largely inconclusive to date in this group, although there is preliminary evidence that less pure factor VIII products may result in a lower rate of induction of inhibitors in severely affected haemophilia patients (Prowse 1992b):

Table 3. Effect of type of factor VIII product on T-helper cell decline in human immunodeficiency virus seropositive haemophilia patients

Product	Type	CD4 cell decline/ul/year
Monoclate	Very High Purity	- 14 to - 100
Hemofil M	Very High Purity	- 5 to - 61
Kogenate	Recombinant	- 39
Various	Intermediate Purity	- 35 to - 98

Table 4. Prevalence of factor VIII inhibitors in patients treated exclusively with selected products

Product	Type	Approx inhibitor prevalence (%) *
Monoclate	Very High Purity	16%
Hemofil M	Very High Purity	9%
Kogenate	Recombinant'	28%
Recombinate	Recombinant	25%
8Y	Intermediate Purity	0%

```
NYBC-VIII-SD      Intermediate Purity     6%
Kryobulin-TIM3    Intermediate Purity     0%
```

(* in severely-affected, previously untreated patients)

The effects of extraneous protein may possibly become more obvious in ongoing trials with recombinant haemoglobin.

3. **Safety**

The main clinical concern here, in the wake or AIDS, is over possible viral infections. While both plasma and recombinant feedstocks may be potentially contaminated with pathogenic viruses, this should in theory be easier to control for recombinant products.

Table 5. Examples of pathogenic viruses of concern

From plasma sources	From rodent recombinant sources
Hepatitis A	Hantaan virus
Hepatitis B	Lymphocytic choriomeningitis virus
Hepatitis C	Rat rotavirus
Human immunodeficiency virus (HIV)	Reovirus type 3
Human B19 parvovirus	Sendai virus

In addition regulatory requirements call for inclusion of virus inactivation procedures during the isolation of proteins from either source. Existing viral inactivation procedures are able to deal with the lipid-enveloped pathogenic virus, but non-enveloped viruses remain an area of concern.

Table 6. Efficacy of existing viral inactivation methods for selected viruses

Virus	Inactivation Technique			
	Pasteurisation	Solvent Detergent	Severe Dry Heat	Steam Heat
Hepatitis A *	?	−	?	?
Hepatitis B	+	+	+	+
Hepatitis C	+	+	+	+
HIV	++	++	++	++
B19 parvovirus	±	−	±	?

(* not lipid-enveloped)

4. Supply

The supply of plasma-derived products is limited by the available supply of (human) plasma, now preferably from voluntary non-renumerated donors. For products such as factor IX and albumin this should not be a problem, except in poorer countries who are in any case unlikely to be able to afford the recombinant products. For other products, antitrypsin, growth factors and plasminogen activator being examples, estimated demands cannot be (fully) met from plasma sources. Biotechnology holds out the promise of fulfilling demand, providing the cost is appropriate, for such products. Development of methods that increase product availability, such as the expression of antitrypsin in the milk of transgenic sheep, improve the likelihood of success for biotechnology.

The market for factor VIII provides an interesting example in that demand for coagulation factor VIII is currently the determining factor in the volume of plasma required by the fractionation industry, plasma being the only source of licensed concentrates. Current use of this product around Europe varies between 0.4 and 5.6 iu per inhabitant, suggesting some patients are undertreated. Furthermore in many parts of the world the availability of factor VIII is minimal, while ongoing trials suggest that optimal therapy of haemophilia requires prophylaxis at doses higher than those used in Europe and America. Recombinant product, which is likely to be licensed soon, may provide a source to fulfil such demands, which are unlikely to be (completely) met by plasma sources.

5. Cost

The costs of developing and trialling recombinant products are large, one recent estimate being $50M for a single product. The risks involved in such investment are considerable, given the product may fail at any stage up to licensing, as has apparently happened recently with a human monoclonal antibody for the treatment of sepsis, particularly where an equivalent proven plasma-derived product exists. As the real costs of recombinant products are likely to be higher than plasma-derived ones, whether customers will pay an additional amount for recombinant products will largely depend on whether they result in improved supply or have a proven clinical advantage. The continued use of streptokinase in the face of recombinant plasminogen activator provides an interesting lesson, as this is a cheaper, albeit more immunogenic product, of similar efficacy to the recombinant alternative.

Comment

The replacement of plasma-derived by any recombinant equivalent will depend largely on comparative costs and their perceived benefit, if any, in terms of supply or efficacy.

Improving on Nature

Biotechnology offers the possibility of improving on nature. Apart from the whole field of gene therapy, there are examples such as B-domainless factor VIII and inhibitor resistant plasminogen activator which nature does not provide. Immunogenicity is a concern here, as is demonstrated by various analogs of factor VIII and leech antistatin.

Table 7. Examples of variant recombinant products

Product	Variant	Effect	Immunogenicity
t-plasminogen activator	a. Tyr 67, Phe 68, Ser 69	Increase half life	?
	b. Ala 296 to 299	Decreased inhibition	?
Factor VIII	a. deletion 796 to 1563	Increased synthesis	+
	b. deletion 743 to 1638	Increased synthesis	(-)
Leech antistatin		Factor Xa inhibitor	+

Finally it should be remembered that in the near future, recombinant technology may provide alternative approaches to simple protein concentrates for the therapy of selective protein deficiencies, prior to the promise of a lifetime cure implicit in gene therapy research. Animal cell lines capable of synthesising the proteins of interest have already been developed as part of the provision of therapeutic recombinant proteins, while methods of encapsulating such cells so as to minimise their immunogenic potential while still allowing release of proteins they synthesise, are under development. It is but a short step from this point to the trial use of encapsulated cell implants for therapy of deficiency states such as diabetes and haemophilia.

References and Further Reading

Brown, M.J. et al (1990): Deletion of a tripeptide sequence of a tissue plasminogen activator prolongs *in vivo* circulation. Thromb. Res. 59, 687-692.

Kunitada, S. et al (1992): Inhibition of clot lysis and decreased binding of tissue-type plasminogen activator as a consequence of clot retraction. Blood 79, 1420-1427.

Mast, A.E. et al (1990): Polyethylene glycol modification of serpins improves therapeutic potential. Biol. Chem. Hoppe-Seyler 371, 101-109.

Prowse, C.V. (1992a): Plasma and recombinant blood products in medical therapy. Publishers: Wiley.

Prowse, C.V. (1992b): The effect of type of factor VIII concentrate used in haemophilia on T-helper cell number and inhibitor incidence. Blood Coagulation and Fibrinolysis 3, 597-604.

Thompson, A. et al ((1990): Clearance of RhD positive red cells with monoclonal anti-D. Lancet 336, 1147-1150.

Recombinant glycoproteins: pitfalls and strategy

Jean Montreuil

Université des Sciences et Techniques de Lille, Laboratoire de Chimie Biologique, UMR n° 111 du CNRS, 59655 Villeneuve d'Ascq Cedex, France

SUMMARY

The knowledge of the role of glycoprotein glycans we have at the present time raises a formidable problem in the field of genetic engineering of human glycoproteins. In fact, prokaryotic cells express only the protein part of a glycoprotein, being devoid of the convenient glycosyltransferase systems. So, the only solution consists to insert the cloned DNA in the genome of eukaryotic cells so that they express a copy of the glycoprotein which is in conformity with the native one. However, the choice of the expression cells as well as the culture conditions deeply influence the glycan biosynthesis. This leads in many cases to a misglycosylation of recombinant proteins of which the consequences are dramatic : increase of hydrophobicity, decrease or inhibition of the secretion level, decrease of the stability towards heat or proteases, shortening of the biological lifetime by increase of the clearance, decrease of the affinity for specific receptors and increase of the antigenicity. The complexity of the metabolic pathways of glycans as well as the fact that the regulation mechanisms of glycan biosynthesis are not well known explain the difficulties and pitfalls encountered in the production of recombinant glycoproteins.

INTRODUCTION

For a long time, glycoconjugates which result from the covalent association of a carbohydrate called *glycan* with a protein or with a lipid, leading to the definition of glycoproteins and glycolipids, have been considered as biomolecules devoid of any biological intelligence. But, due to a series of discoveries and, in particular, due to the demonstration that glycans were recognition signals, glycoconjugates have acquired, in the past 20 years, their "lettres de noblesse". In addition, the production and clinical application of recombinant glycoproteins (rGP) for therapeutic administration in humans is an area of intensive scientific and medical effort. This explains why a growing number of biotechnology companies and of university scientists are focusing on sugars as the next class of molecules to be exploited in medicine. That's why A. Pollack could write in the Herald Tribune of 22nd of August 1990 an article entitled " A spoonful of sugars makes the dividends go up. Sugar : pharmaceutical companies discover the virtues of a spoonful" and in which he claimed : "People say that in five years will be more companies with "glyco" in their name than companies with "gene" in their name today".

The successful introduction in human therapy of recombinant products such as insulin, growth hormone and α-interferon led, during the last decade, many pharmaceutical companies to extend the production of recombinant proteins to numerous compounds like : tissue plasminogen activator (t-PA), erythropoietin (EPO), granulocyte macrophage colony - stimulating factor (GM-CSF), interleukin-2 (IL-2), β-interferon (β-IFN), γ-interferon (γ-IFN), α_1-antitrypsin, soluble CD-4, glucocerebrosidase, human chorionic gonadotropin, follicle stimulating hormone, factors VII, VIII, IX and XIII, antithrombin III, protein C. But, one element that has not been fully appreciated at the beginning is the omission that these proteins were glycosylated in their natural state. For having neglected the carbohydrate part of these compounds led to some errors of appreciation of the activity of recombinant glycoproteins due to the fact that the activity was measured *in vitro* using enzymatic or biological assays. This was a big mistake, as shown in Table I which clearly demonstrates that, if the desialylated erythropoietin remains active *in vitro*, it loses its activity *in vivo*. Only in recent years, the functional importance of the glycans for the *in vivo* efficiency of the recombinant glycoproteins became widely recognized and it is now clear that the glycosylation of recombinant proteins can affect their pharmacokinetics, biodistribution and antigenicity.

Table I - Relative activities of native and recombinant erythropoietin, before and after desialylation.

	Activity (in p. cent)	
	in vitro	in vivo
Native	107	100
Desialylated	99	0
From Psi-3 cells	140	25
Desialylated	240	0

GLYCOPROTEINS : STRUCTURE AND FUNCTIONS.

Glycoproteins result from the classical processes of translation of the genome message at the polysomal level, leading to a peptide chain to which carbohydrate moieties are linked in a second step through covalent bonds. The glycosylation is carried out by enzymes called *glycosyltransferases*, in the absence of any template.
Glycosylation of proteins represents one of the most important of the post-translational events because of the universality of the phenomenon. In fact, most proteins are glycosylated and, in addition, the glycoproteins are widely distributed in animals, plants, micoorganisms and viruses.

Structure of glycoprotein glycans

Glycan - protein linkage.
Glycans are conjugated to peptide chains through two types of primary linkages : N-glycosyl and O-glycosyl linkages leading to the definition of two classes of glycoproteins : *N-glycosylproteins* and *O-glycosylproteins*. Both types of linkages may co-exist in a given glycoprotein which is called *N,O-glycosylprotein*. Up to now, the only N-glycosidic bond characterized so far in glycoproteins is the N-acetylglucosaminyl-asparagine linkage : GlcNAc(β1-N)Asn. On the contrary, the O-glycosidic type offers a wide variety of linkages since all of the kinds of hydroxylated amino-acids may be implicated in the linkage. However, the most distributed ones in animals are *i)* the N-acetyl-α-galactosaminyl serine and threonine : GalNAc(α1-3)Ser/Thr, in the so-called glycans of the *mucin-type*; *ii)* the β-xylosyl serine : Xyl(β1-3)Ser, in the proteoglycans.

Glycan primary structure.
The concept of the common inner-core. The carbohydrate moiety of N- and O-glycosylproteins derives from the substitution of oligosaccharide structures common to all glycans of a given class of glycoproteins. These non-specific and invariant structures are conjugated to the peptide chain and

constitute the *inner-core*. The most common inner-cores characterized so far in glycans are described below : core A exists in the O-glycosylproteins of the mucin type, core B in proteoglycans and core C is common to all N-glycosylproteins :

          Gal(β1-3)GalNAc(α1-3)Ser or Thr   A

          Gal(β1-3)Gal(β1-4)Xyl(β1-3)Ser   B

Man(α1-3)
  \
    Man(β1-4)GlcNAc(β1-4)GlcNAc(β1-N)Asn   C
  /
Man(α1-6)

The concept of the antenna. The glycan structures derive from the substitution of the invariant inner-cores by a wide variety of oligosaccharidic structures which carry the specificity and bear the variable fraction of the glycans. On the basis of their morphology, their flexibility and their recognition signal property, the term *antennae* has been proposed for the outer arms substituting the inner-core.

Glycan structures. Some pictures of glycoprotein glycans are given in Fig. 1. Structure A is a typical example of a glycan of mucin-type O-glycosylproteins. Structures B and D are glycans of N-glycosylproteins. Structure B is called of the *oligomannosidic type* and is synthetized, in particular, by yeasts. Structures C to E are named of the *N-acetyllactosaminic type* because of the presence of a variable number of N-acetyllactosamine Gal(β1-4)GlcNAc residues substituting the pentasaccharidic inner-core, leading to the so-called bi-antennary (B,C), tri-antennary (E) and till hexa-antennary structures.

       NeuAc(α2-3)Gal(β1-3)
            \
             GalNAc(α1-3)Ser or Thr A
            /
       NeuAc(α2-6)

Man(α1-2)Man(α1-2)Man(α1-3)
          \
Man(α1-2)Man(α1-3) Man(β1-4)GlcNAc(β1-4)GlcNAc(β1-N)Asn B
      \   /
       Man(α1-6)
       /
Man(α1-2)Man(α1-6)

NeuAc(α2-3 or 6)Gal(β1-4)GlcNAc(β1-2)Man(α1-3)
                \
                 Man(β1-4)GlcNAc(β1-4)GlcNAc(β1-N)Asn C
                /
NeuAc(α2-3 or 6)Gal(β1-4)GlcNAc(β1-2)Man(α1-6)

```
NeuAc(α2-3 or 6)Gal(β1-4)GlcNAc(β1-2)Man(α1-3)
                                              \
                                               Man(β1-4)GlcNAc(β1-4)GlcNAc(β1-N)Asn    D
                                              /       | (α1-6)
         Gal(β1-4)GlcNAc(β1-2)Man(α1-6)                Fuc
              | (α1-3)
              Fuc


NeuAc(α2-3 or 6)Gal(β1-4)GlcNAc(β1-4)
                                    \
                                     Man(α1-3)
                                    /        \
NeuAc(α2-3 or 6)Gal(β1-4)GlcNAc(β1-2)          Man(β1-4)GlcNAc(β1-4)GlcNAc(β1-N)Asn    E
                                              /
NeuAc(α2-3 or 6)Gal(β1-4)GlcNAc(β1-2)Man(α1-6)
```

Fig. 1 - Classical structures of glycans of the mucin-type (A) and of the N-glycosylproteins of the oligomannosidic type (B) and of the N-acetyllactosaminic type (C to E). Gal : galactose, GlcNAc : N-acetylglucosamine, Man : mannose, Fuc : fucose, NeuAc : acide N-acetylneuraminic acid.

Some glycans carry both oligomannosidic and N-acetyllatosaminic structures : they are said of the *hybrid type*.

It is worth-while to note *i)* that the same peptide chain may carry together, in addition to O-linked glycans as above mentioned, glycans of the oligomannosidic, of the N-acetyllactosaminic and of the hybrid type; *ii)* that yeast and insect cells are able to synthetize glycans of the oligomannosidic type only, and that the higher animals are able to synthetize all types of glycoprotein glycans.

Spatial conformation of glycans.
The two most important concepts to keep in mind about the three-dimensional structure of glycans are the following : *i)* antennae are mobile in space and may adopt, in the case of a biantennary structure, the so-called Y-, T-, bird- and broken wing - conformations. This concept fits perfectly to the concept of glycans acting as recognition signals; *ii)* glycans cover an important surface of the protein, principally in the case of tri- and tetra-antennary structures which adopt the so-called *umbrella-conformation* which plays a protective role towards the peptide chain.

Biological role of glycans.

Little by little the role of glycoprotein glycans has been defined and, in many cases, we know now why proteins are glycosylated and that glycans :
- increase the solubility of proteins,
- induce and maintain the peptide chain in a biologically active three-dimensional conformation,
- protect the peptide chain against proteolytic attack,
- control the proteolysis of polyproteins,
- decrease the immunogenicity of proteins,
- are tissue antigen epitopes,
- control the lifetime of circulating glycoproteins and cells,
- are recognition signals for biomolecules and micro-organisms,
- intervene in the social life of cells : in cell recognition and adhesion and in cell contact inhibition,
- are markers of differentiation and of cancerisation.

Moreover, we know now that the glycan structure of cell membrane glycoconjugates is profoundly altered in cancer cells. This molecular transformation could be related to the appearance of surface neo-antigens and could be a factor of metastatic diffusion.

RECOMBINANT GLYCOPROTEINS : THE PROBLEMS.

At the moment, the glycosylation of recombinant proteins remains a formidable problem because *i)* of the diversity of glycan structures, glycans being markers of Evolution; *ii)* of the complexity of the biosynthetic pathway, particularly that of the N-glycosylation; *iii)* of the tremendous and still unexplained microheterogenicity of the glycans of a given glycoprotein : for example, in ovomucoid which possesses only one potential glycosylation site, more than 30 different glycan structures have been characterized. On the front of such a complexity of the biosynthesis pathways, the following question arises : "How are so complicated mechanisms controlled ?". Answer is brief and clear :" We don't known !". We don't known how is controlled the gene expression of the enzymes implicated in glycan biosynthesis, nor the enzyme activity : phospho- dephospho systems, adenylribosylation, inositol triphosphate regulation, nor the cell compartmentation of events.

Concerning the recombinant glycoproteins, it is evident that the glycosylation of proteins can be realized only by using cells able to synthetize the right glycan to the right place in the peptide chain. This eliminates *a priori* the use of prokaryotic cells which are devoid of the biosynthesis equipment. But, what kind of eukaryotic cells to choose ?

On the basis of some examples, we shall try to demonstrate how difficult is the problem posed by the necessity to produce recombinant glycoproteins of which the glycans conform with those of the native compound. In fact, glycosylation of recombinant proteins depends on a series of factors which are, at the moment, defined on purely empirical bases.

Factors affecting the glycosylation

Glycosylation depends on the nature of the cell used for the production and of its enzymatic equipment. In Table II are described the performances of some animal cells used for producing recombinant glycoproteins.

Table II - Structural features of N-linked glycans from recombinant glycoproteins

	Type of cells			
	CHO	BHK-21	C-127	Ltk-
α-1,6-Fuc	+	+	+	+
α-2,6-NeuAc	-	-	+	+
α-2,3-NeuAc	+	+	+	+
Tri/tetra-antennary	+	+	+	+
Lactosamine repeats	+	+	+	+
Gal(α1-3)Gal	-	-	+	+
Bisecting GlcNAc	-	-	+	+

In this regard, the examples of antithrombin III is demonstrative. In fact, native anti-thrombin III extracted from human serum contains N-acetylneuraminic acid predominantly α-2,6-linked to the terminal galactose residues and lacks fucose at the proximal N-acetylglucosamine residue, but contains fucose α-1,3-linked to the peripheral N-acetylglucosamine residues. The recombinant glycoprotein produced by CHO or BHK cells contains all of the N-acetylneuraminic acid residues in α-2,3-linkage. In addition, glycans are almost completely fucosylated and contain a higher amount of triantennary structures.

Glycan structure depends on the physiological state of the cell.
Glycan structure depends on the induction protocol used to stimulate cells and on the differentiation and physiological state of the cells. For example, γ-IFN contains two potential N-glycosylation sites at Asn-25 and Asn-97. When secreted from primary T-lymphocytes, *i)* Asn-25 linked glycans bear biantennary structure monosialylated and α-2,3-monofucosylated on the peripheral N-acetylglucosamine residues; *ii)* Asn-97 linked glycans bear non-fucosylated and sialylated biantennary structure. When secreted from proliferating T-lymphocytes, *i)* Asn-25 linked glycans are persialylated and fucosylated in α-1,6-position of the proximal N-acetylglucosamine residue; *ii)* Asn-97 linked glycans are 50 p. cent of the N-acetyllactosaminic type and 50 p. cent of the oligomannosidic type.

Glycosylation depends on the cell growth conditions.
The following cell culture conditions influence the glycosylation of proteins :
- Cells attached to a solid substrate or cells in suspension
- Chemical nature of the solid support
- Cell culture in roller bottles or in suspension
- Cell density
- Components of the media : growth and differentiation factors, glucose level, dissolved oxygen and CO_2
- Temperature
- Length of the culture
- Lengthened keeping of cells in liquid nitrogen.

For example, rt-PA from CHO cells cultured in roller tubes has less extensive sialylation than material produced by suspension culture. It has also been reported that scaling up from pilot scale to manufacturing scale altered the biological properties of rt-PA which is cleared more rapidly. In some cases, modification of culture conditions of CHO cells resulted in activation of fucosyltransferases leading to the onco-foetal antigen sialyl Le^x, NeuAc(α2-3)Gal(β1-4)[Fuc(α1-3)]GlcNAc on the N-linked glycans of recombinant glycoproteins which were not fucosylated when cultivated in a different culture medium. In our laboratory, G. Spik has observed that HepG2 cells which originally synthetize serotransferrin with biantennary glycans, synthetize tetraantennary glycans after keeping for 3 years in liquid nitrogen.

Consequences of the misglycosylation of recombinant glycoproteins.

What happens when the protein is not or unsatisfactory glycosylated ? To answer the question, the most common methods for examining the role of glycans and the effects of the non-glycosylation are to produce the protein :
1 - in prokaryotic cells which are devoid of the glycosylation machinery,
2 - in eucaryotic cells *i)* in the presence of the N-glycosylation inhibitor tunicamycin or of the O-glycosylation inhibitor α-benzyl-N-acetylgalactosaminide, *ii)* in a cell line defective in O-glycosylation, *iii)* in carrying out site-directed mutagenesis experiments on particular glycosylation sites, *iv)* by using cells of different origins since glycosylation capability is species and tissue specific, *v)* by using different clones of the same cell line which may differ in their glycosylation characteristics.
Application of this strategy led to the establishment of some relationships between structure and properties of recombinant glycoproteins. In this regard, it has been observed that glycosylation has the potential to affect the level of expression, the physico-chemical, pharmacokinetics and immunological properties, the biological activity, the clinical efficacy and the stability of recombinant glycoproteins.

1 - Effect on solubility. As a general rule, due to the hydrophobic OH groups of monosaccharides and to the ionisable carboxyl groups of sialic acids, glycans enhance the solubility of proteins. Consequently, a decreased glycosylation or sialylation could affect the solubility of a glycoprotein, the negative consequence of which leads to low recoveries during isolation and purification and to increased formation of aggregates.

2 - *Effect on the stability of the protein moiety.* Glycans intervene in the folding and in the maintenance of peptide chain in a biologically active conformation. In this regard, a classical example concerns the IgG which lose their capacity to bind the Fc receptor after modification of their glycans which interact and reinforce the association between the two halves of the molecule.

3 - *Effect on the resistance to proteolytic attack.* Due to a shield effect, glycans protect the peptide chain against proteolytic enzymes and the most common example is that of the mucins which lose their resistance to proteases after desialylation. So, misglycosylation and, in particular, missialylation could decrease the resistance of recombinant proteins to proteolysis.

4 - *Effect on the control of proteases of maturation.* Glycans control the maturation of peptide chains by specific proteases as it has been demonstrated about an inactive polyprotein from the hypophysis of the batracian *Xenopus*. Proteolysis of the glycosylated peptide chain leads to pituitary hormones like ACTH, MSH, endorphin. On the contrary, the proteolytic attack has random effect on the non-glycosylated polyprotein produced in presence of tunicamycin and leads to the formation of physiologically inactive peptides. Consequently, the processing of the peptide chain leading to the active forms of t-PA, β– and γ-IFN and EPO could be perturbed in case of misglycosylation leading to less active or inactive derivatives.

5 - *Effect on glycoprotein antigenicity.* Glycans influence the antigenicity of glycoproteins by two ways :
i) - Glycoproteins are oft weakly antigenic but removal or modification, by desialylation for example, of glycans enhances their antigenicity. For instance, α_1-acid glycoprotein is weakly antigenic but, after removing the sialic acid residues, it becomes strongly antigenic. In the same way, a misglycosylated or a missialylated glycoprotein could be antigenic as it has been observed in the case of yeast derived GM-CSF and of CHO cell derived β-IFN.
ii) - The second mechanism is linked to the antigenicity of glycans themselves *i)* if the glycan induces the production of antibodies which could alter the safety in the case of a strong allergic response and the efficiency of the recombinant glycoprotein if neutralising antibodies are produced , *ii)* if neutralising antibodies pre-exists in the plasma. For example, glycoproteins produced by C127 cells bear the structure Gal(α1-3)Gal at the non-reducing termini of glycans. Now, humans have natural circulating antibodies that recognize this epitope and which consequently neutralize the recombinant glycoprotein bearing this structure.

6 - *Effect on the secretion of glycoproteins.* Secretion of rGP carrying non-orthodox glycans may be affected by several mechanisms :
i) - Since the N-glycosylation is a co-translational phenomenon, glycans may be needed for correct protein folding. This is not the case for yeast-derived rGM-CSF.
ii) - Glycans oft intervene in the formation of protein oligomers, an event that may be required for further intracellular transport. In fact, it is well known that glycoprotein secretion is mediated by cellular components which have been recognized as a "cellular quality control system" which is located into the endoplasmic reticulum and which regulates the expression of proteins. Misglycosylated or misfolded proteins may promote their binding to a 78 kDa protein called "glucose regulatory protein " or GRP-78 which has been identified to the immunoglobulin binding protein or BIP which is a native component of the ER. In this regard, it has been observed that the secretion of poorly glycosylated recombinant factor VIII, rt-PA and von Willebrand factor is inhibited through association with BIP.
iii) - Poorly glycosylated proteins may be rapidly destroyed by intracellular proteases.

iv) - Decrease of the solubility of improperly glycosylated proteins may result in aggregation or precipitation inside the cell.

7 - Effect on the clearance of r-proteins. It is well established that glycans may affect *in vivo* the biological activity of glycoproteins by controlling the clearance of circulating glycoproteins by two distinct glycan - dependent mechanisms : the first one is specific receptor mediated or membrane lectin - mediated, the second one is kidney - mediated.

<u>Receptor - mediated clearance.</u> Clearance depending on membrane lectins as been established in 1968 when Ashwell *et al.* demonstrated that enzymatic removal of terminal sialic acid residue signes the sentence of death of circulating glycoproteins. In fact, the asialoglycoprotein receptor of hepatocyte membrane rapidly binds and internalizes glycoproteins that have glycans terminated with galactose residues. This means that, if their glycans are not or not enough sialylated, recombinant glycoproteins will be removed from blood stream. In a similar manner, the active mannose and N-acetylglucosamine receptors of macrophages, particularly in the liver and spleen, recognize and clear glycoproteins with glycans terminated with N-acetylglucosamine or mannose residues.
Consequently, these specific receptors can affect the serum lifetime and the biodistribution of therapeutic glycoproteins. This is, for example, the case of recombinant glycoproteins expressed in yeast or insect cells only able to synthetize glycans of the oligomannosidic type and which are rapidly uptaken by macrophages or of missialylated EPO which requires a high sialic acid content to prevent premature clearance. In this regard, the lifetime of recombinant glycoproteins can be prolonged by desialylation followed by the oxidation of terminal galactose residues by galactose oxidase (attempts with EPO) or by substitution of the same residues by N-acetylneuraminic acid derivatives towards which neuraminidase is inactive, like 9-amino-N-acetylneuraminic acid residues transfered by sialyltransferases (attempts with antithrombin III).

<u>Kidney clearance</u>. Another common pathway for the clearance of serum glycoproteins is by filtration through the glomerular tubules of the kidney into urine. Proteins with a molecular weight less than 30 kDa are subject to elimination in this manner. The glycans, by increasing the molecular size of the protein, tend to reduce the clearance *via* this pathway and also by the negative charge density.
Non-glycosylated rGP such as a_1-antitrypsin, EPO and GM-CSF have been found to have significantly shorter circulatory half-lives when compared to their glycosylated counterparts. Likewise, a form of rEPO with biantennary glycans is cleared from circulation more rapidly than rEPO with tetra- antennary chains.

In conclusion, many factors must be taken into consideration when selecting an expression system for the large-scale production of a therapeutic protein. One consideration of importance is the glycosylation potential of the host-cell. Unfortunately; at the moment, it is impossible to predict the ideal glycosylation for a therapeutic protein. In addition, only a very limited number of recombinant glycoproteins have had their glycans characterized in detail. Thus, it is difficult to anticipate the exact structures of the oligosaccharides that will be attached by a cell line.
Nonetheless, a few general principles are becoming apparent for some of the more common expression systems, as well as other factors that may affect the nature of the glycosylation of a protein by a specific cell.
1 - *E. coli* lacks the biosynthetic machinery to carry out either N- or O-glycosylation. This deficiency has a negative impact on the physical and biological properties of a protein product :
- Abnormal folding of miscount polypeptide chain
- Increased hydrophobicity leading to greater difficulties is handling
- Increased antigenicity
2 - *Yeast* glycosylates Asn and Ser/Thr residues with oligomannosidic type glycans. Consequently, the glycans have a bad effect on the circulatory lifetime and biodistribution of the product. In fact, cells of

the reticulo-endothelial system will rapidly clear the glycoproteins *via* binding to the Man/GlcNAc receptor and internalisation. In addition, another potential problem that may be encountered with yeast-derived glycoproteins is the antigenicity of the mannan chains.

3 - **Insect** cells generally transfected by using baculovirus vectors lack the glycosyltransferases to synthesize N-acetyllactosamine type glycans. Highly processed glycan is converted to Man_3GN_2 which directs the protein to the reticulo-endothelial system.

4 - Many *mammalian cells* are capable of synthetizing the common classes of glycans depending on the cell line employed. The most widely employed mammalian cell line for expression of human recombinant proteins is CHO cell line. In fact, the glycosylation pattern of CHO cell - derived proteins appears to be compatible with therapeutic use in human. However, the most serious biosynthetic deficiency is the inability of CHO cells to synthetize α-2,6-linked neuraminic acid residues, but the α-2,3-linked sialic acid residues could be cleaved with neuraminidases and replaced *in vitro* by α-2,6-linked neuraminic acid residues using an α-2,6-sialyltransferase.

RECOMBINANT GLYCOPROTEINS : TO A CONSISTENT STRATEGY.

It is now evident that the control of glycoprotein glycan biosynthesis making the carbohydrate moieties of a given recombinant glycoprotein identical to those of the native one could be obtained on the three following conditions :

1 - Methods of isolation of the different glycoprotein glycoforms have to be improved. In fact, sooner or later the Drug Administrations and the Patent Offices will ask the following question : "In your mixture of glycoforms, which is the most or the only active one ?"

2 - Methods of glycan structure determination have to be miniaturized on the basis of the use of mass spectrometry and NMR analysis, because the native, as well as the recombinant glycoproteins, are generally obtained in few quantity and oft present an important microheterogeneity.

3 - The mechanisms of regulation and control of glycan biosynthesis must be defined in details. This is the only way to become able to sculpture and to chisel the recombinant glycoprotein glycans so that they will conform with the native ones on Cartesian bases and no longer on empirical bases laying on the following fundamental principle : " The more it fails, the more chances we have that it will succeed".

REFERENCE (REVIEWS)

Allen, H.J. & Kisailus, E.C. (1992) : *Glycoconjugates*. Ed. Marcel Dekker, New York.

Cumming, D.A. (1991) : Glycosylation of recombinant protein therapautics : control and functional implications. *Glycobiology* **1**, 115-130.

Enfors. S.O. (1992) : Control of in vivo proteolysis in the production of recombinant proteins. *Trends Biotechnol.* **10**, 310-315.

Goochee, C.F., Gramer, M.J., Andersen, D.C., Bahr, J.B. & Rasmussen, J.R. (1991) : The oligosaccharides of glycoproteins : bioprocess factors affecting oligosaccharide structure and their effect on glycoprotein properties. *Biotechnology* **9**, 1347-1355.

Liu, D.T.Y. (1992) : Glycoprotein pharmaceuticals : scientific and regulatory considerations and the US Orphan Drug Act. *Trends Biotechnol.* **10**, 114-120.

Montreuil, J. (1982) : Glycoproteins. In *Comprehensive Biochemistry*, ed. A. Neuberger & L.L.M. van Deenen, pp. 1-188. Amsterdam : Elsevier.

Montreuil, J. (1984) : Spatial structure of glycan chains of glycoproteins in relation to metabolism and function . Survey of a decade of research. *Pure Appl. Chem.* **56**, 859-877.

Montreuil, J. (1984) : Spatial conformation of glycans and glycoproteins. *Biol. Cell*, 115-132.

Nishi, T. & Itoh, S. (1992) : Qualitative improvement of therapeutic glycoproteins by glycotechnology. *Trends Glycosci. Glycotechnol.* **4**, 336-344.

Rademacher, T.W., Pareklh R.B. & Dwek, R.A. (1988) : Glycobiology. *Ann. Rev. Biochem.* **57**, 785-838.

Seamon, K. (1991) : Evaluation of recombinant glycoproteins. *Glycoconjug. J.* **8**, 3-5.
Stanley, P. (1992) : Glycosylation engineering. *Glycobiology* **2**, 99-107.
Vlak, J.M., Schlaeger, E.J. & Bernard, A.R. (1991) : Proceedings of the B*aculovirus* and recombinant protein production workshop, *Interlaken*, March 29 - April 1 1991. Ed. Roche, Basel.

Résumé

Le rôle que jouent les glycannes des glycoprotéines dans l'activité biologique de ces dernières posent de redoutables problèmes dans le domaine de la production des glycoprotéines recombinantes. En effet, les procaryotes ne possédant pas la machinerie enzymatique complexe de glycosylation des protéines, seules les cellules eucaryotiques sont capables d'exprimer des glycoprotéines recombinantes qui soient les copies conformes de leurs homologues naturelles. Le choix des cellules d'expression reste toutefois difficile car la structure des glycannes dépend étroitement du choix des cellules et des conditions de leur culture. Une glycosylation imparfaite peut avoir des conséquences néfastes : augmentation de l'hydrophobicité et baisse de la sécrétion, diminution de la stabilité vis-à-vis des protéinases, diminution du temps de vie des molécules circulantes par augmentation de la clearance, erreurs d'adressage et augmentation de l'antigénicité. La complexité de la biosynthèse des glycannes et l'ignorance dans laquelle nous sommes de sa régulation rend singulièrement complexe le problème de la conformité des glycannes des glycoprotéines recombinantes.

Purification and physicochemical properties of recombinant human serum albumin

A. Sumi, W. Ohtani, K. Kobayashi, T. Ohmura, K. Yokoyama, M. Nishida and T. Suyama

Central Research Laboratories, The Green Cross Co., 2-25-1, Shodai-Ohtani, Hirakata, Osaka 573, Japan

INTRODUCTION

Two major problems are expected to arise in the future in connection with plasma proteins. The first problem is the lack of source materials. The second problem is the transmission of viral diseases such as hepatitis, HIV or other unidentified viruses. Genetic engineering is the best approach to solve these problems. Plasma derived human serum albumin (pHSA) is one of the most useful plasma proteins. However, many difficulties are met in attempting to produce albumin commercially using genetic engineering. Two hurdles must be cleared in order to develop recombinant human serum albumin (rHSA). One is cost and the other is quality. As to cost, one gram of pHSA costs a few dollars. Our goal is to produce rHSA at least as economically as pHSA. To reduce the cost of rHSA, high productivity of albumin in culture and highly efficient, high-yield purification methods are necessary. As to quality, albumin is typically administered in multiples of ten grams. If purity of rHSA is 99.999 per cent (this level is sufficient for the other recombinant protein preparations), impurities of the order of one mg will be injected into the human body. So impurities from yeast must be reduced to a minimum. Furthermore, purified rHSA must be identical to natural plasma albumin. In this paper, we report on purification methods for rHSA from culture solution and the physicochemical properties of purified rHSA.

MATERIALS AND METHODS

Recombinant albumin

Recombinant albumin was secreted by yeast (Pichia pastoris). Culture of this yeast was performed using the fed-batch method with methanol as carbon source.

Purification of recombinant albumin

The purification method for recombinant albumin is shown in Fig. 1.

Assay of yeast components

To detect yeast impurities at a high level of sensitivity, an antibody against the yeast components was prepared. After culturing the non-albumin producing yeast, yeast components were partially purified from the culture supernatant. These yeast components were used to immunize rabbits. An EIA test was carried out using this antibody (*Ohtani et al.,* 1988). The detection limit of this EIA system was 1ng/ml.

Flow Chart of Purification

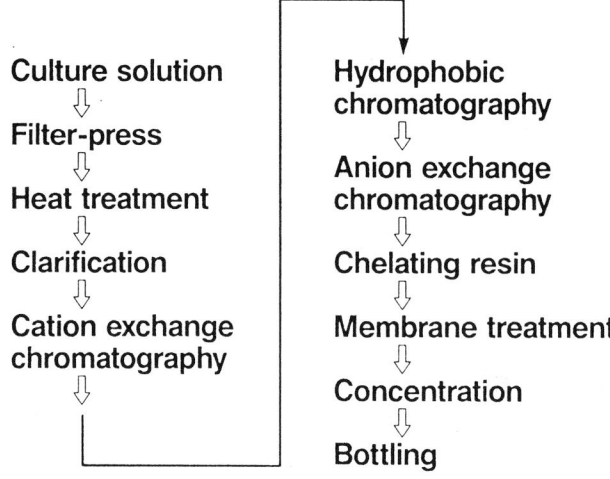

Fig. 1 Flow Chart of Purification Method

RESULTS

PURITY OF RECOMBINANT ALBUMIN

The purity of recombinant albumin purified by this method was almost 100 per cent as determined by SDS-PAGE, Immuno-blotting and HPLC gel permeation chromatography. Typical results of these analyses are shown in Fig. 2. The electrophoresis pattern of recombinant albumin was a single band. No contaminating bands were detected. Furthermore, the position of recombinant albumin was identical to that of plasma albumin. In HPLC analysis, the gel permeation elution profile of recombinant albumin was a single peak with no contaminating peaks, although a small peak containing dimer was observed. Elution profiles and retention times of recombinant albumin were consistent with those of plasma albumin.

To detect yeast impurities at a high level of sensitivity, the level of yeast components was measured by EIA. No yeast components were detected in purified recombinant albumin at a concentration of 250 mg/ml. As the detection limit of this EIA system was 1ng/ml, the purity of recombinant albumin was above 99.9999996 per cent. Contaminant DNA was assayed by the threshold method. With purified recombinant albumin, no DNA was detected in an extract of 2 ml of 25 per cent albumin. Since the detection limit of this system was 4 pg/2 ml of 25 per cent albumin, contaminant DNA was less than 100 pg/dose.

Analysis of r-HSA by Electrophoresis and Gel Permeation Chromatography

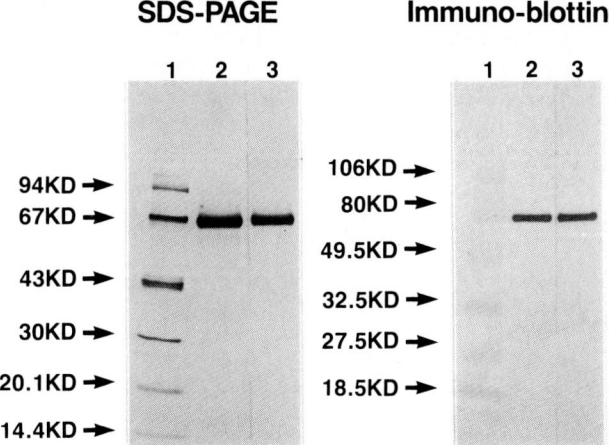

Lane 1: Molecular weight marker
Lane 2: plasma albumin
Lane 3: recombinant albumin

HPLC gel permeation chromatography

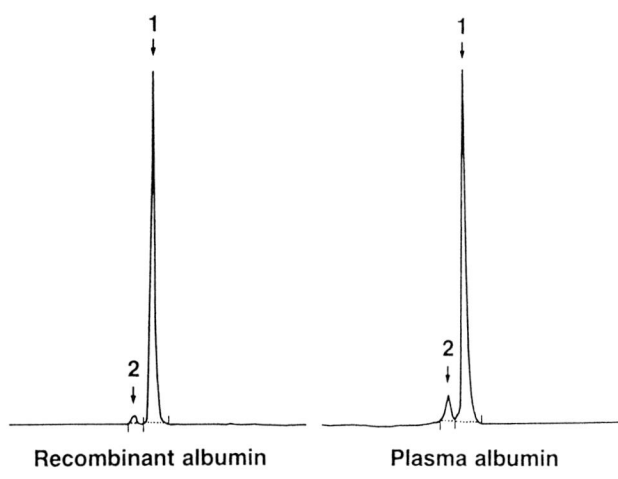

Peak 1: albumin monomer
Peak 2: albumin dimer

Fig. 2 Analysis of rHSA by Electrophoresis and Gel Permeation Chromatography

COMPOSITION AND STRUCTURE

To ascertain the composition and structure of recombinant albumin, the amino acid analysis was examined and the CD spectrum measured. The amino acid composition and N and C terminal sequence of recombinant albumin were identical to those of plasma albumin. These results were consistent with the values estimated from c-DNA. The peptide mapping pattern of recombinant albumin is shown in Fig. 3. Albumin was degradated by lysil-endopeptiase, then each peptide was separated by reverse-phase HPLC. As shown in Fig. 3, the elution profile of recombinant albumin was consistent with that of plasma albumin. To examine the higher structure of recombinant albumin, the CD spectrum of albumin was measured. As shown in Fig. 4, the CD spectrum of recombinant albumin was identical in shape and magnitude to that of plasma albumin in the region of 350 nm to 195 nm.

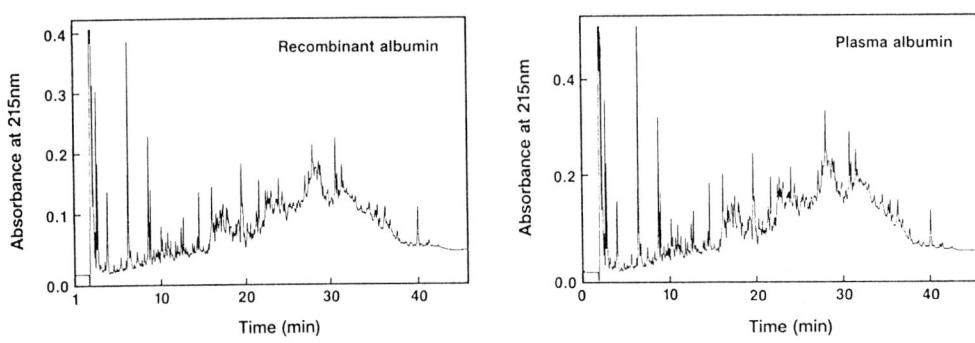

Fig. 3 Peptide Mapping Pattern of Albumin

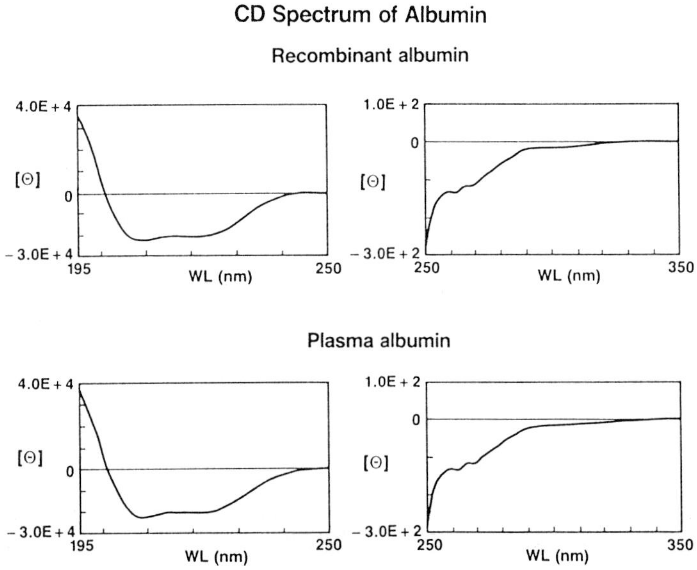

Fig. 4 CD Spectrum of Albumin

BIOLOGICAL CHARACTERIZATION

One of the most important biological functions of albumin is ligand binding. Albumin binds various materials. The binding ability of albumin to three typical materials was examined. Bilirubin was selected to represent pigment (*Nakamura & Lee*, 1977), Warfarin (*Sun et al.,* 1984) was used to represent drugs and lauric acid to represent fatty acids (*Ashbrook et al.,* 1975; *De Witt*, 1958). The binding of these three materials was analyzed by a Scatchard plot model. Binding constants and the number of binding sites of these three materials to recombinant albumin were consistent with those of plasma albumin. Binding curves of lauric acid to albumin are shown in Fig. 5 as an example.

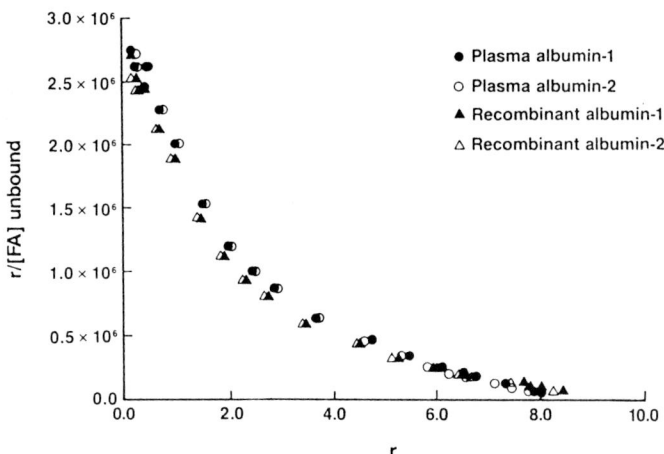

Fig. 5 Binding Curves of Lauric Acid to Albumin

PRE-CLINICAL STUDY

Preliminary data was collected during a pre-clinical study conducted in animals. The half-life of recombinant albumin in dog blood was almost identical to that of plasma albumin (recombinant albumin: 6.3 ± 0.5 day , plasma albumin: 6.0 ± 0.7 day). The following hemodynamic parameters were tested in dogs: blood pressure; central venous pressure; pulmonary artery pressure; cardiac output; blood gas; respiration; electrocardiogram. At doses of 0.5 and 1.5 g/kg, the same results were obtained for recombinant albumin as for plasma albumin.

The results of a pyrogen test using rabbits showed no temperature rise up to a dosage of 2.5 g/kg. An acute toxicity test of recombinant albumin demonstrated no toxicity in monkeys and rats up to a dosage of 12.5 g/kg.

DISCUSSION

A large part of the purification method established involved column chromatography and membrane treatment. This means that it is possible to purify recombinant albumin using automated methods. This is very significant for reducing the production cost of recombinant albumin. As far as high-sensitivity assays showed, levels of contaminants such as yeast components and DNA were below the detection limit in recombinant albumin purified by this method. Physicochemical properties of recombinant albumin were the same as those of plasma albumin as far as tests revealed. The identical results for amino acid analysis (amino acid composition, N-terminal sequence, C-terminal sequence and peptide mapping) indicated that the primary structure of recombinant albumin was consistent with that of plasma albumin. Moreover, it was suggested by the results of CD spectrum data that the secondary structure of recombinant albumin was also the same as that of plasma albumin. Ligand (Warfarin, Bilirubin and lauric acid) binding assays gave similar results. The binding affinities and the number of binding sites of recombinant albumin with bilirubin, warfarin and lauric acid were similar to those of plasma albumin, indicating biological equivalency between the two HSAs.

A pre-clinical trial in animals was conducted. Measurement of half-life in dog blood and hemodynamic parameters gave the same results for both HSAs. A pyrogen test of recombinant albumin using rabbits was negative.

An acute toxicity test of recombinant albumin demonstrated no toxicity in monkeys and rats. These results indicate that recombinant albumin prepared by our method is as safe as plasma albumin.

REFERENCES

Ashbrook, J.D., Spector, A.A., Santos, E.C., Fletcher, J.E. (1975): Long chain fatty acid binding to human plasma albumin. *J. Biol. Chemistry* 250 (6) 2333-2338.

De Witt, S.G. (1958): Interaction of human serum albumin with long chain fatty acid anions. *J. Am. Chem. Soc.* 80, 3892-3898.

Sun, S.F., Kuo, S.W., Nash, R.A. (1984): Study of binding of Warfarin to serum albumins by high-performance liquid chromatography. *J. Chromatography* 288, 377-388.

Nakamura, H. & Lee, Y. (1977): Microdetermination of unbound Bilirubin in icteric newborn sera: an enzymatic method employing peroxidase and glucose oxidase. *Clinica Chimica Acta* 79, 411-417.

Ohtani, W., Ohmizu, A., Sumi, A., Ohmura, T., Uemura, T., Yokoyama, K. (1988): Study on recombinant hepatitis B vaccine: development of ELISA methods for detection of contaminating yeast components in the vaccine and humoral anti-yeast component antibody developed in humans and guinea-pigs. *Yakugaku Zasshi* 108 (4) 339-344.

SUMMARY

A purification method for recombinant albumin has been established. The purity of recombinant albumin obtained by this purification method exceeds 99.999999 per cent. Furthermore, a large part of this purification method involves column chromatography and membrane treatment. This means that it is possible to purify albumin using automated methods. This is very significant for reducing production costs. Pysicochemical properties of purified recombinant albumin were identical to those of plasma albumin as far as tests showed. The pre-clinical animal study with recombinant albumin gave the same results as for plasma albumin. From these results, it was concluded that recombinant albumin prepared in this way has a high level of safety and quality.

VI. Other plasmatic proteins

VI. *Autres protéines plasmatiques*

…

Dye-affinity purification and assessment of the biosafety of human plasma transthyretin destined to clinical uses

V. Regnault[1], L. Vallar[1], C. Geschier[1,2], C. Rivat[1] and J.-F. Stoltz[1,2]

[1]INSERM, [2]Laboratoire d'Hématologie, Faculté de Médecine et CRTS, Brabois, 54500 Vandœuvre-lès-Nancy, France

ABSTRACT

A dye-affinity chromatography procedure on Remazol Yellow GGL-Sepharose has been developed in order to allow large-scale preparation of human plasma transthyretin for substitutive therapy. A by-product of the chromatographic purification of albumin using the Spherodex-Spherosil process was chosen as starting material and the optimum working conditions for the fixation and the elution of the transthyretin were defined. The dye leaching from the affinity sorbent was quantitatively studied by a sensitive enzyme immunoassay. The stability of the biological activity of the purified protein was investigated after heat treatment for virus inactivation and over months when the heated transthyretin was stored at 4°C, 20°C or 37°C.

INTRODUCTION

Human plasma transthyretin (TTR), a multifunctional tetrameric protein actively involved in the transport of thyroxine and retinol binding protein (Raz et al., 1969), is widely recognized as a sensitive marker to have pronostic value with regard to complications and outcome in various pathologic situations (Cano et al., 1987; Cynober et al., 1991). Variant transthyretins have been related to different patterns of amyloid involvement, in particular familial amyloidotic polyneuropathy (Saraiva et al., 1984) also characterized by decreased plasma TTR levels (Saraiva et al., 1983). Substitutive therapy using purified TTR in association or not with a specific removal of the abnormal TTR by an extracorporeal immunoadsorption procedure (Regnault et al., 1992) may be anticipated. The value of Remazol Yellow GGL as a biomimetic ligand for the affinity chromatography of TTR from serum has been previously established (Copping et al., 1982; Birkenmeier et al., 1984). However, the application of this technique is hindered by interference with classical fractionation of plasma and contamination of the final product with albumin and IgG. To circumvent these problems, a procedure was developed from a by-product of the chromatographic purification of albumin using the Spherodex-Spherosil process (Stoltz et al., 1987) which contains high levels of TTR, trace-amounts of albumin and no IgG. The central concern for manufacturers of therapeutic products is the biosafety of the final entity (Stoltz et al., 1992). The dye leakage was investigated by means of a sensitive enzyme immunoassay (Regnault et al., 1992). With the goal of preparing a virus-safe protein, the possibility of heat treatment while preserving the biological activity of TTR was assessed.

MATERIALS AND METHODS

<u>Preparation of the dye-sorbent</u> : A 250 g amount of packed Sepharose CL-4B (Pharmacia, Sweden), 25 g of NaCl and 2.5 g of Remazol Yellow GGL (Vilmax, Argentina) were mixed and made up to a volume of 450 ml with distilled water. The mixture was stirred for 30 min, then

50 ml of 0.25 M NaOH were added. After overnight agitation, the sorbent was washed with distilled water until the absorbance at 400 nm reached zero. It was stored at 4°C, either in distilled water containing 0.2 g/l NaN_3 or in a 20 % ethanol aqueous solution.

Dye-affinity chromatography of TTR : The fraction (termed here DNaCl) eluted with 1 M NaCl in the first chromatographic step of the purification of human albumin by the Spherodex-Spherosil process was dialysed against 0.1 M sodium phosphate buffer, pH 7.4 and then applied to the dye-sorbent equilibrated with the same buffer. TTR was eluted with 10 % ethanol in water, concentrated by ultrafiltration using a membrane with a 10,000 MW cut-off and dialysed against 9 g/l NaCl in water.

Heat treatment : The purified TTR, adjusted to a concentration of about 50 g/l in a 9 g/l NaCl solution, was heated in a water-bath at 60°C for 10 h.

TTR assay : The TTR concentration was determined by rocket immunoelectrophoresis according to Laurell (1966) using a specific antiserum and a serum as standard (Behring, Germany).

Thyroxine binding capacity : A 10 µl volume of sample containing TTR at a concentration of 100 mg/l was incubated with 10 µl of [^{125}I]thyroxine (1.85 MBq/ml, 55.5 MBq/µg, Amersham, UK) and 1 µl of bromophenol blue for 2 h at room temperature. A 1 µl aliquot of the mixture was subjected to native PAGE using Phastgel gradient (8-25 %) and a Phastsystem apparatus (Pharmacia). Electrophoresis was stopped when bromophenol blue reached the anode buffer strip. The gel was sliced in lanes and each lane in various length sections. Each slice was assayed for radioactivity in a gamma counter.

Dye assay : Microtiter plates (Costar) were coated with a 1 µg/ml Remazol Yellow GGL-ovalbumin conjugate in 50 mM sodium carbonate, pH 9.6 (100 µl/well) at 4°C overnight. All washes were done with 130 mM NaCl, 5 mM Na_2HPO_4 and 1 mM KH_2PO_4, pH 7.2 containing 0.05 % Tween 20 (PBS-Tween). The plates were blocked with 125 µl of 0.5 % gelatin (cold water fish skin, Sigma, USA) in PBS for 3 h at 37°C. During this time, four volumes of sample or standard were added to one volume of biotinylated anti BSA-Remazol Yellow GGL rabbit immunoglobulins (prepared in our laboratory) and incubated for 2 h at 37°C. A 100 µl aliquot of each mixture was then added to the wells and incubated for 2 h at 37°C. The streptavidin-peroxidase complex was incubated for 15 min at 37°C. After extensive washes with PBS-Tween and 140 mM sodium acetate-citrate, pH 6.0, color was developed with 100 µl of 0.1 mg/ml TMB, 0.01 % H_2O_2 in acetate-citrate. The enzyme reaction was stopped with 25 µl of 2 M H_2SO_4 and the absorbance was measured at 450 nm in an ELISA reader.

RESULTS

Optimization of the dye-affinity purification of TTR

The influence of several parameters on the fixation and the elution of TTR was studied. The binding capacity of the sorbent assessed by the amount of TTR eluted per ml of gel is dependent on the washing volume to elute non-bound proteins and the total amount of TTR applied to the sorbent. Conversely the chromatographic results are unchanged whatever the residence time (calculated as the ratio of the sorbent volume to the flow-rate) and the TTR level in the DNaCl fraction.

Optimum effectiveness of the sorbent is obtained with a 2 column volume washing before elution of TTR with ethanol and when the amount of TTR loaded is about 1 g per litre of gel (Fig. 2). In these working conditions the dye-affinity purification resulted in the isolation of a 80 % pure TTR (the main contaminant being albumin) with a 70 % chromatographic recovery at a pilot scale. The overall recovery in relation to cryoprecipitate-free plasma was about 30 % and the greatest losses occured during the pretreatment of plasma (Table 1).

The binding capacity of the sorbent was not altered when it was stored in a 20 % ethanol aqueous solution (a bacteriostatic and non toxic solution) between uses in order to prevent bacterial contamination. Moreover, the efficiency of the purification remained constant over ten procedures (Fig. 3).

Table 1 : *Purification of human plasma transthyretin*

fraction	recovery (%)	overall recovery (%)	mg of TTR per mg of protein	apparent purification	overall apparent purification
plasma	100	100	0.0039		
S II+III	48	48	0.0044	1.1	1.1
DNaCl	89	43	0.0292	6.6	7.5
TTR	70	30	0.8333	28.5	214.0

Results are mean of 5 experiments. S II+III : Cohn supernatant II+III

The biological activity of the TTR was assessed throughout the purification procedure by means of its thyroxine binding capacity. As can be seen in Fig. 1, TTR effectively bound [^{125}I]thyroxine since two separated radioactivity peaks were observed in the samples containing both TTR and thyroxine, one in the slice containing TTR (slice 2) and one major in the anodal slice corresponding to free thyroxine. When calculated as a molar ratio, one molecule of thyroxine was bound per molecule of TTR. The thyroxine binding capacity of TTR was preserved during the dye-affinity chromatography.

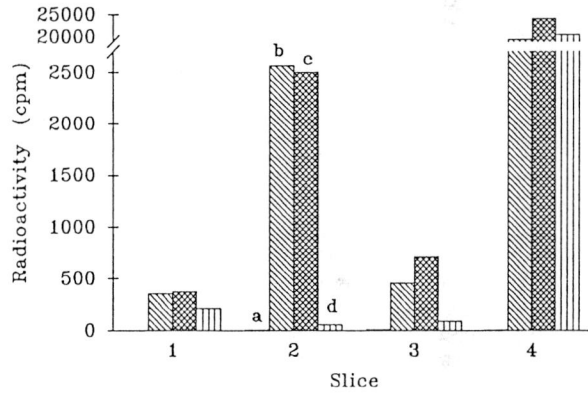

Fig. 1 : *Thyroxine binding capacity.* a : TTR alone, b : DNaCl fraction, c : purified TTR, d : thyroxine alone.

Dye leakage

The competitive enzyme immunoassay developed to monitor the dye column leaching is sensitive to 1 ng/ml and allows the accurate detection of both free dye and dye complexed to TTR (Regnault et al., 1992).

The stability of the dye-sorbent was studied by measuring the amount of dye leached in several buffers with pH values ranging from 1 to 14. In the pH range 4-10, as well as in the solutions used for the TTR chromatographic purification procedure (0.1 M sodium phosphate, pH 7.4 and 10 % ethanol) the leakage was of the same order of magnitude, a minimal value of about 5 µg of dye per g of sorbent for a 24-h incubation time.

The dye leakage was found to be increased in protein-containing fractions during the chromatographic procedure. When the sorbent was stored in 0.1 M sodium phosphate, pH 7.4 containing 0.2 g/l NaN$_3$, the amount of dye leached in the flow-through DNaCl fraction is six-fold higher than in the phosphate buffer alone and about ten-fold more important in the TTR ethanol eluate than in the ethanol solution. Similar leakage values (expressed as the amount of dye per ml) are measured in these two protein fractions although the TTR concentration is significantly different.

The dye leakage was assayed in TTR ethanol fractions obtained by applying various volumes of a DNaCl fraction to identical dye-sorbent columns. The dye concentration in the eluates remained relatively unchanged whereas the TTR recovery increased as the amount of TTR loaded increased. As the increase is not linear the ratio µg of dye per g of TTR decreases and levels out for amounts of TTR loaded greater than 1-1.5 g per litre of sorbent (Fig. 2).

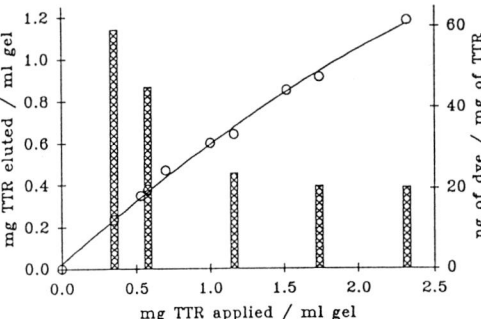
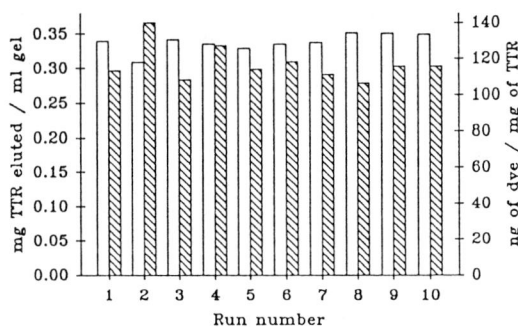

Fig. 2 : *Influence of the amount of TTR loaded on the binding capacity of the sorbent and the dye leakage*. Volumes of DNaCl (TTR concentration of 1.16 mg/ml) ranging from 3 to 20 ml were applied to the dye-sorbent (1.6 x 5 cm) at a flow-rate of 50 ml/h. Dye was assayed in the eluted TTR dialysed against NaCl (bars).

Fig. 3 : *Dye leakage over runs*. Each run was achieved by applying 10 ml of a DNaCl fraction (TTR level of 0.5 mg/ml) to the sorbent (1.6 x 5 cm) at a flow-rate of 50 ml/h. The sorbent stored in 20 % ethanol was washed before each run with ten column volumes of phosphate buffer. Dye was assayed in the dialysed TTR (hatched bars).

Although the dye-sorbent was washed with ten column volumes of phosphate buffer before use, the dye leakage was shown to be two-fold higher when the sorbent was stored in 20 % ethanol rather than in phosphate buffer (Fig. 2 and Fig. 3).

The dye leakage was investigated over ten identical chromatographic runs. The sorbent was stored in 20 % ethanol between uses. The amount of dye leached as well as the binding capacity of the sorbent remained constant over runs (Fig. 3).

<u>TTR pasteurization</u>

The possibility of heat treatment for the purified TTR while preserving its biochemical and functional characteristics was investigated. Heating in solution at 60°C for 10 h without stabilizers had no significant effect on the measured contents of TTR, Remazol Yellow GGL dye or total protein. In native PAGE analysis, only one band with anodal mobility was observed for heated or unheated TTR. The thyroxine binding capacity of TTR was totally preserved during the pasteurization step (Fig. 4). The stabilities of the biological activity of heated and unheated purified TTR stored at 4°C, 20°C or 37°C were compared over a 6-month period. As shown in Fig. 4, the thyroxine binding capacity was retained in the same manner over this period for the heated and unheated TTR. The thyroxine

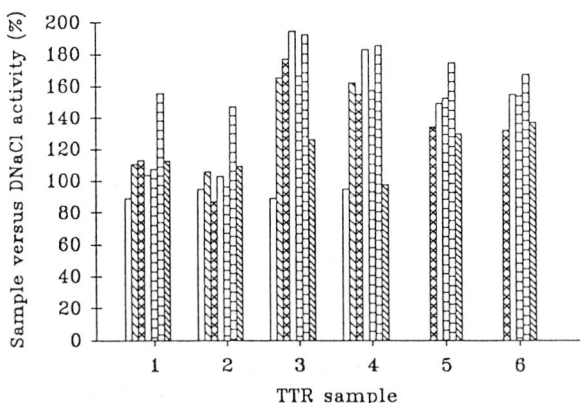

Fig. 4 : *Stability of the biological activity of the purified TTR*. All TTR samples came from the same purified TTR pool (concentration of 47 g/l). Unheated TTR samples (1, 3, 5) and heated TTR samples (2, 4, 6) were stored respectively at 4°C, 37°C and 20°C. The thyroxine binding capacity was evaluated monthly (different bars) over a 6-month period. Left empty bar : initial activity.

binding capacity of the purified TTR was evaluated in relation to the thyroxine binding capacity of the initial DNaCl fraction stored at 4°C. Storage at more elevated temperatures (20°C or 37°C) increased the thyroxine binding capacity of the TTR. However, the biological activity of the purified TTR was stable at these temperatures over a 6-month period.

DISCUSSION

The use of affinity chromatography methods for large-scale preparation procedures of therapeutic plasma proteins is connected with considerations on the quality, safety and scale-up criteria required for such technology and products.

Dye-affinity chromatography of TTR from an unexploited by-product of plasma fractionation combines two main advantages, the low cost of production of the ligand and the non interference with plasma valorization. The by-product used as starting material was chosen since it contains high levels of TTR, trace-amounts of albumin and no IgG. It must be noted that other by-products of human plasma fractionation contains significant levels of TTR and could also be usable.

The optimization of the procedure conditions its large scale application. As TTR is only delayed in its passage through the dye-sorbent, the chromatographic recovery is influenced by the washing volumes. One major safety concern for affinity chromatography is the unavoidable leakage of ligand. Dye leakage is dependent on the presence of proteins in the chromatographed solutions. It could be assumed that the dye-TTR interaction is responsible for the increase in dye leakage. However, the dye level in eluting fractions is not correlated with the TTR concentration. The dye increase in protein-containing solutions is thus due to a multifactorial phenomenon. Increasing the amount of TTR loaded resulted in a non linear increase in the amount of TTR eluted and consequently in a decrease of the chromatographic yield. As the dye leakage remained relatively unchanged whatever the amount of TTR eluted, the quantity ratio of dye to protein reaches a plateau when the amount of TTR loaded increases. Optimum chromatographic working conditions are thus obtained with 1 g of TTR loaded per litre of sorbent. These conditions allows optimum effectiveness of the sorbent in relation to the total amount of TTR applied and minimal leakage of dye. In order to avoid bacterial contamination affinity supports can be stored in 20 % ethanol with no loss of binding capacity. However, this storage condition leads to an increase in dye leakage even if the sorbent is extensively washed before use.

In the above-mentioned optimum working conditions the purification procedure can be easily scaled-up since the results obtained at a pilot scale closely correlate with analytical results. Moreover, the sorbent can be used several times in highly reproducible conditions with regard to chromatographic timing and recovery as well as dye leakage.

The dye-affinity chromatography procedure developed resulted in a 80 % pure protein. Although the current trend is to prepare highly purified proteins, the purity of TTR is convenient for substitutive therapeutic purposes since the main contaminant is albumin.

Biological products prepared from large pools of human plasma may contain endogenous viruses. The possibility of including a viral inactivation step in the purification procedure is therefore a major safety concern for manufacturers of plasma-derived proteins. Heat treatment is an attractive method due to its simplicity and efficiency. The virus inactivation in human albumin preparations heated in solution in the presence of suitable stabilizers at 60°C for 10 h has been established. Heat treatment often required addition of stabilizers to preserve the biological activity of the therapeutic protein. The biological activity of the purified TTR assessed by means of its thyroxine binding capacity is not altered during heating in solution at 60 °C for 10 h without stabilizers indicating a great stability of the functional properties of the protein. Moreover heat treatment has no effect on the stability of the biological activity of TTR over a 6-month period. Interestingly, storage of the purified protein at room or more elevated temperatures induces an increase in its thyroxine binding capacity. Throughout the purification procedure and when the isolated TTR is stored at 4°C, the thyroxine assay results are consistent with a single thyroxine binding site for the TTR tetramer. The data obtained after storage at room temperature or at 37°C indicated 1.5 to 2 thyroxine binding sites. It must be emphasized that the thyroxine binding can occur in two sites in the internal channel of the TTR tetramer.

The dye-affinity chromatography method developed using Remazol Yellow GGL and a by-product of the chromatographic purification of albumin by the Spherodex-Spherosil process is suitable for large-scale preparation of a therapeutic TTR and investigations have now to be performed to elucidate the potential toxicity of the dye ligand. Moreover, if results of the virus removal and inactivation during the pretreatment of plasma and during the first step of the chromatographic purification of albumin using the Spherodex-Spherosil process have already been reported (Stoltz et al., 1992), model virus studies are required as a preliminary screen of the virucidal potency of the dye-affinity chromatography and the heat treatment steps before starting clinical trials in humans.

REFERENCES

Birkenmeier, G., Tschechonien, B., Kopperschläger, G. (1984): Affinity chromatography and affinity partition of human serum pre-albumin using immobilized Remazol Yellow GGL. *FEBS Lett.*, 174, 162-166.

Cano, N., Di Costanzo-Dufetel, J. (1987): Transthyrétine (préalbumine) sérique. *Nutr. Clin. Metabol.* 1, 7-15.

Copping, S., Byfield, P.G.H. (1982): Prealbumin : extraction from serum by Remazol Yellow GGL-Sepharose. *Biochem. Soc. Trans.* 10, 104-105.

Cynober, L., Prugnaud, O., Lioret, N., Duchemin, C., Saizy, R., Giboudeau, J. (1991): Serum transthyretin levels in patients with burn injury. *Surgery* 109, 640-644.

Laurell, C.B. (1966): Quantitative estimation of proteins by electrophoresis in agarose gel containing antibodies. *Anal. Biochem.* 15, 45-52.

Raz, A., Goodman, D.S. (1969): The interaction of thyroxine with human plasma prealbumin and with the prealbumin-retinol-binding protein complex. *J. Biol. Chem.* 244, 3230-3237.

Regnault, V., Costa, P.M.P., Teixeira, A., Rivat, C., Stoltz, J.F., Saraiva, M.J.M., Costa, P.P. (1992): Specific removal of transthyretin from plasma of patients with familial amyloidotic polyneuropathy : optimization of an immunoadsorption procedure. *Int. J. Artif. Organs* 15, 249-255.

Regnault, V., Rivat, C., Vallar, L., Geschier, C., Stoltz, J.F. (1992): Purification of biologically active human plasma transthyretin by dye-affinity chromatography : studies on dye leakage and possibility of heat treatment for virus inactivation. *J. Chromatogr.* 584, 93-100.

Regnault, V., Vallar, L., Rivat, C., Stoltz, J.F., Boschetti, E. (1992): A sensitive enzyme immunoassay for the detection of a synthetic affinity ligand, the reactive yellow 13 dye. *J. Immunoassay* in press.

Saraiva, M.J.M., Costa, P.P., Goodman, D.S. (1983): Studies on plasma transthyretin (prealbumin) in familial amyloidotic polyneuropathy, Portuguese type. *J. Lab. Clin. Med.* 102, 590-603.

Saraiva, M.J.M., Birken, S., Costa, P.P., Goodman, D.S. (1984): Amyloid fibril protein in familial amyloidotic polyneuropathy, Portuguese type. *J. Clin. Invest.* 74, 104-119.

Stoltz, J.F., Rivat, C., Geschier, C., Colosetti, P., Sertillanges, P., Tondon, J., Regnault, V. (1987): Purification chromatographique de l'albumine plasmatique humaine à l'échelle pilote. *Bio-Sciences* 6, 103-106.

Stoltz, J.F., Rivat, C., Regnault, V. (1992): Considerations on the technical and legal requirements involved in the use of affinity chromatography for clinical and biological applications. *LC-GC Int.* 5, 23-26.

Stoltz, J.F., Rivat, C., Geschier, C., Sertillanges, Ph., Grandgeorges, M., Liautaud, J., Dumont, L. (1992): Validation des capacités d'inactivation des virus d'un procédé de purification de l'albumine plasmatique humaine par chromatographie. *Ann. Pharm. Franç.* in press.

Résumé

Une technique d'affinité utilisant le colorant Jaune Remazol GGL comme ligand biomimétique a été développée pour la préparation à grande échelle de transthyrétine plasmatique humaine destinée à un usage thérapeutique. Une fraction non exploitée de la purification chromatographique de l'albumine par le procédé Spherodex-Spherosil a été choisie comme matériel de départ et les conditions optimales de fixation et d'élution de la transthyrétine ont été définies. Le colorant relargué du support d'affinité a été quantifié par une technique immunoenzymatique très sensible. La stabilité de l'activité biologique de la protéine purifiée a été évaluée après une étape de chauffage pour l'inactivation des virus potentiellement présents et sur une période de 6 mois durant laquelle la transthyrétine traitée à la chaleur a été conservée à 4°C, 20°C ou 37°C.

Preparation of fibrin glue and its clinical application

C. Chao, X. Wang, S. Chen and T. Zhang

Laboratory of Plasma Products, Shanghai Institute of Biologic Products, Ministry of Public Health, China

Abstract

The fibrin glue was composed of the concentrates of fibrinogen, thrombin and aprotinin which were prepared from cryoprecipitate, Cohn fraction III and bovin lung respectively. 1 ml reconstituted fibrinogen solution contained 83.3 mg clottable protein (therefor 74.1 mg fibrinogen and 19.1 mg fibronectin), 20-40 U factor XIII and 88.3 ug plasminogen. The human thrombin was 400-500 U/ml or 5-10 U/ml for different application. The activity of bovin aprotinin was more than 3200 UKIU/ml, which could inhibit fibrinolysis up to 144 hrs in vitro.

The product had been used in virous fields of surgery, and reached an ideal effect on hemostasis in cardiovascular surgery, adhesion in middle ear reconstrucive procedure and closure of cerebrospinal rhinorrhea. The clinical application also showed that the fibrin glue could enhance wound healing. In more than 200 cases the glue had not any side effects.

Identification by HPLC of a hyperglycemic peptide induced by temperature in rat and human serum

Rhizlane Bouguerne[1], Jean-Louis Guéant[1], Catherine Masson[1], Fabienne Bois[1], Philippe Guimelly[2], Jean-Claude Michalski[3] and Jean-Pierre Nicolas[1]

[1]INSERM U.308, Equipe de Biochimie-Immunologie, B.P. 184, 54505 Vandœuvre Cedex, France. [2]Laboratoire de Biochimie, Faculté de Pharmacie, Université de Nancy I, France. [3]Laboratoire de Chimie Biologique, URA CNRS, Université des Sciences et Techniques, Lille, France

SUMMARY

Heated rat serum is responsible for hyperglycemia when it is injected intraperitoneally in rats. The involvement of a peptidic temperature induced factor could explain this effect. We have identified this factor and compared its physicochemical properties in rat serum and in human serum, using size exclusion-HPLC, chromatofocusing and reversed-phase HPLC. The properties were similar in both sera : the molecular mass was of the order of 5 kDa and the isoelectric point was estimated to be about 3.4. In both cases, the peptide was eluted in presence in 90 - 100 % (vol/vol) of acetonitrile in reversed-phase HPLC. The composition of the purified material demonstrated that this factor contained 10 % carbohydrates.

INTRODUCTION

Blood glucose level is increased in normal rats and in tumor-bearing rats subjected to local hyperthermia (Beer Gabel & Yerushalmi, 1981). Hyperglycemia is observed notwithstanding areas which are heated. In addition, serum from locally heated rats elevates blood glucose level of recipients animals when injected intraperitoneally (Bois et al, 1984). The same results have been obtained with rabbits (Yerushalmi et al, 1982).
The involvement of a serum temperature induced factor for explaining this hyperglycemia has been suggested since serum heated in vitro and injected to normal rats was also responsible for hyperglycemia (Bois et al, 1984). This factor of rat heated serum has a molecular size lower than 10 kDa in Sephacryl S300 gel permeation chromatography (Bois et al, 1984).
In the present work, we describe the presence of this factor in human as well as in rat serum and we compare the behaviour of the human and of the rat factor in reversed-phase HPLC and chromatofocusing.

MATERIALS AND METHODS

<u>Collection of sera</u> : aliquots of human blood were collected from healthy individual donors of peripheral venipuncture. The rat samples were collected from anesthetized Wistar rats by intra-heart puncture. Rats were anesthetized intraperitoneally with sodium pentobarbital. The serum were

separated by centrifugation at 1500 x g for 15 min at + 4° C and stored in aliquots at - 20° C.

Preparation of heated sera : a pool of the human and rat serum samples was placed for 15 min in a water bath at 44° C. The temperature was measured with a teflon-coated termocouple. The serum was cooled to reach the room temperature.

Serum fractionation : the serum (50 ml rat heated serum and 48 ml human heated serum per purification) was fractionated by gel permeation chromatography using a preparative column (100 x 5 cm I.D.) packed with Sephacryl S300 (Pharmacia Fine Chemicals, Uppsala, Sweden) and eluted with 0.05 M phosphate buffer, pH 7.4 containing 1 M NaCl at a flow rate of 1.5 ml/min. The column was previously calibrated for estimation of molecular size using Dextran blue 2000. ^3H_2O and (^{125}I) iodinated standards proteins (IgG and HSA) as described (Bois et al, 1984). The distribution coefficients of IgG and HSA were 0.371 ± 0.022 and 0.449 ± 0.023, respectively (n = 10). The 200 collected fractions were arbitrarily pooled into 5 aliquots according to their relative molecular masses (Mr). The Mr range fof aliquots I, II, III, IV and V was 1500-300, 300-60, 60-11, 11-2 and 2-0.3 kDa respectively. The aliquots were then concentrated 20-fold and desalted by diafiltration using a Diaflo membrane (type YM2, exclusion limit 2000, Amicon, Corp., Lexington, MA, USA) in a Micro-ultrafiltration system 8MC (Amicon Corp.). A part of each aliquot (1 ml) was tested for hyperglycemic effect in rats by intraperitoneal injection.

HPLC analysis was performed at room temperature using a two pump gradient system (Waters Associates, Milford, MA, USA) as described recently (Bois et al, 1984; Guéant et al, 1986). The eluate was detected at 280/250 nm and collected in 1 ml fractions. The HPLC system was interconnected with teflon tubing. The active fraction (IV) was filtered through a Lichrospher Diol preparative column (30 x 25 cl I.D.) (Merck, Darmstadt, FRG) in 0.02 M Tris HCl buffer pH 7.5 containing 1 M urea at a flow-rate of 10 ml/min. The detection was at 254 and a 280 nm (no difference of the elution profile was observed with these two wawelength). Each peak was collected concentrated and desalted by diafiltration as described above. A part of the collected samples was tested for hyperglycemic effect in rats.

Chromatofocusing :this step was performed with a column Mono P (20 x 5 cm I.D.) (Pharmacia). The column was washed with 0.025 M Bis-Tris buffer pH 6.3 (HCl). The pH gradient was obtained by eluting the column with a Polybuffer/Pharmalyte solution prepared by mixing 10 ml of Polybuffer $^{TM}74$ (Pharmacia), 2 ml of Pharmalyte 2-2.5 (Pharmacia) in 150 ml water. The Polybuffer Pharmalyte solution was adjusted to pH 2 with 0.1 M HCl prior to its use. The flow-rate was 1.0 ml/min. The collected peaks were tested for the hyperglycemic effect after adjusting the pH to 7.4. The absence of hyperglycemic effect of the mobile phase was attested by injecting the Bis-Tris buffer and the Pharmalyte Polybuffer solution to rats.

Reversed-phase HPLC : the active fraction was poured onto a C18 reversed phase affinity column (5 x 0.5 cm I.D.) (Pharmacia Fine Chemicals, Uppsala, Sweden), eluted consecutively with 2 ml distilled water containing 0.01 % TFA (v/v) and with a 0-100 % gradient of acetonitrile containing 0.01 % TFA (v/v) in a total volume of 32 ml at a flow rate of 0.2 ml/min. Fractions collected from reversed-phase HPLC were evaporated to dryness. They were resuspended in 1 ml water and used to test the hyperglycemic effect in recipients rats.

Test of hyperglycemic effect in recipient rats : the samples (1 ml) were injected intraperitoneally to rats. The animals fasted for 17 h were sacrificed 24 h after the injections. Blood was collected as described above (intra-heart). Blood samples were immediately centrifuged and stored at + 4° C. The determination of glucose blood level was made on all serum samples, by the glucose oxydase method (PAP 250, Biomerieux, Lyon, France).

A preliminary experiment was performed as described above with 21 groups of 5 rats in order to determine the optimal delay for detecting the hyperglycemia. Each group was sacrified with a delay warying from 2 hours to 16 days after injection of heated serum.
Electrophoresis polyacrylamide disc gel electrophoresis was performed according to the method of Fairbanks et al. (Fairbanks et al, 1971). The gels were prepared as described by Swank and Munkres (Swank and Munkres, 1971). The sample contain 10 µg proteins and 10 % sucrose (w:v) in a total volume of 30 µg. The gels were stained with Coomassie brillant blue. The Mr of the peptide was estimated with calibrated myoglobin peptids (Pharmacia).
Amino acid and carbohydrate analysis: amino acids were analysed with a Technicon NC-2P system. Purified peptide was hydrolysed for 24 h at 105° C in te vapour of 5.6 M HCl in vacuum. The molar carbohydrate composition of the glycoprotein was determined according to the method of Zanetta et al (Zanetta et al, 1972) modified as follows, the purified peptide was subjected to acid methanolysis in 1 ml MeOH containing 0.5 M HCl for 24 h at 80° C. The sample was cooled to room temperature and the methanolysate was extracted twice with 1 ml hexane. The upper phase containing mostly amino acids was discarded and the lower phase was concentrated under a nitrogen flow. The residue was treated with 10 µg of dichloromethane and 10 µg of trifluoroacetic anhydride ; derivatives were identified by gas chromatography.

RESULTS AND DISCUSSION

The hyperglycemia induced by heated rat serum was optimal 24 h after serum injection (Fig. 1).
The hyperglycemia was not observed when the same experiment was performed with non heated serum. This demonstrated that neither animal manipulation nor anesthesia were responsible for the hyperglycemic effect. The hyperglycemia of recipient rats was maximal at 24 h and decreased 5 days after injection of heated serum : normal glycemia was recovered 15 days after the injection (Fig. 1).

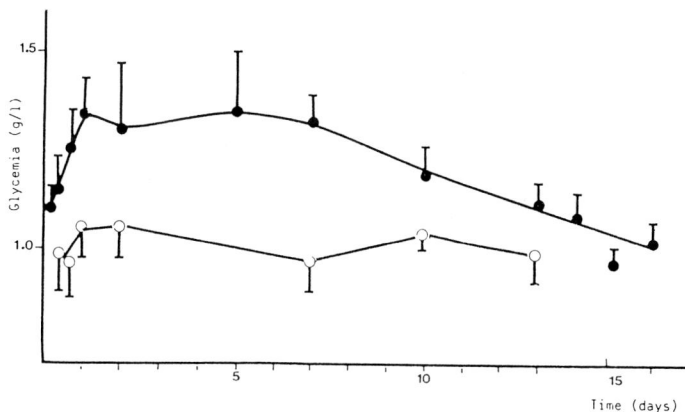

Fig. 1. Kinetic of glycemia in recipient rats after intraperitoneal injection of 1 ml serum. Data are mean ± standard deviation and each point represents the mean from glycemia observed in 5 recipient rats after injection heated serum while open circles correspond to control data obtained with non heated serum.

The aliquot IV obtained from Sephacryl S300 gel permeation chromatography of heated rat serum was responsible for a hyperglycemia in rats. This aliquot corresponded to a molecular mass range of 2-12 kDa. This has been previously observed by us (Bois et al, 1984). The same result was obtained with heated human serum, showing that human serum contained also a temperature-induced factor having a hyperglycemic effect. The hyperglycemic effect of the aliquot IV from human serum was similar to that of the aliquot IV from rat serum, with a respective hyperglycemia of 1.36 ± 0.10 g/l (n = 10) and 1.37 ± 0.13 g/l (n = 10). This effect corresponded respectively to a 32 % and 35 % increase of glycemia when comparing the results with the glycemia of recipient rats injected with a control aliquot IV obtained from non heated serum. The glycemia of recipient rats injected with control aliquot IV was at 1.03 ± 0.07 g/l (n = 5) and 1.01 ± 0.06 g/l (n = 5) respectively with samples from non heated rat serum and non heated human serum. Glycemia obtained with aliquots I, II, III and V from both non heated sera ranged from 0.96 ± 0.15 g/l to 1.05 ± 0.09 g/l (n = 3) for each sample tested.

The aliquot IV of rat heated serum was eluted in 3 peaks, in size exclusion-HPLC, with respective retention times of 9.5, 14.5 and 16.2 min. A similar elution profile was obtained with the aliquot IV from human heated serum (Fig. 2A and Fig. 2D). The test for hyperglycemic in recipient rats showed that the temperature-induced factor was present in the second eluted peak. This was observed for the rat sample as well as the human sample. From this result, it may be concluded that both factors have nearly the same molecular size. The retention time was close to that observed for glucagon in this size exclusion-HPLC column. We estimated that the Mr was of the order of 5 kDa when calibrating the column with reference molecules (chymotrypsinogen, ribonuclease and glucagon). The second eluted peak was not observed when injecting non heated rat serum and non-heated human serum in size exclusion-HPLC. This confirmed previous data from our group (Bois et al, 1984). Three peaks were observed in the chromatofocusing elution profile of the hyperglycemic fraction obtained from size exclusion-HPLC of the rat sample. Four peaks were obtained with the corresponding fraction of the human sample. The hyperglycemic effect was observed in the peak eluted at pH 3.35 and 3.50 respectively for the rat and the human sample. One may therefore assume that this peptide is anionic in blood.

The hyperglycemic fraction obtained from chromatofocusing was studied in reversed phase-HPLC in order to check the purity and the hydrophobicity of the factor. Two peaks were eluted in the acetonitrile-TFA gradient, with the rat sample as well as with the human sample (Fig. 2C and Fig. 2 F). The second eluted peak was the only one which provoked hyperglycemia in recipient rats. It was eluted with 97 % and 91 % of acetonitrile, respectively for the rat sample and for the human sample. The main part of this purified sample was used to verify the hyperglycemic effect in triplicate. The remaining proteic amount of the temperature induced peptide purified from human serum was too small for performing a SDS-PAGE. The purified sample from rat serum was identified as a main band corresponding to a Mr of 5 kDa in SDS-PAGE. Minor bands were also observed with respective Mr of 2.5 and 18.2 kDa and represented less than 7 % of the electrophoretic pattern. The amino acid composition of the rat purified sample is given in Table 1. It shows that the peptide contained a proportion of hydrophobic amino acids in order of 40 %. The peptide contained 10 % carbohydrates corresponding to 71.4 % mannose and 28.6 % N-acetylglucosamine residues. Unfortunatly, the amount of purified peptide was not sufficient to perform the amino acid sequence.

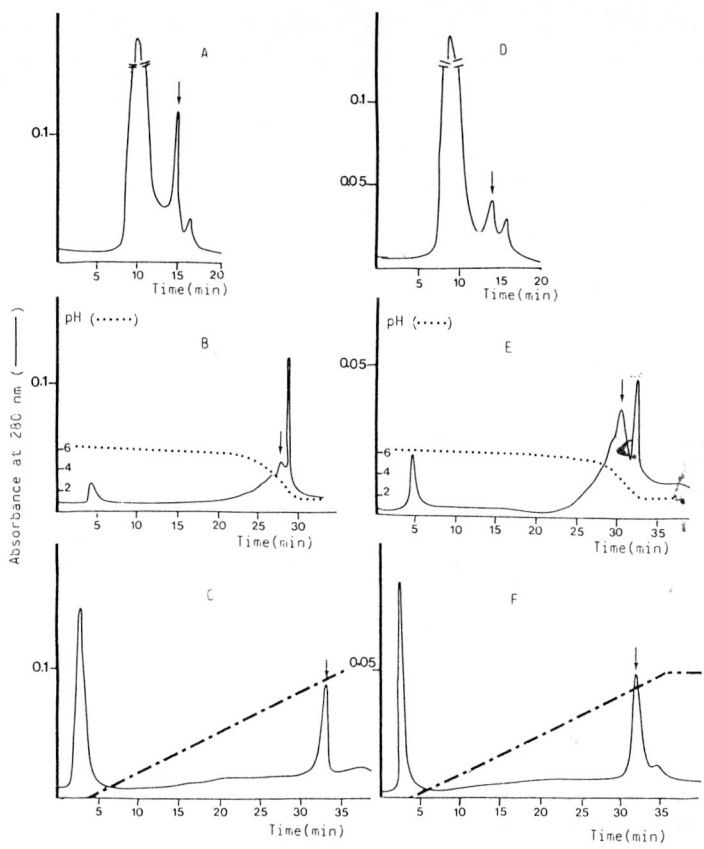

Fig. 2. Elution profiles of the hyperglycemic temperature induced peptide in HPLC. (A,D) : Size exclusion-HPLC of a seric fraction of the seric factor obtained from gel permeation were injected in a Lichrospher Diol column (Merck) eluted with Tris HCl buffer at a flow-rate of 10 ml/min. (B,E) : Chromatofocusing (column Mono P) of the active fractions collected from the step (A,D). (C,F) : Reversed-phase HPLC (C18) of the fraction obtained in step (B,E). The peaks corresponding to the hyperglycemic factor are indicated by arrows.

Table I : Amino acid composition of the temperature-induced peptide purified from rat serum

Amino acid	Residues per mole
Lysine	3
Histidine	2
Arginine	1
Aspartic acid	5
Threonine	3
Serine	5
Glutamic acid	6
Glycine	8
Alanine	4
Valine	2
Leucine	2
Total	41

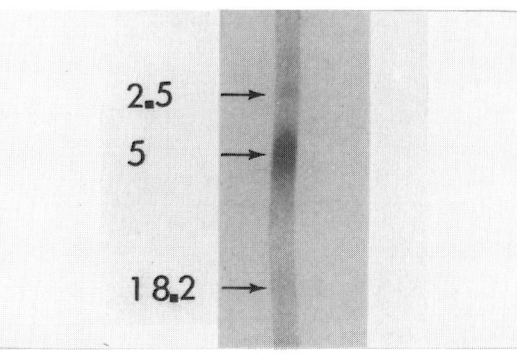

Fig. 3. SDS-PAGE of the purified peptide. A main band was identified with a Mr of 5 kDa Migration direction was from bottom to top.

Increasing dilutions of heated rat serum (1:2, 1:4, 1:1.6, 1:3.2 and 1:6.4) in 0.15 mol/l sodium chloride were injected in 6 groups of 5 rats. The hyperglycemic effect was still observed with sample diluted 1:3.2. No hyperglycemic effect was observed with undiluted heated human serum while a hyperglycemic effect was obtained with heated rat serum diluted 1:3.2. This suggested that the concentration of temperature induced factor was at least 3-fold lower in human serum than in rat serum. This could also explain that the final proteic amount of temperature induced factor was 3-fold lower when the factor was purified from human serum than when purified from rat serum.

In conclusion, we have identified a temperature-induced factor in serum heated in vitro. This factor is a peptide which is present in human as well as in rat serum. It has a Mr in order of 5 kDa and an isoelectric point of about 3.4. These physicochemical properties are similar for both rat and human peptides.

REFERENCES

Beer Gabel, M., and Yerushalmi, A. (1981). Bull. Cancer 68: 321
Bois, F., Beer Gabel, M., Guéant, J.L., Masson, C., and Nicolas, J.P. (1984). Biomedicine and Pharmacotherapy 38: 404
Yerushalmi, A., Shpirer, Z., Hod, I., Gottespeld, F., and Bass, D.D. (1982). J. Radiat. Oncol. Biol. Phys. 9: 77
Guéant, J.L., Khanfri, J., Gérard, H., Frémont, S., Gérard, A., Grignon, G., and Nicolas, J.P. (1986) FEBS 207: 280
Fairbanks, G., Steck, T.L., and Walalch, D.F.H. (1971). Biochemistry 10: 2606
Swank, R.T., and Munkres, K.D. (1971). Anal. Biochem. 39: 462
Zanetta, J.P., Breckenridge, W.C., and Vincendon, G. (1972). J. Chromatogr. 69: 291

Le sérum de rat chaufffé in vitro provoque une hyperglycémie chez des rats le recevant en intrapéritonéal. Cet effet impliquerait un facteur peptidique induit par élévation de température. Nous avons isolé et caractérisé ce facteur à partir de sérum de rat et humain, par Diol-CLHP, chromatofocalisation et phase inverse-CLHP. Les propriétés du facteur sont identiques dans les 2 sérums : la masse moléculaire est de l'ordre de 5 kDa et le point isoélectrique est à 3.4, le peptide est élevé à plus de 90 % d'acétonitrile en phase inverse-CLHP. L'étude de sa composition montre qu'il contient environ 10 % de glucides.

Author index
Index des auteurs

Alexandre P., 97
Armand J., 75

Bailly M., 13
Berglöf J.H., 31
Berntorp E., 69
Birkenmeier G., 201
Bois F., 309
Boschetti E., 3, 175
Bouguerne R., 309
Boyeldieu D., 57
Brands L., 81
Briquel M.-E., 97
Brunko P., 215
Burnouf T., 91, 249
Burnouf-Radosevich M., 249
Burton S.J., 19

Chabbat J., 131
Chao C., 307
Chen S., 307
Chen Chunsheng, 137

Das P.C., 109
Davies J.R., 143, 155
De Jonge E., 49
Dellacherie E., 43
De Wit J.H.C., 125
Dietze H., 201
Drummond O., 87
Dumont L., 175, 267

Eriksson B., 69
Evans D.R., 63
Evans H.E., 63
Ezzedine M., 115

Fanget B., 75
Feldman P.A., 63
Ferguson J., 87
Fournier P., 183

Gattel P., 75, 183
Geschier C., 97, 175, 207, 267, 301
Girot P., 3
Glavind S., 103
Graafland H., 163
Grandgeorge M., 75, 175, 183, 267
Guéant J.-L., 309
Guerrier L., 3
Guimelly P., 309

Hakkennes C.T., 81
Hämäläinen E., 261

Hansen E., 103
Harris L., 63
Herrington R.W., 143, 155
Hiemstra H., 81
Hoff H.S., 109
Horaud F., 229
Horowitz B., 237
Horowitz M.S., 237
Huart J.-J., 91, 249
Hubert P., 43

Ingerslev J., 103

Jørgensen J., 103

Kamath M.V., 151
Knevelman A., 125
Kobayashi K., 293
Koenderman A.H.L., 81
Koops K., 109

Lambrecht B., 255
Larrieu M.-J., 131
Laurian Y., 131
Lawny F., 115
Liautaud J., 175, 267
Linssen P.H.J.M., 49
Li Shujin, 137
Löf A.L., 69
Lowe C.R., 25
Luo Liang, 137
Lutsch C., 75

MacGregor I., 87
MacLaughlin L., 87
Mandjiny S., 189
Marrs S.B., 169
Masson C., 69, 309
Michalski J.C., 91, 309
Micucci V., 143, 155
Mohr H., 255
Montreuil J., 283
Morgenthaler J.-J., 221
Muller E.J., 81

Naylor G., 155
Nicolas J.-P., 309
Nicoud R.M., 13
Nishida M., 293
Nourichafi N., 207

Ohmura T., 293
Ohtani W., 293
Östlin A., 69
Over J., 49, 81

Pla J., 183
Prince A.M., 237
Prowse C.V., 87, 275

Radema H., 49
Ray V., 151
Regnault V., 43, 97, 301
Ribeyron J., 175
Rivat C., 43, 97, 175, 267, 301
Rucheton M., 163

Sertillanges P., 267
Smith K., 75
Smit Sibinga C.T., 109
Stefas I., 163
Stewart D.J., 37
Stoltz J.-F., 97, 175, 207, 267, 301
Streiff F., 175
Sultan Y., 57
Sumi A., 293
Suomela H., 261
Suyama T., 293
Svinhufvud L., 69

Ter Hart H.G.J., 81
Thomas J.A., 25
Turner P.J., 143, 155

Ubrich N., 43

Vallar L., 301
Van Duren N., 81
Van Leeuwen M.A.W., 49
Van Weperen J.J., 109
Van Wijngaarden L., 109
Véron J.-L., 75, 183, 267
Verroust F., 131
Vijayalakshmi M.A., 115, 189
Voute N., 3

Wallevik K., 103
Wang X., 307
Watklevicz C., 237
White B.R., 155
Winge S., 69

Yap H.B., 143, 155
Yokoyama K., 293
Young I.F., 143, 155

Zhang T., 307
Zhao Shuliang, 137
Zhong Lu, 137
Zhou Quing, 137

Colloques INSERM
ISSN 0768-3154

Other *Colloques* published as co-editions by John Libbey Eurotext and INSERM

153 Hormones and Cell Regulation (11th European Symposium). *Hormones et Régulation Cellulaire (11ᵉ Symposium Européen).*
Edited by J. Nunez and J.E. Dumont.
ISBN : John Libbey Eurotext 0 86196 104 8
INSERM 2 85598 324 X

158 Biochemistry and Physiopathology of Platelet Membrane. *Biochimie et Physiopathologie de la Membrane Plaquettaire.*
Edited by G. Marguerie and R.F.A. Zwaal.
ISBN : John Libbey Eurotext 0 86196 114 5
INSERM 2 85598 345 2

162 The Inhibitors of Hematopoiesis. *Les Inhibiteurs de l'Hématopoïèse.*
Edited by A. Najman, M. Guignon, N.C. Gorin and J.Y. Mary.
ISBN : John Libbey Eurotext 0 86196 125 0
INSERM 2 85598 340 1

164 Liver Cells and Drugs. *Cellules Hépatiques et Médicaments.*
Edited by A. Guillouzo.
ISBN : John Libbey Eurotext 0 86196 128 5
INSERM 2 85598 341 X

165 Hormones and Cell Regulation (12th European Symposium). *Hormones et Régulation Cellulaire (12ᵉ Symposium Européen).*
Edited by J. Nunez, J.E. Dumont and E. Carafoli.
ISBN : John Libbey Eurotext 0 86196 133 1
INSERM 2 85598 347 9

167 Sleep Disorders and Respiration. *Les Evénements Respiratoires du Sommeil.*
Edited by P. Lévi-Valensi and D. Duron.
ISBN : John Libbey Eurotext 0 86196 127 7
INSERM 2 85598 344 4

169 Neo-Adjuvant Chemotherapy. *Chimiothérapie Néo-Adjuvante.*
Edited by C. Jacquillat, M. Weil, D. Khayat.
ISBN : John Libbey Eurotext 0 86196 150 1
INSERM 2 85598 349 5

171 Structure and Functions of the Cytoskeleton. *La Structure et les Fonctions du Cytosquelette.*
Edited by B.A.F. Rousset.
ISBN : John Libbey Eurotext 0 86196 149 8
INSERM 2 85598 351 7

Colloques INSERM
ISSN 0768-3154

172 The Langerhans Cell. *La Cellule de Langerhans.*
Edited by J. Thivolet, D. Schmitt.
ISBN : John Libbey Eurotext 0 86196 181 1
INSERM 2 85598 352 5

173 Cellular and Molecular Aspects of Glucuronidation. *Aspects Cellulaires et Moléculaires de la Glucuronoconjugaison.*
Edited by G. Siest, J. Magdalou, B. Burchell
ISBN : John Libbey Eurotext 0 86196 182 X
INSERM 2 85598 353 3

174 Second Forum on Peptides. *Deuxième Forum Peptides.*
Edited by A. Aubry, M. Marraud, B. Vitoux
ISBN : John Libbey Eurotext 0 86196 151 X
INSERM 2 85598 354 1

176 Hormones and Cell Regulation (13th European Symposium). *Hormones et Régulation Cellulaire (13ᵉ Symposium Européen).*
Edited by J. Nunez, J.E. Dumont, R. Denton
ISBN : John Libbey Eurotext 0 86196 183 8
INSERM 2 85598 356 8

179 Lymphokine Receptors Interactions. *Interactions Lymphokines-récepteurs.*
Edited by D. Fradelizi, J. Bertoglio
ISBN : John Libbey Eurotext 0 86196 148 X
INSERM 2 85598 359 2

191 Anticancer Drugs (1st International Interface of Clinical and Laboratory responses to anticancer drugs). *Médicaments anticancéreux (1ʳᵉ Confrontation internationale des réponses cliniques et expérimentales aux médicaments anticancéreux).*
Edited by H. Tapiero, J. Robert, T.J. Lampidis
ISBN : John Libbey Eurotext 0 86196 223 0
INSERM 2 85598 393 2

193 Living in the Cold (2nd International Symposium). *La Vie au Froid (2ᵉ Symposium International).*
Edited by A. Malan, B. Canguilhem
ISBN : John Libbey Eurotext 0 86196 234 9
INSERM 2 85598 395 9

Colloques INSERM
ISSN 0768-3154

194 Progress in Hepatitis B Immunization. *La Vaccination contre l'épatite B.*
Edited by P. Coursaget, M.J. Tong
ISBN : John Libbey Eurotext 0 86196 249 4
INSERM 2 85598 396 7

196 Treatment Strategy in Hodgkin's Disease. *Stratégie dans la maladie de Hodgkin.*
Edited by P. Sommers, M. Henry-Amar, J.H. Meezwaldt, P. Carde
ISBN : John Libbey Eurotext 0 86196 226 5
INSERM 2 85598 398 3

198 Hormones and Cell Regulation (14th European Symposium). *Hormones et Régulation Cellulaire (14e Symposium Européen).*
Edited by J. Nunez, J.E. Dumont
ISBN : John Libbey Eurotext 0 86196 229 X
INSERM 2 85598 400 9

199 Placental Communications : Biochemical, Morphological and Cellular Aspects. *Communications placentaires : aspects biochimique, morphologique et cellulaire.*
Edited by L. Cedard, E. Alsat, J.C. Challier, G. Chaouat, A. Malassiné
ISBN : John Libbey Eurotext 0 86196 227 3
INSERM 2 85598 401 7

204 Pharmacologie Clinique : Actualités et Perspectives. (6e Rencontres Nationales de Pharmacologie clinique).
Edited by J.P. Boissel, C. Caulin, M. Teule
ISBN : John Libbey Eurotext 0 86196 225 7
INSERM 2 85598 454 8

205 Recent Trends in Clinical Pharmacology (6th National Meeting of Clinical Pharmacology).
Edited by J.P. Boissel, C. Caulin, M. Teule
ISBN : John Libbey Eurotext 0 86196 256 7
INSERM 2 85598 455 6

206 Platelet Immunology : Fundamental and Clinical Aspects. *Immunologie plaquettaire : aspects fondamentaux et cliniques.*
Edited by C. Kaplan-Gouet, N. Schlegel, Ch. Salmon, J. McGregor
ISBN : John Libbey Eurotext 0 86196 285 0
INSERM 2 85598 439 4

Colloques INSERM
ISSN 0768-3154

207 Thyroperoxidase and Thyroid Autoimmunity. *Thyroperoxydase et auto-immunité thyroïdienne.*
Edited by P. Carayon, T. Ruf
ISBN : John Libbey Eurotext 0 86196 277 X
INSERM 2 85598 440 8

208 Vasopressin. *Vasopressine.*
Edited by S. Jard, R. Jamison
ISBN : John Libbey Eurotext 0 86196 288 5
INSERM 2 85598 441 6

210 Hormones and Cell Regulation (15th European Symposium). *Hormones et Régulation Cellulaire (15ᵉ Symposium Européen).*
Edited by J.E. Dumont, J. Nunez, R.J.B. King
ISBN : John Libbey Eurotext 0 86196 279 6
INSERM 2 85598 443 2

211 Medullary Thyroid Carcinoma. *Cancer Médullaire de la Thyroïde.*
Edited by C. Calmettes, J.M. Guliana
ISBN : John Libbey Eurotext 0 86196 287 7
INSERM 2 85598 440 0

212 Cellular and Molecular Biology of the Materno-Fetal Relationship. *Biologie cellulaire et moléculaire de la relation materno-fœtale.*
Edited by G. Chaouat, J. Mowbray
ISBN : John Libbey Eurotext 0 86196 909 1
INSERM 2 85598 445 9

215 Aldosterone. Fundamental Aspects. *Aspects fondamentaux.*
Edited by J.P. Bonvalet, N. Farman, M. Lombes, M.E. Rafestin-Oblin
ISBN : John Libbey Eurotext 0 86196 302 4
INSERM 2 85598 482 3

216 Cellular and Molecular Aspects of Cirrhosis. *Aspects cellulaires et moléculaires de la cirrhose.*
Edited by B. Clément, A. Guillouzo
ISBN : John Libbey Eurotext 0 86196 342 3
INSERM 2 85598 483 1

217 Sleep and Cardiorespiratory Control. *Sommeil et contrôle cardio-respiratoire.*
Edited by C. Gaultier, P. Escourrou, L. Curzi-Dascalora
ISBN : John Libbey Eurotext 0 86196 307 5
INSERM 2 85598 484 X

Colloques INSERM
ISSN 0768-3154

218 Genetic Hypertension. *Hypertension génétique.*
Edited by J. Sassard
ISBN : John Libbey Eurotext 0 86196 313 X
　　　INSERM 2 85598 485 8

219 Human Gene Transfer. *Transfert de gènes chez l'homme.*
Edited by O. Cohen-Haguenauer, M. Boiron
ISBN : John Libbey Eurotext 0 86196 301 6
　　　INSERM 2 85598 497 1

220 Medicine and Change: Historical and Sociological Studies of Medical Innovation. *L'innovation en médecine : études historiques et sociologiques.*
Edited by Ilana Löwy
ISBN : John Libbey Eurotext 2 7420 0010 0
　　　INSERM 2 85598 508 0

221 Structures and Functions of Retinal Proteins. *Structures et fonctions des rétino-protéines.*
Edited by J.L. Rigaud
ISBN : John Libbey Eurotext 0 86196 355 5
　　　INSERM 2 85598 509 9

222 Cellular and Molecular Biology of the Adrenal Cortex. *Biologie cellulaire et moléculaire du cortex surrénal.*
Edited by J.M. Saez, A.C. Brownie, A. Capponi, E.M. Chambaz, F. Mantero
ISBN : John Libbey Eurotext 0 86196 362 8
　　　INSERM 2 85598 510 2

223 Mechanisms and Control of Emesis. *Mécanismes et contrôle du vomissement.*
Edited by A.L. Bianchi, L. Grélot, A.D. Miller, G.L. King
ISBN : John Libbey Eurotext 0 86196 363 6
　　　INSERM 2 85598 511 0

224 High Pressure and Biotechnology. *Haute pression et biotechnologie.*
Edited by C. Balny, R. Hayashi, K. Heremans, P. Masson
ISBN : John Libbey Eurotext 0 86196 363 6
　　　INSERM 2 85598 512 9

Colloques INSERM
ISSN 0768-3154

226 Calculation of health expectancies: harmonization, consensus achieved and future perspectives. *Calcul des espérances de vie en santé : harmonisation, acquis et perspectives*
Edited by J.-M. Robine, C.D. Mathers, M.R. Bone, I. Romieu
ISBN : John Libbey Eurotext 2 7420 0009 7
　　　 INSERM 2 85598 514 5

228 Non-Visual Human-Computer Interactions. *Communication non visuelle homme-ordinateur.*
Edited by D. Burger, J.C. Sperandio
ISBN : John Libbey Eurotext 2 7420 0014 3
　　　 INSERM 2 85598 540 4

230 From Research in Oncology to Therapeutic Innovations. *De la recherche oncologique à l'innovation thérapeutique.*
Edited by P. Tambourin, M. Boiron
ISBN : John Libbey Eurotext 2 7420 0016 X
　　　 INSERM 2 85598 542 0

LOUIS-JEAN
avenue d'Embrun, 05003 GAP cedex
Tél. : 92.53.17.00
Dépôt légal : 516 — Juin 1993
Imprimé en France